Solar-Energy-Absorbing Substances and Oxidative Stress and Inflammatory Diseases

Solar-Energy-Absorbing Substances and Oxidative Stress and Inflammatory Diseases

By

George Sosnovsky,

C. Thomas Gnewuch

and Mikołaj Jawdosiuk

Cambridge Scholars Publishing

Solar-Energy-Absorbing Substances and Oxidative Stress and Inflammatory Diseases

By George Sosnovsky, C. Thomas Gnewuch and Mikołaj Jawdosiuk

This book first published 2017

Cambridge Scholars Publishing

Lady Stephenson Library, Newcastle upon Tyne, NE6 2PA, UK

British Library Cataloguing in Publication Data
A catalogue record for this book is available from the British Library

ISBN (10): 1-4438-5062-4
ISBN (13): 978-1-4438-5062-9

Acclinis falsis animus meliora recusat
The mind charmed by false appearances refuses to admit better things
Quintus Horatius Flaccus, 65–8 B.C.

Nullus est liber tam malus ut non aliqua parte prosit
No book is so bad that some parts of it could not be useful
Gaius Plinius Secundus, Pliny the Elder, 23–79 A.D.
Gaius Plinius Caecilus Secundus, Pliny the Younger, 61–114 A.D.

In vitium ducit culpae fuga, si caret arte
When we try to avoid a fault, we are led to the opposite unless we be very careful
Quintus Horatius Flaccus, 65–8 B.C.

Non multa, sed multum
Not multifarious, but many
Gaius Plinius Caecilus Secundus, Pliny the Younger, 61–114 A.D.

Feci quod potui faciant meliora potentes
I have done what I could let those who can do better

TABLE OF CONTENTS

ABSTRACT

Critical evaluations are presented on myths and facts about solar-energy-absorbing substances, including sunscreen agents, their influence on skin cancers and other cancers and diseases, and beliefs that have been promulgated over the years about the prevention of skin cancers by using sunscreen agents, i.e., the use of solar-energy-absorbing substances that actually are known to undergo photophysical and photochemical reactions generating toxic oxygen species and other maladies in biological systems. A general consensus is emerging that the use of sunscreen agents cannot prevent the photoinitiation of malfunctioning of many biological systems, such as immunosuppression, DNA degradations, and malignant melanomas, just to mention a few. On the contrary, sunscreens and their formulation components could be involved in enhancing the negative solar-energy-induced effects by skin penetration and transport of xenobiotics through the skin and by their own adverse properties, such as estrogenic environmental effects. This review encompasses a wide range of topics that are relevant to understanding the complexities of biological effects that are generated by solar radiations. The main areas include the photochemistry of skin components urocanic acid and melanins, allergic reactions caused by sunscreen agents and ingredients in commercial sunscreen products, radiation-induced damages to the human skin including DNA components, glycations, immunosuppression and related systems, cancerous dermatologic changes, human skin cancers induced by solar radiations and mechanisms of anticancer drugs, mechanisms of photoexcitations and energy dissipations, formation and reactions of reactive oxygen species (ROS), photochemistry of organic and inorganic sunscreen agents, exogenous and endogenous antioxidants as possible sunscreen ingredients, and as oral medications either for the prevention or cure of various diseases including cancers. Critical appraisals are presented of clinical studies involving vitamins and nonsteroidal anti-inflammatory agents, including Aspirin™, for either alleviating, mitigating, or even curing of various inflammatory diseases including cancers. Finally, we scrutinize the intertwining of reactive oxygen species with processes of infection, chronic inflammation, chronic pain, pruritus, cancer, and other inflammatory diseases. We have attempted to avoid an overly specialized presentation of topics throughout this work in order to enable a non-specialist reader to follow the most advanced topics.

ACKNOWLEDGMENTS

The authors are sincerely grateful to Professor Lucedio Greci, Dipartimento di Scienze e Tecnologie Chimiche, Università Politecnica delle Marche, Ancona, Italy; Professor Kálmán Hideg, Department of Organic and Medicinal Chemistry, University of Pécs, Hungary. The authors are also grateful to Mrs. Lydia Dyer and to Professor Andrew Kakabadse of the Henley Business School, England, for recommending and advocating the manuscript to Cambridge Scholars Publishing Ltd, England, which has led to its acceptance for publication. We are happy for the assistance of Dr. Sharbil J. Firsan in editing and proofreading the manuscript for this edition of the book.

INTRODUCTION

Solar radiation is of paramount importance for the sustenance of all living species on this planet, whereby it provides the energy for the maintenance of health, livable climatic conditions, and illumination for visual perception. It also mediates the photosynthesis of plant materials from carbon dioxide and water in the presence of chlorophyll, at the same time generating the essential molecular oxygen gas.

About 5000 to 2500 years before the present (B.P.), the peoples of ancient civilizations, e.g., the Egyptians, Assyrians, Babylonians, Aztecs, Incas, and ancient Greeks were overwhelmed by the power of sunlight and deified and worshipped the sun as the sun god Ra or Re in Egypt [1–3] and Helios in Greece [2]. However, in Greece about 2400 B.P. [2], the philosopher Anaxagoras dared to declare that the god Helios is simply a big fiery rock, and the famous physician Hippocrates advocated exposure to sunrays for ameliorating physical and even mental health problems. Similarly in the Roman Empire about 1800 B.P. [2], the physician Galen(us) was prescribing heliotherapy, and the practice of "sunbathing" was widely accepted during the Greco-Roman era. Since the decline of the Roman Empire, photo/(helio)-therapy and exposure to solar radiation for health and cosmetic purposes, with some interruptions during the Middle Ages, continued unabated to the present, and, at the beginning of the last century, the general opinion prevailed that solar light has a beneficial effect on health. However, during the past two centuries, publications sporadically appeared [2] on the detrimental effects of solar radiation on humans and various other species in vivo and in vitro, and, in the middle of the last century to the present, it was firmly established [1–9] that there are harmful consequences of either prolonged or frequent exposures to solar and other sources of ultraviolet radiation. The serious effects of the interaction of ultraviolet light with components of the human skin were shown to result in dermatological changes of the skin, leading ultimately to the development of skin cancers [1–9]. As a matter of fact, the ultraviolet part of solar radiation has been considered a "perfect carcinogen" and implicated in the carcinogenesis of human skin [4, 5].

The realization by the 1920s that solar radiation is the cause of erythema, i.e., the reddening, inflammation, and the "sunburn" effect of the human skin, led to the commercial development of the so-called sunscreens. The first compounds selected for sunscreen applications were benzyl salicylate and benzyl cinnamate. These compounds were readily available at that time because they had been synthesized and patented on several occasions since 1869 for various pharmaceutical applications [10]. The commercial sunscreen products were marketed for the first time in 1928 in the United States [11, 12]. By the way, the word sunscreen is a misnomer, a catchword. The compounds are in reality ultraviolet-light-energy-absorbing substances. Nevertheless, the catchword is still used for simplicity's sake. Over the past eighty years, a large number of various compounds have been synthesized and evaluated for sunscreen use; however, only about fifty compounds are registered internationally [5, 11–13] to be used in lotion, cream, and spray "formulations" for protection against solar radiation. In the United States, these products are sold to the public as "over-the-counter" drugs [13].

Incidentally, during the same period, skin cancer cases, in particular melanomas, have grown at an alarming rate [5, 9]. Thus, in the 1930s, dermatologic cancers were practically unknown, in spite of the fact that large portions of the population were working on farm fields, exposed all day to solar radiation. At present, melanomas are the fastest growing cancers [5, 9]. Concomitant with these developments, the sales of sunscreen products worldwide also progressed at a brisk pace to more than three billion dollars annually [10]. There have been several hypotheses advanced to explain the rapid growth of melanoma cases, such as the depletion of the ozone layer, the enlargement of the "ozone hole," and the substantial increase of xenobiotics in the atmosphere, attributable to industrial pollution and the use of motor vehicles worldwide [14, 15]. In the meantime, it has been shown in a number of investigations that, on irradiation with ultraviolet light, many sunscreen compounds can cause allergic and toxic reactions on the human skin [16, 17], and undergo photochemically induced transformations, such as isomerizations, dimerizations, derivatizations, degradations, and reactions with molecular oxygen to give reactive oxygen species (ROS), which can cause the so-called oxidative stress in biological environments [5, 14, 18, 19].

In the present review, we critically evaluate various deleterious factors evoked by solar ultraviolet radiations in naturally occurring and synthetic ultraviolet-light-energy-absorbing substances, including sunscreens [4–9, 16–20]. The ultimate goal is to be able to assess the possible merits and demerits of currently used radiation "filters" and the reasons for the unprecedented growth of dermatological cancers.

SCOPE AND LIMITATIONS

The aim of this book is to establish a compelling general pattern for photochemical transformations of ultraviolet-light-energy-absorbing substances, in particular, in the presence of molecular oxygen, resulting in harmful reactive oxygen species that can cause mutations, carcinogenesis, and ultimately skin cancers. Comparatively little information is available in the scientific literature on the possible enhancement of the carcinogenic properties of ultraviolet radiations by sunscreen agents.

In the past fifty years, a steep increase has occurred in the number of publications on the harmful effects of ultraviolet radiations and the protective properties of sunscreens and other substances. Hence, it is impossible to make an exhaustive collection of references on the many interrelated and relevant topics for the present review. Instead, a selective search has been conducted with emphasis on data that have been published mainly during the past two decades. Efforts were made to include as much as possible review articles and monographs about the most relevant topics, since these publications contain more exhaustive collections of references. In this process, it was unavoidable that some worthy articles may have been overlooked.

In cases of biological evaluations, credence was placed first on the results of tests obtained on humans, then on in vivo tests obtained with the so-called "animal models", and last on in vitro tests. Furthermore, it was felt that interpretations of test data obtained on animals should be treated with caution when drawing conclusions on analogous conditions in humans. The results obtained using UVC radiation were seldom included since this radiation, to date, is effectively absorbed by the ozone layer, and, hence, is not involved in interactions with the human body. However, this radiation has been used to establish principles and to study biological mechanisms.

The present review uses chemical structures and schemes extensively, in contrast to many other relevant publications that tend to be descriptive. A number of related areas are excluded because they are outside its scope. Nevertheless, a few comments are warranted on some of the excluded topics. Thus, there exist a large number of non-malignant dermatologic diseases, which either are caused by solar ultraviolet radiations or are ameliorated or aggravated by radiations [6, 14, 15]. The photodermatoses can have various origins, such as genetic, metabolic, degenerative, xenobiotically induced, and idiopathic, i.e., of unknown origin [14].

The skin disease psoriasis is treated with UVA in conjunction with methoxypsoralenes. The naturally occurring psoralenes are fucocoumarins, and are known to have tumorogenic properties [5–9, 15]. Nevertheless, it appears that this PUVA therapy is the best available treatment for the alleviation of this uncomfortable condition, while taking into account the possible risk for developing skin cancers.

Psoralenes have also been extensively employed, unwittingly, in cosmetics and sunscreen formulations for rapid suntanning effects in commercial suntan parlors [5–9, 15–21]. The radiations employed in these cases can be as high as 100% UVA radiation, with a 12 times higher dose than is present in solar radiation [9]. It appears that, under these circumstances, there would be a high risk of developing skin cancers. Nevertheless, about twenty-five million Americans seem to be oblivious to this risk, and are increasingly participating in these practices [9].

One of the beneficial attributes of solar radiation is the generation and regulation of vitamin D_2 and D_3 levels in humans [22–29]. The exposure of the skin to solar radiation results in the conversion of 7-dehydrocholesterol to vitamin D, which, in conjunction with the parathyroid hormone, regulates the homeostasis of calcium cations. It was found that an application of sunscreen agents to the skin causes a reduction of the formation of vitamin D. However, this reduction was believed to have no serious consequences since, although the levels of vitamin D were lowered, there was no noticeable effect on the serum parathyroid function and the calcium concentration, and it was assumed that the small amount of vitamin D required daily by the human body is provided by diets containing milk, egg yolk, butter fat, and fish. This simple assumption turns out to be only partially correct, since many persons cannot attain the required levels of about 1000 IU per day of vitamin D_3 by diet and occasional exposure to sunlight [30].

As a consequence, many health-related problems, including various cancers and other diseases, have been attributed to the vitamin D deficiencies. These problems are reflected in the following surprising and alarming statistics. Thus, for example, in the USA, the economic burden that is attributable to vitamin D insufficiencies, caused by inadequate UV radiation exposures was estimated at $40–50 billion in 2004, whereas the economic burden for the excess of UV irradiation exposures was estimated at $6–7 billion [26–28]. An extensive literature exists on all these topics, which are beyond the scope of our review [27].

Photodynamic therapy is well established in clinical oncology for the treatment of various cancers, including dermatologic cancers [30]. In this therapy, photosensitizers are used for absorption by cancer cells. On irradiation with a suitable light, the sensitizer molecules are promoted to excited singlet and triplet states, which readily interact with molecular oxygen to give toxic reactive oxygen species, causing the destruction of cancerous cells. This radiation method is closely related to the present review topic; however, the details of photodynamic therapy will not be discussed further.

Excluded from this review are at-length discussions of regulatory procedures for sunscreen products in various countries, formulations of sunscreen products, analytical quality controls, and marketing [31].

In the cited references, the authors use three nomenclatures—nitroxides, nitroxyls, and aminoxyls—for spin-labeled compounds containing the following free radical functional group:

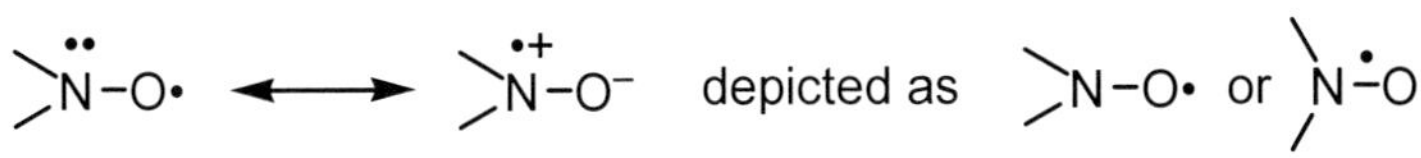

The nomenclature of this functional group in compounds is always –oxyl, e.g., the compound TEMPOL is 4-hydroxy-2,2,6,6-tetramethylpiperidine-1-oxyl. The International Union of Pure and Applied Chemistry (IUPAC) has recommended the name aminoxyls.

References

1. Breasted J. J. (1964) *A History of Egypt*, Bantam Books, Classic Edition, New York.
2. Giacomoni P. U. (2001) Women (and men) and the sun in the past. In: *Sun Protection in Man*, pp 1–10, Giacomoni, P. U. (ed.), Elsevier Science, Amsterdam.
3. Hockberger P. E. (2002) A history of ultraviolet photobiology for humans, animals and microorganisms. *Photochem. Photobiol.* **76**: 561–579.
4. IARC (1992) Solar and Ultraviolet Radiation. In: *IARC Monographs on the Evaluation of Carcinogenic Risks to Humans*, Vol. 55, pp 1–316, International Agency for Research on Cancer, Lyon.
5. Vainio H. and Bianchini F. (eds.) (2001) Sunscreens. In: *IARC Handbooks of Cancer Prevention*, Vol. 5, International Agency for Research on Cancer, WHO, Lyon.

6. Tyrell R. M. (1994) The molecular and cellular pathology of solar ultraviolet radiation. *Mol. Aspects Med.* **15**: 1–77.
7. Brash D. E. and Ponten J. (1998) Skin precancers. In: *Cancer Surveys* Vol. 32: Precancer: Biology, Importance and Possible Prevention, pp 69–113, Imperial Cancer Research Fund.
8. Ponten J. (1998) Cell biology of precancers. In: *Cancer Surveys* Vol. 32: Precancer: Biology, Importance and Possible Prevention, pp 5–35, Imperial Cancer Research Fund.
9. Wang S. Q., Setlow R., Berwick M., Polsky D., Marghoob A. A., Kopf A. W. and Bart R. S. (2001) Ultraviolet A and melanoma: a review. *J. Am. Acad. Dermatol.* **44**: 837–846.
10. Gomberg M. and Buchler C. C. (1920) The preparation of benzyl esters and other benzyl derivatives from benzyl chloride. *J. Am. Chem. Soc.* **42**: 2059–2072.
11. Roelandts R. (2009) History of photoprotection. In: *Clinical Guide to Sunscreens and Photoprotection*, pp 1–10, Lim H. W. and Draelos Z. D. (eds.), Informa Healthcare, New York.
12. Urbach F. (2001) The historical aspects of sunscreens. *J. Photochem. Photobiol. B.* **64**: 99–104.
13. Food and Drug Administration. (1999) Sunscreen Drug Products for Over-the-Counter Human Use; Final monograph. *Fed. Regist.* (98) **64**: 27666–27693.
14. Fuchs J. (1992) *Oxidative Injury in Dermatopathology*, Springer Verlag, Berlin.
15. Edlich R. F., Winters K. L., Lim H. W., Cox M. J., Becker D. G., Horowitz J. H., Nichter L.S., Britt L. D. and Long W. B. (2004) Photoprotection by sunscreens with topical antioxidants and systemic antioxidants to reduce sun exposure. *J. Long-Term Eff. Med. Implants* **14**: 317–340.
16. Schauder S. and Ippen H. (1997) Contact and photocontact sensitivity of sunscreens. Review of a 15-year experience and of the literature. *Contact Dermatitis* **37**: 221–232.
17. Schauder S. (2001) Dermatologische Verträglichkeit von UV-Filtern, Duffstoffen und Konservierungsmitteln in Sonnenschutzpräparaten. *Bundesgesundheitsblatt-Gesundheits-forschung-Gesundheitsschutz* **44**: 471–479.
18. Sies H. (ed.) (1991) *Oxidative Stress: Oxidants and Antioxidants*, Academic Press, New York.
19. Scharffetter-Kochanek K., Wlaschek M., Brenneisen P., Schanen M., Blandschun R. and Wenk J. (1997) UV-induced reactive oxygen

species in photocarcinogenesis and photoaging. *Biol. Chem.* **378**: 1247–1257.

20. Gasparro F. P. (ed.) (1997) *Sunscreen Photobiology Molecular, Cellular and Physiological Aspects*. Springer Verlag, Berlin, and Landes Bioscience, Georgetown, TX. Printed in Germany.
21. Cyr W. H. and Miller S. A. (2001) Sunlamps and sunbeds: safety and regulatory issues. In: *Sun Protection in Man*, pp 691–704, Giacomoni, P. U. (ed.), Elsevier, Amsterdam.
22. Holick M. F. (2001) A perspective on the beneficial effects of moderate exposure to sunlight: bone health, cancer prevention, mental health and well being. In: *Sun Protection in Man*, pp 11–37, Giacomoni, P. U. (ed.), Elsevier, Amsterdam.
23. Holick M. F. (2008) Sunlight, UV-radiation, vitamin D and skin cancer: How much sunlight do we need. In: *Sunlight, Vitamin D and Skin Cancer*, pp 1–15, Reichrath J. (ed.), Springer Science + Business Media, LLC, New York, and Landes Bioscience, Austin, TX.
24. Bischoff-Ferrari H. A. (2008) Optimal serum 25-hydroxy vitamin D levels for multiple health outcomes. In: *Sunlight, Vitamin D and Skin Cancer*, pp 1–15, Reichrath J. (ed.), Springer Science+Business Media, LLC, New York, and Landes Bioscience, Austin, TX.
25. Bischoff-Ferrari H. and Lim H. W. (2009) Effect of photoprotection on vitamin D and health. In: *Clinical Guide to Sunscreens and Photoprotection*, pp 117–237, Lim H. W. and Draelos Z. D. (eds.), Informa Healthcare, New York.
26. Grant W. B. (2008) Solar ultraviolet irradiance and mortality. In: *Sunlight, Vitamin D and Skin Cancer*, pp 16–30, Reichrath J. (ed.), Springer Science+Business Media, LLC, New York, and Landes Bioscience, Austin, TX.
27. Reichrath J. (ed.) (2008) *Sunlight, Vitamin D and Skin Cancer*, Springer Science+Business Media, LLC, New York, and Landes Bioscience, Austin, TX.
28. Ainsleigh H. G. (1993) Beneficial effects of sun exposure on cancer mortality. *Prev. Med.* **22**: 132–140.
29. Tang J. Y., Fu T., Lau C., Oh D. H., Bikle D. D. and Asgari M. M. (2012) Vitamin D in cutaneous carcinogenesis. *J. Am. Acad. Dermat.* **67**: 803–814.
30. Gnewuch C. T. and Sosnovsky G. (2002) Critical appraisals of approaches for predictive designs in anticancer drugs. *Cell. Mol. Life Sci.* **59**: 959–1023.
31. Shaath N. (ed.) (2005) *Sunscreens. Regulations and Commercial Development*, 3rd ed., Taylor and Francis, Boca Raton.

CHAPTER ONE

PHOTOCHEMISTRY OF THE HUMAN SKIN

A. Human Behavioral Practices with Sunscreen Applications. Predictive Significance of the Sun Protection Factor (SPF) in the Onset of Erythema and Other Biological Entities

It has been estimated that less than five percent of the total solar radiation energy is received by the earth's surface as ultraviolet radiation. This radiation has a pronounced and often long-lasting effect on mammals and plant species. The degree of the effectiveness of solar radiation on the earth inhabitants will depend on some of the conditions under which the sun rays impinge on the "human target", such as the intensity and the wavelength of the radiation, the duration of the exposure, the time of day the exposure occurs, the season, the geographic location, the atmospheric conditions such as clouds and fog, the pollution caused by xenobiotics, the prevailing extent of the ozone layer, the altitude above sea level, the vicinity of reflecting surfaces, e.g., water, snow, and sand, and a number of behavioral practices of the "human target", i.e., duration and type of outdoor activities, the type of clothing worn, the use of medication, which may migrate to the skin surfaces, and the use of UV light absorbing materials, e.g., sunscreens.

Furthermore, the intensity of the UVA and UVB radiations can be differently affected by some of the listed factors in wintertime as compared to summertime, whereby the intensity of UVB radiation will be diminished to a greater degree in wintertime than that of UVA radiation [1, 2]

Ideally, sunscreen application should occur before the first prolonged full body exposure to the sun is contemplated, initially for only short periods, and, preferably, not during the highest intensity of solar radiation. Clearly, this type of practice is a utopian ideal, since, in most cases, the use of ultraviolet filters follows after some degree of discomfort has been experienced, and in the worst cases, the photodamage is clinically detectable. At this stage, severe damage to the skin tissue may have already occurred. The damage can be either of a reversible or irreversible nature, depending on the prevailing conditions during the sustained solar exposure. The damage can remain latent for long periods of time before a skin disease can be diagnosed.

A further problem is the mode of application of sunscreens to the skin [3–11]. Thus, even in cases where the sunscreen lotion or cream is applied to the skin prior to a full exposure to solar radiation, it is very difficult, if not impossible, to assure an application resulting in a film of perfect evenness and required thickness to achieve the desired protection, since there are no practical means to measure such a requirement. Although there exist photographic methods [8] that can be used [12] in clinical tests to insure a uniformity of sunscreen application to the skin, these methods would be impractical for use by the public "in the field". Thus, in practice, the casual applications of either a spray, which primarily dissipates into the surroundings, or a lotion or cream, will result in a film of uneven thickness, leaving either uncovered or thinly covered areas on the skin, which permit an effective penetration into the skin tissue by ultraviolet rays. Furthermore, the present system of labeling commercial products by manufacturers conveys, unsurprisingly, overly optimistic messages about the safety and effectiveness of their products. These messages include nonirritating, nonallergenic, premature aging prevention, sunburns and irritation, and even cancer prevention properties, which is clearly unsubstantiated in cases of basal cell carcinoma (BCC) and melanoma [3]. In addition, the present system of rating sunscreen preparations for effectiveness by assigning sun protection factors (SPFs), ranging from about 2 to 30 and higher, are primarily a guide for the prevention of a sunburn effect caused by UVB radiation [3, 11], while neglecting the more serious effects of solar radiation caused by the deeper penetrating UVA rays [3]. Thus, the public inadvertently develops a sense of full reliance on the safety and protecting properties of commercial sunscreen preparations [3]. Nevertheless, in order to have some idea about adequate protection against solar radiation by sunscreen products, the FDA in the U.S.A. has issued a recommendation to apply 2 mg/cm^2 of sunscreen agents to the skin [4, 10]. This guideline could be useful provided the public intuitively knows how much of a given sunscreen agent to apply to the skin in order to achieve the desired effect. In actual practice, however, it has been found that the quantities of sunscreen agents on the skin amounted to only 0.5 mg/cm^2 or less, i.e., a much lower dose than that recommended by the FDA [5–9]. Since the relationship between the percentage of absorbed UV radiation by the sunscreen at the skin and the SPF is not linear but logarithmic, the following result can be derived for the effective SPF [5, 6]. Thus, if the listed SPF for a sunscreen agent is 15, the effective SPF at a 0.5 mg/cm^2

coverage of the skin would be 5–6 times less, i.e., about 2.5–3 [4, 5]. Therefore, even in the unlikely event the whole skin was uniformly covered by the sunscreen product, the protection would be rated as poor and no better than the hereditary protection rendered by urocanic acid and melanins at no cost.

Under these conditions, it was estimated by the Environmental Working Group in the U.S.A. that the SPF of 15 actually results in a SPF value of about 2 with a UV transmission, i.e., the amount of radiation that reaches the skin, of about 50%. The same considerations in the case of SPF 30 result in an actual SPF value of 2.3 with a UV transmission of 43%. For an SPF 50, the actual SPF value would be 2.6 with a UV transmission of 38%, and an SPF 100 would be reduced to an actual SPF value of 3.2 with a UV transmission of 21%.

Concerning the SPF ratings of commercial sunscreen products by the manufacturers, it has become general practice in recent years to rate the sunscreen products with SPF values higher than 30, implying a superior product quality with higher SPF values. As a matter of fact, SPF values above 30 have only a psychological effect on the customer without a gain in quality, since it was shown by a plot [**Fig. 1A-1**] of the reduction of the erythemogenic radiation against SPF values to flatten at SPF 30, where 97% of the erythemogenic UV radiation has been absorbed, and the change from 97% to 99% was shown clinically to be irrelevant [13]. Therefore, in some countries, the labeling of commercial sunscreen products is restricted by authorities to SPF 30 and 30+. In 2011, the FDA allowed the use of SPF 50+ in spite of insufficient evidence that sunscreens with values above SPF 50 are of benefit [13]. The use of SPF 50+ is practiced in many other countries.

SPF values are obtained on the basis of the so-called minimal erythema dose (MED), i.e., the smallest dose of radiation that, at 24 hours, causes a minimally perceptible, but well defined, erythema after one single irradiation of the skins of volunteers. Since volunteers are used, one could expect that the MED would depend on the type of skin, pigmentation, and other factors, such as food intake by the volunteer, medications, and other conditions. Hence, various individual persons could have somewhat different MEDs. Therefore, for SPF calculations, an average MED value is used [13]. The sun protection factor (SPF) values are obtained by the following equation [13]:

$$\text{SPF} = \frac{\text{MED obtained in the absence of suscreen}}{\text{MED obtained with the tested suscreen}}$$

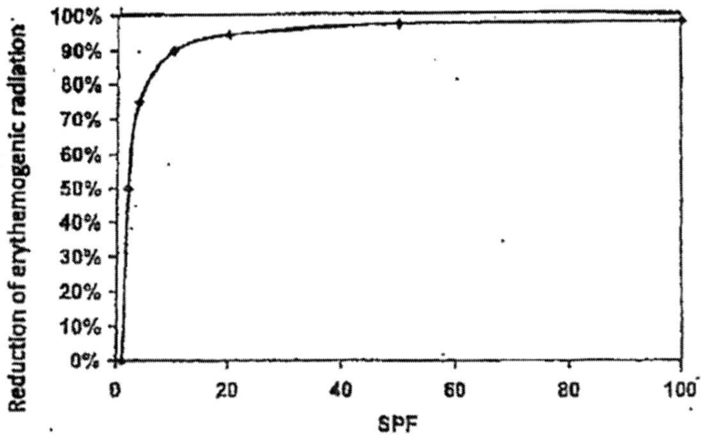

Fig. 1A-1. The logarithmic relationship between the percentage of filtered UV radiations and sun protection factor (SPF).

The values of the sun protection factor that are found on commercial products are indicative of the capacity of a given sunscreen product to provide protection against the sunburn effect (erythema) that is caused by irradiation of the skin with sunlight. Thus, e.g., an SPF of 20 as shown on the commercial product label would imply to the user that one could stay in the sun 20 times longer using the sunscreen than without the product application, provided, however, that the sunscreen is uniformly applied to the skin at 2 mg/cm^2. Since the UVB radiation, covering the 280–315 nm range of the UV spectrum, is about 1000 times more erythemogenic than the UVA2 (range 315–340 nm) and the UVA1 (range 340–400 nm), and, although the UVA radiations comprise more than 95% of the sunlight, the tests used for arriving at the SPF factors are conducted by using lamps emitting simulated solar radiation composed primarily of the UVB and some UVA, i.e., UVA2 radiations. Hence, SPF values are essentially useful as indicators of protection against sunburn, i.e., dermatitis, erythema [13].

The sun protection factor is inadequately understood by users and in scientific aspects, such as limitations of the implied protection, overestimation of protection, and the degree of UVA protection that determines the quality of protection. Furthermore, while the SPF is an indicator of the quantity of protection, the protection against the onset of reactive oxygen species (ROS) formation, that always occurs upon UV irradiation of sunscreens and excipients on the human skin, and the degree of immunoprotection and warning of the onset of other maladies are uncertain [14–16].

In numerous publications over the years, the use of sunscreen preparations has been described for the prevention of the onset of damages to biological entities induced by solar radiations, such as immunosuppression, DNA damages resulting in thymine dimer formations, oxidative damages to the DNA caused by reactive oxygen species (ROS), and skin cancers, just to mention a few [17–19]. As will be seen in subsequent sections of this review, highly divergent results have been frequently reported by various authors on the same topic. Thus, e.g., in the case of some skin cancers, the applications of sunscreens have been found to be either (a) effective (b) ineffective or (c) contributing to the initiation of cancers. These divergencies can be explained on the basis of recent scientific recognitions. Thus, the question is whether the onset of the erythema, its prevention by application of sunscreens, and the use of the SPF as a predictive device for the estimation of the preventative qualities of sunscreens, could also be applied to the estimation of the onset of damages to other biological systems. In such cases, it would mean that persons with different MEDs would experience the onset of erythema to coincide with the onsets of damages to various biological systems, and the SPFs of sunscreens could be used as indicators for possible durations of exposure by the skin to UV radiations of sunlight [17–19]. However, in recent years, it was shown that the onset of erythema is not an indicator for the onset of damages to other biological systems. Furthermore, it was found that the onset of damages to biological systems other than erythema, such as damages to the DNA, immunosuppression, and oxidative damages by ROS often occur before the onset of the erythema. Hence, the SPFs of sunscreens are of no value for estimating the possible duration of protection by sunscreen against the UV radiation induced damages to those biological systems [17–19]. This whole area is exceedingly complex in detail, and has been extensively investigated [19–21]. (See **Section 2F**.)

UVA and UVB radiations can cause immunosuppression even at suberythemal doses. The photoinduced immunosuppression is of concern since it is believed that, as a consequence of immunosuppression, mutation of the p53 gene can occur resulting in loss of apoptosis control by the gene. Furthermore, the Langerhans cells contact hypersensitivity (CHS) and other biologically important entities are affected [22, 23]. Furthermore, there are great concerns about the endocrine disruptive properties of UV energy absorbing substances present in sunscreens and cosmetic products. These adverse effects have been studied in vitro and in vivo with mice, rats, rainbow trouts, minnows, and human volunteers [24]. (For further biological properties of sunscreens, see **Section 2F**.)

It appears that the sun protection factor has no relevance to these events, since, on the basis of SPF values, it might be possible to estimate the period of exposure to the sun without a visible erythema, while no information can be obtained about the possible onset of the immunosuppression and other biological events that may occur prior to the erythema [17–23]. Hence, it seems to be unlikely that the exceedingly complex initiation pathways leading to cancers, in particular skin melanoma, could be prevented by using sunscreen agents. Nevertheless, a successful in vivo study with human volunteers was reported [25] using 0.5 and 1.0 mg/cm^2 of sunscreens with SPF 70–100 for protection against photodamage and skin cancers, whereas no protection was obtained by using sunscreens with SPF 30 and 50 [25].

UVA and UVB radiations induce structural and cellular changes in the tissues of the human skin by forming radicals and reactive oxygen species (ROS), whereby UVA radiations at 320–400 nm induce the formation of radicals and ROS in the lower parts of the dermis [26, 27].

The UV radiation induced harmful oxidative reactions are not unique to sunscreen products, since compounds of various classes with similar conjugated chromophores can undergo such reactions. Of particular importance is being aware that a large number of orally administered drugs and their metabolites readily migrate to the human skin and are exposed to UV radiations.

The extent of radical and ROS formation and the protection of the human skin by sunscreen agents can be quantitatively measured in vivo at the human skin by electron paramagnetic resonance spectrometry (ESR) and expressed as the radical sun protection factor (RSP).

The RSP can be similarly used as the SPF for the determination of increases in time for sun exposure of the skin with sunscreen to generate the same number of radicals and ROS as compared to unprotected skin [26, 27].

Another sun protection factor, the p53 labeling index, is obtained in vivo by an assessment of the sunscreen effectiveness in preventing the UV radiation induced DNA damage [28].

The use of SPF numbers on commercial sunscreen products should be abandoned. Instead, a device should be developed similar to the UV Color Index of the World Health Organization (WHO) that would enable the sunscreen user to assess by color changes the degree of solar radiation at prevailing exposure conditions.

References

1. Dummer R. and Maier T. (2002) UV protection and skin cancer. *Recent Results Cancer Res.* **160**: 7–11.
2. Vainio H. and Bianchini F. (eds.) (2001) Sunscreens. In: *IARC Handbooks of Cancer Prevention*, Vol. 5, International Agency for Research on Cancer, Lyon.
3. Wang W. Q., Setlow R., Berwick M., Polsky D., Marghoob A. A., Kopf A. W. and Bart R. S. (2001) Ultraviolet A and melanoma: a review. *J. Am. Acad. Dermatol.* **45**: 837–846.
4. De Fine Olivarius F., Wulf H. C., Crosby J. and Norval M. (1999) Sunscreen protection against *cis*-urocanic acid production in human skin. *Acta Derm. Venereol.* **79**: 426–430.
5. Pinnell S. (2003) Cutaneous photodamage, oxidative stress and topical antioxidant protection. *J. Am. Acad. Dermatol.* **48**: 1–19.
6. Wulf H. C., Stender I. M. and Look-Anderson J. (1997) Sunscreens used at the beach do not protect against erythema: a new definition of SPF is proposed. *J. Photochem. Photoimmunol. Photomed.* **13**: 129–132.
7. Brown S. and Diffey B. L. (1986) The effect of applied thickness on sunscreen protection: in vivo and in vitro studies. *Photochem. Photobiol.* **44**: 509–513.
8. Stenberg C. and Larko O. (1985) Sunscreen application and its importance for the sun protection factor. *Arch. Dermatol.* **121**: 1400–1402.
9. Bech-Thomsen N. and Wulf H. C. (1993) Sunbather's application of sunscreen is probably inadequate to obtain the sun protection factor assigned to the preparation. *Photodermatol. Photoimmunol. Photomed.* **9**: 242–244.
10. Department of Health and Human Services, Food and Drug Administration. (1999) Sunscreen Drug Products For Over-The-Counter Human Use; Final Monograph. *Fed. Regist.* **64**: 27666–27693, (2007) Sunscreen Drug Products for Over-the-Counter Human Use; Proposed Amendment of Final Monograph. *Fed. Regist.* **72**: 49069–49122, and (2011) Labeling and Effectiveness Testing; Sunscreen Drug Products for Over-the-Counter Human Use. *Fed. Regist.* **76**: 35620–35665.
11. Edlich R. F., Winters K. L., Lim H. W., Cox M. J., Becker D. G., Horowitz J. H., Nichter L.S., Britt L. D. and Long W. B. (2004) Photoprotection by sunscreens with topical antioxidants and systemic an-

tioxidants to reduce sun exposure. *J. Long-Term Eff. Med. Implants* **14**: 317–340.

12. Grencis P. W. and Stokes R. (1999) An evaluation of photographic methods to demonstrate the uniformity of sunscreen applied to the skin. *J. Audiov. Media Med.* **22**: 171–177.
13. Bens, G. (2008) Sunscreens. In: *Sunlight, Vitamin D and Skin Cancer*, pp 137–161, Reichrath J. (ed.), Springer Science+Business Media, LLC, New York, and Landes Bioscience, Austin, TX.
14. Osterwalder U. and Herzog B. (2009) Sun protection factors: worldwide confusion. *Br. J. Dermatol.* **161**: 13–24.
15. Rohr M., Klette E., Ruppert S., Bimzcok R., Klebon B., Heinrich U., Tronnier H., Johncock W., et al. (2010) In vitro sun protection factor: still a challenge with no final answer. *Skin Pharmacol. Physiol.* **23**: 201–212.
16. Giacomoni P. U., Teta L. and Najdek L. (2010) Sunscreens: the impervious path from theory to practice. *Photochem. Photobiol. Sci.* **9**: 524–529.
17. Heenen M., Giacomoni P. U. and Golstein P. (2001) Erythema, a link between UV-induced DNA damage, cell death and clinical effects? In: *Sun Protection in Man*, pp 277–285, Giacomoni, P. U. (ed.), Elsevier, Amsterdam.
18. Young A. R. (2007) Damage from acute vs chronic solar exposure. In: *Biophysical and Physiological Effects of Solar Radiation on Human Skin*, pp 3–23, Giacomoni P. U. (ed.), The Royal Society of Chemistry, Cambridge.
19. Halliday G. M. and Rana S. (2007) The effects of solar radiation on the immune response in humans. In: *Biophysical and Physiological Effects of Solar Radiation on Human Skin*, pp 127–163, Giacomoni P. U. (ed.), The Royal Society of Chemistry, Cambridge.
20. Giacomoni P. U. (ed.) (2007) *Biophysical and Physiological Effects of Solar Radiation on Human Skin*, The Royal Society of Chemistry, Cambridge.
21. Halliday G. M. and Hönigsmann (2009) Sunscreens, photoimmunosuppression, and photoaging. In: *Clinical Guide to Sunscreens and Photoprotection*, pp 101–116, Lim H. W. and Draelos Z. D. (eds.), Informa Healthcare, New York.
22. Poon T. S., Barnetson R. S. and Halliday G. M. (2003) Prevention of immunosuppression by sunscreens in humans is unrelated to protection from erythema and dependent on protection from ultraviolet A in the face of constant ultraviolet B protection. *J. Invest. Dermatol.* **121**: 184–190.

23. Wolf P., Hoffmann C., Quehenberger F., Grinschgl S. and Kerl H. (2003) Immune protection factors of chemical sunscreens measured in the local contact hypersensitivity model in humans. *J. Invest. Dermatol.* **121**: 1080–1087.
24. Krause M., Klit A., Blomberg J. M., Seeborg T., Frederiksen H., Schlumpf M., Lichtensteiger W., Skakkebaek N. E and Drzewiecki K. T. (2012) Sunscreens: are they beneficial for health? An overviev of endocrine disrupting properties of UV-filters. *Int. J. Androl.* **35**: 424–436.
25. Ou-Yang H., Stanfield J., Cole C., Appa Y. and Rigel D. (2012) High-SPF sunscreens (SPF $\geq$ 70) may provide ultraviolet protection above minimal recommended levels by adequately compensating for lower sunscreen user application amounts. *J. Am. Acad. Dermatol.* **67**: 1220–1227.
26. Herrling T., Jung K. and Fuchs J. (2006) Measurements of UV-generated free radicals/reactive oxygen species (ROS) in skin. *Spectrochim. Acta, Part A* **63**: 840–845.
27. Jung K., Seifert M., Herrling T. and Fuchs J. (2008) UV-generated free radicals (FR) in skin: their prevention by sunscreens and their induction by self-tanning agents. *Spectrochim. Acta, Part A* **69**: 1423–1428.
28. Lens M., Bielfeldt S., Bataille V. and Wilhelm K. P. (2008) p53 labeling index in assessing the efficacy of a sunscreen in protection against UV-induced damage. *Int. J. Dermatol.* **47**: 1234–1239.

B. Urocanic Acid. Structure, Photochemistry, and Initiation of Immunosuppression in Humans

Urocanic acid (UCA) with an absorption maximum (λ_{max}) at 277 nm, the amino acids tyrosine (λ = 275 nm) and tryptophan (λ = 280 nm), DNA (λ = 260 nm and with partial absorption to about 360 nm), and melanins (covering a wide range of 350–1200 nm) are the major ultraviolet light absorbers in the stratum corneum and epidermis of the human skin. The so-called "blood-borne chromophores" hemoglobin, oxyhemoglobin, bilirubin, and β-carotene in the dermis are the major absorbers of solar energy with wavelengths longer than 320 nm [1, 2]. Urocanic acid and melanins are considered the natural endogenous sunscreens, with protection properties against the UVB radiation from 280 to 320 nm and against the UVA radiation from 320 to 400 nm. Thus, it could be assumed that urocanic acid and melanins have been predestined by evolutionary events to protect, in particular, the vital DNA from damaging solar radiations. Questions arise about the efficiency of these natural UV absorbers and to what extent urocanic acid and the melanins could sustain the effects that are produced by urocanic acid absorption of solar radiation energy [**Fig. 1B-1**].

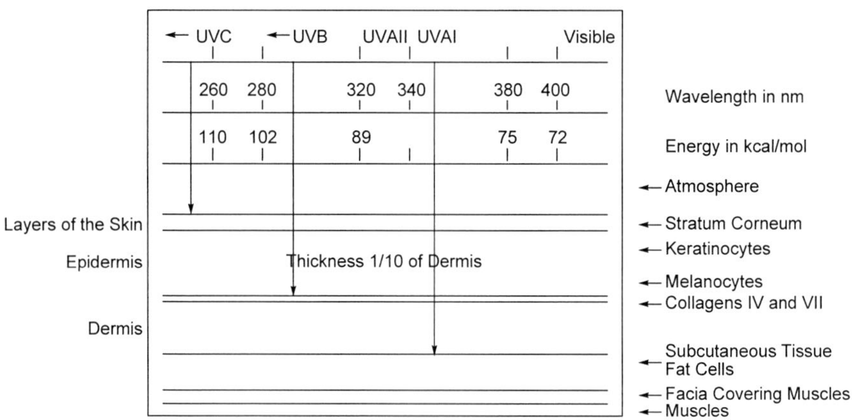

Fig. 1B-1. A sketch of the human skin and UV radiations. The bandwidth of UVA is twice that of UVB. Bandwidths of UVA = 320–380 (400) nm. UVA II = 320–340 nm, UVA I = 340–380 nm. UVB = 280 (290)–320 nm. UVC = 190 (200)–290 nm. Melanocytes can be reached by 10–14% UVB and 20–50% UVA. Dermis can be reached only by 60% UVA.

Natural urocanic acid (3-(1*H*-imidazol-4-yl)-2-propenoic acid, **2**) is a metabolite of histidine (**1**) produced by a deamination reaction mediated by the enzyme histidinase [3, 4] [**Sch. 1B-1**].

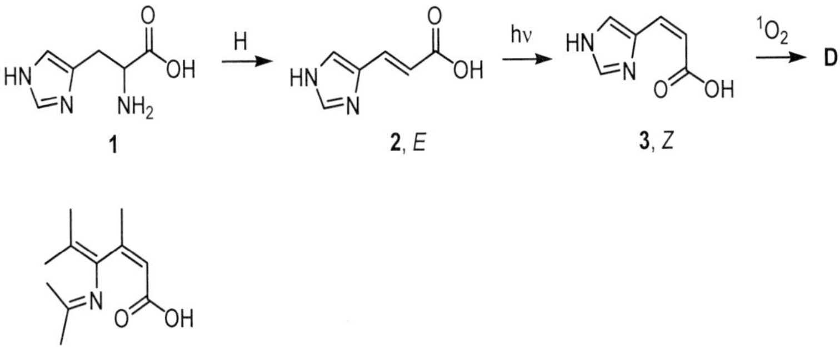

Sch. 1B-1. Formation and transformation of urocanic acid. H = histidine enzyme. D = degradation. Conjugated chromophore of urocanic acid (**4**).

Urocanic acid itself is a substrate for the enzyme urocanase which is absent in the human skin. On solar irradiation, UCA appears on the human skin dissolved in the sweat and is deposited on the skin surface [1, 3]. The incident solar radiation is reflected at the human skin to about 5% because of a change in the reflective index between the air (n = 1.0) and stratum corneum (n ≈ 1.55) [1]. This reflectance is always about 5% over a wide spectral range between 250–3000 nm, and is independent of the tan of human skin. The penetration of the ultraviolet radiations of 280, 300, 350, and 400 nm wavelengths in fair Caucasian skin corresponds to a depth of 1.5, 6.0, 60, and 90 μm, respectively [1]. The naturally occurring urocanic acid has a trans/*E* configuration [2]. Irradiation of the trans/*E* isomer with ultraviolet light results in isomerization to the cis/*Z* configuration, until a photostationary state is reached [3–12], corresponding to about equal quantities of both isomers [7]. *cis*/(*Z*)-Urocanic acid accumulates in the stratum corneum, but may also diffuse into deeper layers of the epidermis [2, 10, 11]. *cis*-Urocanic acid has been recognized as the initiator of the UV light induced immunosuppression that results in further impairment of various biological systems, such as degradation of DNA and initiation of autoimmune diseases and skin cancers, and malfunctioning of other biological entities. The whole area is extremely convoluted, and has been extensively investigated and reviewed [13–27]. Urocanic acid is structured as a conjugated chromophore (**4**) containing carbon–carbon, carbon–oxygen, and carbon–nitrogen double bonds. The double bonds contain the bonding π electrons which can undergo, on irradiation with ultraviolet light, a π,π* transition to give an excited state species. In addition, the nonbonding electrons on the oxygen and nitrogen atoms will undergo n,π* transitions to give excited state species. (For more details, see **Section 3D and Scheme 3D-1**.) Hence, it would be expected that, on irradiation with ultraviolet light, urocanic acid would be elevated to singlet and triplet excited states, which could be quenched by molecular oxygen on and in the skin to give reactive oxygen species (ROS). Thus, irradiation of urocanic acid with ultraviolet light produces singlet oxygen ($^1O_2$) and superoxide anion radical $O_2^{\cdot -}$ [4, 7–9]. The ensuing reactions of singlet oxygen with urocanic acid result in "self-destruction" of urocanic acid, and prolonged irradiation results in formation of degradation products, such as carbon dioxide, ammonia, glycine, urea, aspartic acid, glutaric acid, fumaric acid, maleic acid, and other fragments [4, 8]. Degradations of urocanic acid with other reactive oxygen species, such as Fenton's reagent, also result in a mixture of products, including three imidazoles [28]. Based on these results, one would scarcely expect good sunscreen properties of urocanic acid. Indeed, it was shown [10] that an application to the skin of a cream containing about 5% of urocanic acid, which would correspond to at least a twenty-fold excess of urocanic acid over that found in normal human skin, resulted in a protection factor of about two. Consequently, the protection properties of urocanic acid against solar radiation are actually quite poor. Surprisingly, urocanic acid is listed [29] as a sunscreen agent. Thus, one could conclude that urocanic acid is not only a mediator of immunosuppressive responses upon irradiation with ultraviolet light, but also a participant in the formation of toxic species, such as singlet oxygen. (For the oxidative reaction of the DNA heterobase guanine with singlet oxygen and other reactive oxygen species, see **Section 2D**.)

A number of studies [30–33] have been conducted in order to establish to what extent the application of exogenous ultraviolet light absorbers to the human skin could either alleviate or even inhibit the effects of the photoisomerization of *trans*/(*E*)-urocanic acid to the cis/*Z* isomer. Thus, in these experiments, organic compounds—such as 4-*tert*-butyl-4'-methoxydibenzoylmethane, 2-hydroxy-4-methoxybenzophenone (oxybenzone), 2-ethylhexyl 4-methoxycinnamate, 2-phenylbenzimidazole-5-sulfonic acid, 3-(4'-methylbenzylidene)-camphor tetraphthalylidene 3,3'-dicamphor-10,10'-disulfonic acid—and inorganic UV absorbers zinc oxide and titanium dioxide have been used as UV light absorbers, either alone or in combinations.

Experiments on human subjects with sunscreens showed that the ability to inhibit *cis*-UCA (**3**) formation was not influenced by the penetration characteristics of the sunscreen [2], or by the skin type [1]. The sunscreen protection factors (SPFs) ranged between 4 and 10, and UV radiations between 280 and 365 nm. The skin was covered with the UV absorbers prior to the irradiations, either with the optimum recommended amount of 2 mg/cm^2 or with a more realistic dose of 0.5 mg/cm^2 which might be expected in 'real life' situations in the field. The UV irradiations were either single or multiple exposures. Naturally, the results were varied and often scattered, depending on the prevailing experimental conditions [30–33]. Nevertheless, it appears that under the most ideal conditions, the isomerization of *trans*/(*E*)-urocanic acid to the cis/*Z* form could be reduced to about 5%, as compared to the irradiation results of the unprotected skin in which case about 50% isomerization occurred. In contrast, under the more realistic conditions that use 0.5 mg/cm^2 coverage of the skin, about 20% isomerization was found [30–33].

In general, the rate of *cis*-UCA formation was substantially decreased with an increase of SPF and the thickness of the sunscreen layer on the skin. A better protection against the immunosuppression effect was found using the so-called "broad spectrum sunscreens", including UVA, UVB, and titanium dioxide filters [30–33]. In some cases, the titanium dioxide UV absorber was found to be either less effective, equal, or superior to the organic UV filters [13]. The difference between these types of UV absorbers is not only the degree of the reflectance scatter and absorbance of light but also the penetration into the epidermis by the organic sunscreens, resulting in a lesser protection than expected [33, 34]. However, the UV absorbers on and in the skin could also undergo photochemical reactions resulting in the formation of reactive oxygen species.

In conclusion, it is important to be aware that the UV light induced, *cis*-urocanic acid initiated immunosuppression occurs at lower radiation doses than those which are required for the onset of erythema, i.e., sunburns, inflammations, since erythema is primarily caused by the UVB radiation and to a much lesser extent by the UVA radiations, while the UVA radiations have a much greater effect than the UVB radiation on the onset of the immunosuppression. Hence, the SPF that is used as indicator for the initiation of erythema cannot be applied for the prediction of the onset of immunosuppression, since one could experience no erythema, but at the same time, unconsciously suffer the onset of immunosuppression [26]. It appears that, even under idealized experimental conditions, the application of sunscreens cannot entirely prevent some photochemical reactions on and in the human skin, whereas under practical conditions prevailing in the field, appreciable isomerization of urocanic acid occurs and other photochemical reactions can be expected.

References

1. Anderson R. R. and Parrish J. A. (1981) The optics of human skin. *J. Invest. Dermatol.* **77**: 13–19.
2. Young A. R. (1997) Chromophores in human skin. *Phys. Med. Biol.* **42**: 789–802.
3. Morrison H. (1985) Photochemistry and photobiology of urocanic acid. *Photodermatol.* **2**: 158–165.
4. Morrison H. and Deibel R. M. (1986) Photochemistry and photobiology of urocanic acid. *Photochem. Photobiol.* **43**: 663–665.
5. Kammeyer A., Teunissen M. B. M., Pavel S., DeRie M. A. and Bos J. D. (1995) Photoisomerization spectrum of urocanic acid in human skin and in vitro: effects of simulated solar and artificial ultraviolet radiation. *Br. J. Dermatol.* **122**: 884–891.
6. Hasegawa H. (1964) Photolysis of urocanic acid. *Nagasaki Igakkai Zasshi* **35**: 1669–1676.
7. Menon E. L., Perera R., Kuhn R. J. and Morrison H. (2003) Reactive oxygen species formation by UV-A irradiation of urocanic acid and the role of trace metals in this chemistry. *Photochem. Photobiol.* **78**: 567–575.
8. Menon E. L. and Morrison H. (2002) Formation of singlet oxygen by urocanic acid by UV irradiation and some consequences thereof. *Photochem. Photobiol.* **75**: 565–569.
9. Haralampus-Grynaviski N., Ransom C., Ye T., Rozanowska M., Wrona M., Sarna T. and Simon J. D. (2002) Photogeneration and quenching of reactive oxygen species by urocanic acid. *J. Am. Chem. Soc.* **124**: 3461–3468.
10. Scharffetter-Kochanek K., Wlaschek M., Brenneisen P., Schauen M., Blaudschun R. and Wenk J. (1997) UV-induced reactive oxygen species in photocarcinogenesis and photoaging. *Biol. Chem.* **378**: 1247–1257.
11. Hanson K. M. and Simon J. D. (1998) Epidermal *trans*-urocanic acid and the UVA-induced photoaging of the skin. *Proc. Natl. Acad. Sci. U. S. A.* **95**: 10576–10578.
12. Scharffetter-Kochanek K., Brenneisen P., Wenk J., Herrmann G., Ma W., Kuhr L., Meewes C. and Wlaschek M. (2000) Photoaging of the skin from phenotype to mechanisms. *Exp. Gerontol.* **35**: 307–316.
13. Hemelarr P. J. and Beijersbergen van Henegouwen G. M. (1996) The protective effect of *N*-acetylcysteine on UVB-induced immunosuppression by inhibition of the action of *cis*-urocanic acid. *J. Photochem. Photobiol.* **63**: 322–327.

14. Kripke M. L. (1984) Skin cancer, photoimmunology and urocanic acid. *Photodermatology* **1**: 161–163.
15. Noonan F. P. and De Fabo E. C. (1992) Immunosuppression by ultraviolet B radiation: initiation by urocanic acid. *Immunol. Today* **13**: 250–254.
16. Fuchs J. (1998) Potentials and limitations of the natural antioxidants RRR-alpha tocopherol, L-ascorbic acid and β-carotene in cutaneous photoprotection. *Free Radical Biol. Med.* **25**: 848–873.
17. Gruner S., Diezel W., Stoppe H., Oesterwitz H. and Henke W. (1992) Inhibition of skin allograft rejection and acute graft-versus-host disease by *cis*-urocanic acid. *J. Invest. Dermatol.* **98**: 459–462.
18. Yarosh D. B., Gettings S. D., Alas L. G., Kibitel J. T., San R. H. C., Wagner V. O. and McEwen G. N. (1992) The biological interaction of *cis*- and *trans*-urocanic acid and DNA. *Photodermatol. Photoimmunol. Photomed.* **9**: 121–126.
19. Yarosh D. B., Alas L., Kibitel J. T. and Ullrich S. (1992) Urocanic acid isomers, immunosuppressive cytokines and the induction of human immunodeficiency virus. *Photodermatol. Photoimmunol. Photomed.* **9**: 127–130.
20. Norval M. (2001) Effects of solar radiation on the human immune system. *J. Photochem Photobiol.* **63**: 28–40.
21. Norval M. (2001) Effects of solar radiation on the human immune system. In: *Sun Protection in Man*, pp 91–115, Giacomoni, P. U. (ed.), Elsevier, Amsterdam.
22. Macve J. C. (2002) The effects of UV waveband and *cis*-urocanic acid on tumor outgrowrh in mice. *Photochem. Photobiol. Sci.* **1**: 1006–1011.
23. Norval M. (2006) The mechanism and consequences of ultraviolet-induced immunosuppression. *Prog. Biophys. Mol. Biol.* **92**: 108–118.
24. Halliday G. M. and Rana S. (2007) The effects of solar radiation on the immune response in humans. In: *Biophysical and Physiological Effects of Solar Radiation on Human Skin*, pp 127–163, Giacomoni P. U. (ed.), The Royal Society of Chemistry, Cambridge.
25. Gibbs N. K. and Norval M. (2008) Recent advances in urocanic acid photochemistry, photobiology and photoimmunology. *Photochem. Photobiol. Sci.* **7**: 655–667.
26. Halliday G. M. and Hönigsmann (2009) Sunscreens, photoimmunosuppression, and photoaging. In: *Clinical Guide to Sunscreens and Photoprotection*, pp 101–116, Lim H. W. and Draelos Z. D. (eds.), Informa Healthcare, New York.

27. Decara J. M., Aguilera J., Abdala R., Sánchez P., Figueroa F. L. and Herrera E. (2008) Screening of urocanic acid isomers in human basal and squamous cell carcinoma tumors compared with tumor periphery and healthy skin. *Exp. Dermatol.* **17**: 806–812.
28. Kammeyer A., Eggelte T. A., Overmars H., Bootsma A., Bos J. D. and Teunissen M. B. (2001) Oxidative breakdown and conversion of urocanic acid isomers by hydroxyl radical generating systems. *Biochim Biophys. Acta* **1526**: 277–285.
29. Vainio H. and Bianchini F. (eds.) (2001) Sunscreens. In: *IARC Handbooks of Cancer Prevention*, Vol. 5, International Agency for Research on Cancer, WHO, Lyon.
30. Fine de Olivarius F., Wulf H. C., Crosby J. and Norval M. (1996) The sunscreening effect of urocanic acid. *Photodermatol. Photoimmunol. Photomed.* **12**: 95–99.
31. Fine de Olivarius F., Wulf H. C., Crosby J. and Norval M. (1999) Sunscreen protection against *cis*-urocanic acid production in human skin. *Acta Derm.-Venereol.* **79**: 426–430.
32. Krien P. M. and Moyal D. (1994) Sunscreens with broad-spectrum absorption decrease the *trans* to *cis* photoisomerization of urocanic acid in the human *stratum corneum* after multiple UV light exposures. *Photochem. Photobiol.* **60**: 280–287.
33. Van der Molen R. G., Out-Luiting C., Driller H., Claas F. H., Koerten H. K. and Mommaas A. M. (2000) Broad-spectrum sunscreens offer protection against urocanic acid photoisomerization by artificial ultraviolet radiation in human skin. *J. Invest. Dermatol.* **115**: 421–426.
34. Smith G. J., Miller I. J., Clair J. F. and Diffey B. L. (2002) The effect of UV-absorbing sunscreens on the reflectance and consequent protection of skin. *Photochem. Photobiol.* **75**: 122–125.

C. Melanins: Structure and Photochemistry

Melanins are heterogeneous, amorphous biopolymers of large molecular weight and high thermal stability [1–7]. Thus, certain melanins can be heated to about 600 °C without noticeable decomposition, and some fossil findings of melanins were estimated to be 150 million years old [2]. In human skin, two melanins are prevalent: the eumelanins composed of units derived from 3,4-dihydroxyphenylalanine (dopa, **2**) and phaeomelanins derived from the sulfur-atom-containing component cysteinyldopa (**11**) [1–13] [**Sch. 1C-1** and **Sch. 1C-2**]. The structures of eumelanins are probably composed, at least in part, of three-dimensional assemblies, whereby the individual layers are arranged in stacks with an interlayer spacing of 3.4 Å [5–7]. Most melanins are insoluble in water and organic solvents, although some melanins can absorb water up to thirty percent of their weight, and phaeomelanins are soluble in aqueous alkali solutions [2]. Melanins are probably the most important biological pigment in mammals, since they are components of the skin, feathers, hair, and fur, and, hence, are part of the protecting properties of the skin against the exterior environment [2, 5]. Melanins are widely distributed in nature not only in mammals but also in birds, reptiles, fish, insects, fungi, bacteria, plants, and other species [2]. Related to melanins are the humic acids, which can be found in soils, plants, and low-grade coals [2]. Some components of humic acids have a resemblance to components in melanins, such as ortho-dihydroxy-aromatic and quinoidal moieties [2]. The one-line electron paramagnetic resonance spectra (EPR) of humic acids are similar to those of eumelanins [2]. Naturally occurring melanins are always bound to proteins [2, 5, 7, 14]. Melanins have ion-exchange properties, and can harbor various metal cations, such as calcium, magnesium, and the all-important transition metal redox cations of copper and iron, which are involved in various redox reactions of melanins [2, 5, 7, 14–19].

Eumelanins contain an abundance of carboxyl, amino, and *ortho*-dihydroxyphenolic groups [**Sch. 1C-1**], which can readily interact with a variety of diamagnetic and paramagnetic cations, forming chelates. Some of these chelates have binding strengths comparable to that of ethylenediaminetetraacetic acid (EDTA). The metal cation chelates of ortho-semiquinones, the persistent oxygen-centered radicals in the eumelanins, are of particular interest for studies with EPR spectroscopy [**Sch. 1C-3**]. The diamagnetic cation chelates, e.g., those of the calcium cation, cause an increase in the intensity of the EPR signal as compared to the uncomplexed ortho-semiquinones, whereas the paramagnetic chelates, such as those of the cupric ion, result in a decrease of the EPR signal intensity.

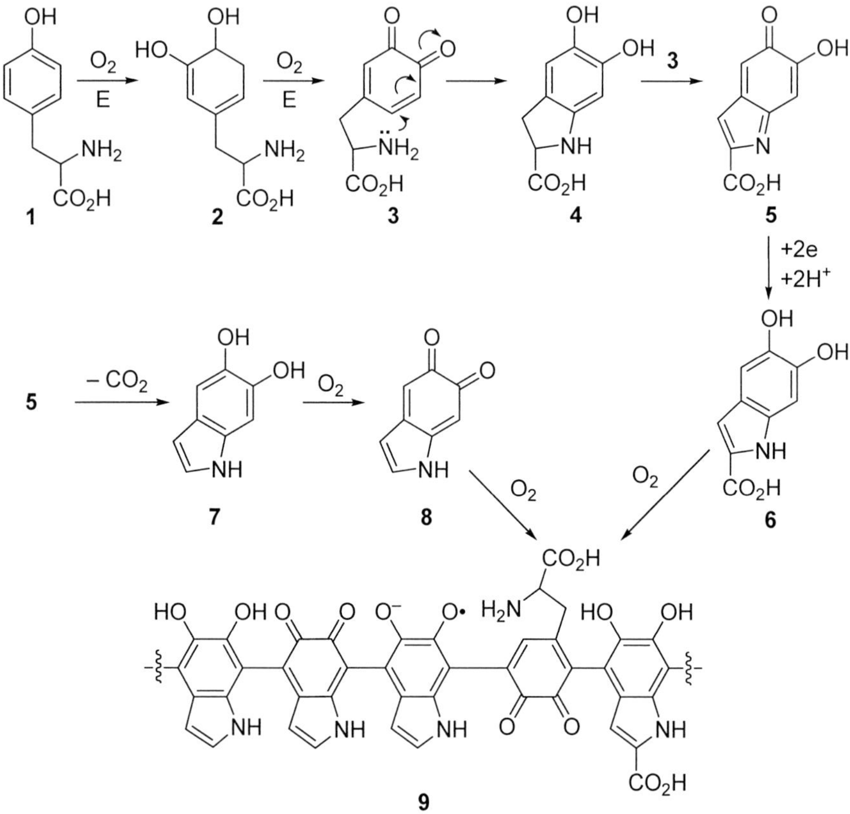

Sch. 1C-1. Formation of eumelanins. Tyrosinase (E), tyrosine(**1**), 3,4-dihydroxy-phenylalanine (dopa) (**2**), dopaquinone (**3**), cyclodopa (**4**), dopachrome (**5**), 5,6-dihydroxyindole-2-carboxylic acid (**6**), 5,6-dihydroxyindole (**7**), 5,6-indoquinone (**8**), and melanin (**9**).

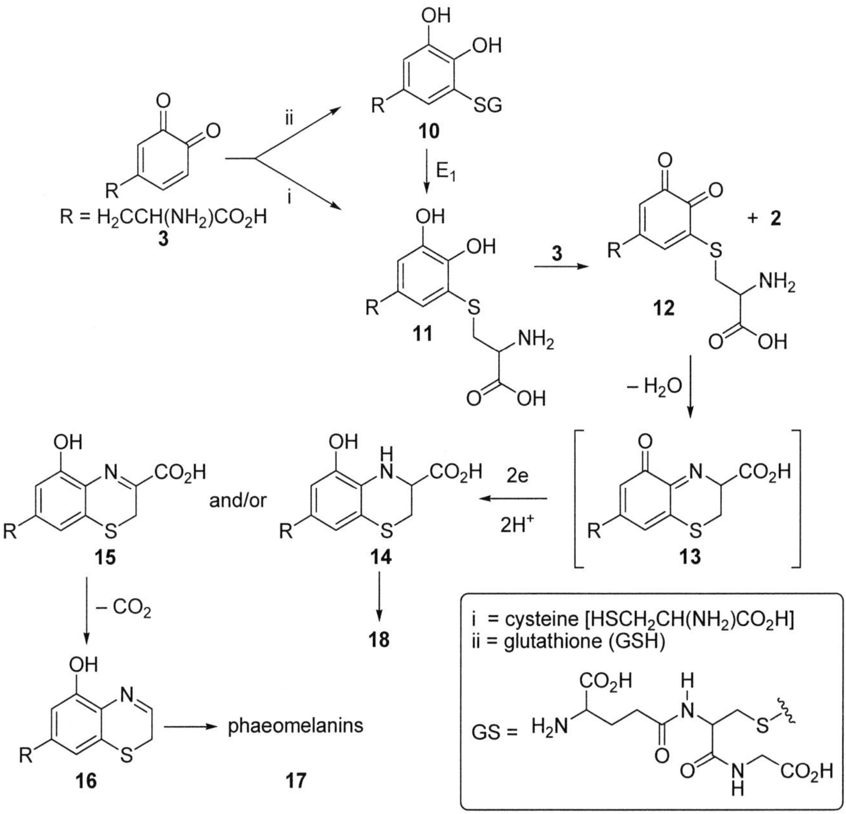

Sch. 1C-2. Formation of phaeomelanins. Tyrosinase (E), γ-glutamyltranspeptidase (E_1), dopaquinone (**3**), 5-glutathion-*S*-yldopa (**10**), 5-cystein-*S*-yldopa (**11**), cysdopaquinone (**12**), cyclocysdopa-*o*-quinoneimine (**13**), dihydrobenzothiazine (**14**), and 2*H*-1,4-benzothiazines (**15**, **16**).

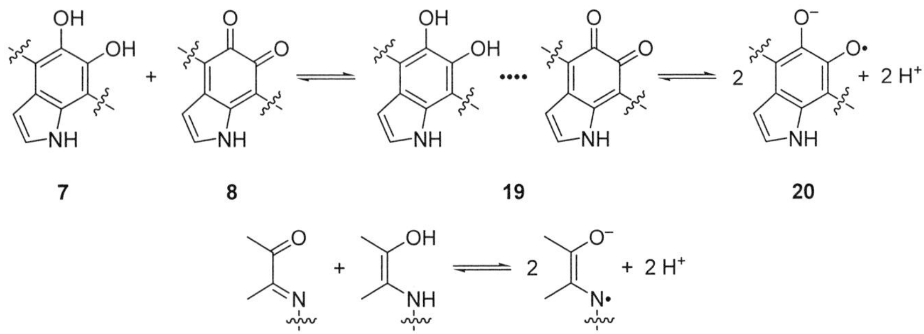

7 8 19 20

13 14 18

Sch. 1C-3. In eumelanin-type polymer: 5,6-dihydroxyindole unit (**7**), 5,6-indoquinone unit (**8**), and quinhydrone unit, a molecular complex, diamagnetic (**19**) in equilibrium with paramagnetic semiquinone unit (**20**). In phaeomelanin-type polymer: ortho-quinonimine unit (**13**) and *ortho*-aminophenol unit (**14**) in equilibrium with semiquinoneimine unit of radical **18**.

The name given to these polymers is obscure. The name is derived from the Greek word melas for black. Eumelanins means actually "good black". However, eumelanins in humans are seldom absolutely black, but all tinges of brown as well, and as far as good is concerned, it will be seen that human melanins have also less desirable qualities. The phaeomelanins according to the Greek name are considered dusky. That is also not entirely correct, since most phaeomelanins have brilliant shades of yellow, brown, orange, and red colorations [2]. Nevertheless, in spite of these incongruities, the name melanin has been retained in the literature as a descriptive term.

About fifty years ago, it was shown by electron paramagnetic resonance spectroscopy (EPR) that melanins have free radical properties derived from organic free radical species [12]. Since that time, extensive studies [1, 5, 8–31] have been conducted for further elaborations on the pioneering seminal work. It was found, by using EPR spectroscopy, that all dopa (**2**) derived melanins have a one-line spectrum that is attributable to an oxygen-centered radical species [1, 5, 10, 11, 14, 16, 26] while cysteinyldopa (**11**) derived phaeomelanins [**Sch. 1C-2**] are characterized by a poorly resolved immobilized three-line spectrum, attributable to a nitrogen-centered radical species, such as **18** [**Fig. 1C-1**] [11–13]. In nature, melanins are often found as copolymers rather than as mixtures of eumelanins and phaeomelanins in various ratios. In such cases, a poorly resolved, highly distorted, three-line spectrum was observed [16]. In addition, in well-documented studies, various parameters have been published, such as line widths, g-values, spin densities, and line shapes of melanin EPR spectra [1, 10–13,15, 26]. It has been estimated that the level of intrinsic radical species in melanin polymers are only about 0.1–0.2%, i.e., the radical species are probably randomly located every 200–1000 units apart in the polymers [1, 10].

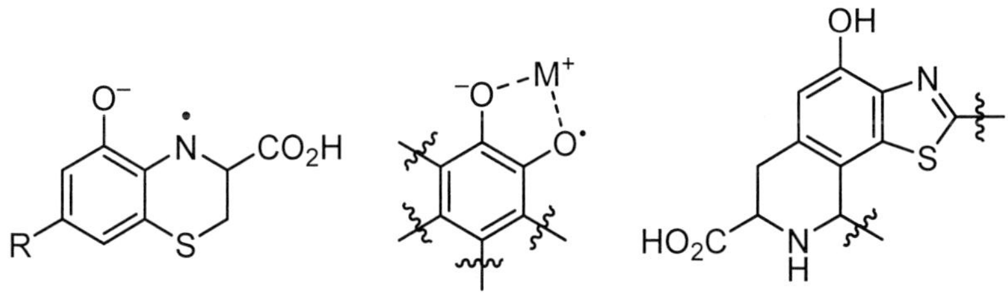

18 **20** **21**

Fig. 1C-1. Semiquinoneimine radical (**18**), five-membered chelates between ortho-semiquinone radical (**20**) and metal ions, and benzothiazoletetrahydroisoquinol unit (**21**) as possible phaeomelanin components.

In most photophysical, photochemical, and photobiological experiments described in the literature, light sources have been used that emit mainly light of wavelengths between 230–600 nm, i.e., light covering the important solar UVA and UVB radiations, and a good part of the visible spectrum [6–10, 18, 21–25, 29]. It is important to be aware that light energies of very short wavelengths are in the range of bond energies of organic compounds [**Fig. 1B-1**].

Eumelanins contain a preponderance of indoquinol (**7**) and indoquinone (**8**) structural elements, which form weak complexes (**19**) [**Sch. 1C-3**]. These diamagnetic quinhydrone complexes (**19**) are in equilibrium with the paramagnetic semiquinone species (**20**) [9, 10, 16, 19, 23]. Since eumelanins always absorb substantial amounts of water, there exists an aqueous aerated environment around the solid-state complexes. Hence, it can be expected, that this environment would have some influence on the reactions of these complexes in eumelanins. The intrinsic stable free radical semiquinone species (**20**) can always be detected by EPR, even in the absence of light irradiation [11, 14].

Over the years, extensive efforts have been made to delineate the structures and mechanisms of formation of the species. The studies have been hampered, of course, by the complete insolubility of eumelanins and poor solubility of phaeomelanins. Therefore, in many cases, harsh degradation methods had to be used, resulting in degradation products, which were not necessarily those of the starting polymer materials. Many studies have been conducted using synthetic melanins, and many conclusions are based on those studies [1–6, 8, 10, 21–29]. Nevertheless, there is a fair understanding of the formation, reactions, and properties of melanins. For the purposes of this review, they are more than adequate.

The formation of eumelanins proceed synthetically, and most likely also in the biological environment, according to **Sch. 1C-1** [1–5], commencing with the oxidative conversion of tyrosine (**1**) in the presence of oxygen to 3,4-dihydroxyphenylalanine (dopa, **2**). The hydroxylation step is mediated by the enzyme tyrosinase, which is actually composed of three isozymes, in conjunction with copper cations [4]. Dopa (**2**) is then converted into dopaquinone (**3**), again catalyzed by tyrosinase in the presence of oxygen. These two oxidative steps, no doubt, proceed by free radical type mechanisms. The cyclization reaction of dopaquinone (**3**) to cyclodopa (**4**) is probably a base-catalyzed unimolecular reaction. The subsequent redox reactions and partial decarboxylation yield 5,6-dihydroxyindol-2-carboxylic acid (**6**), 5,6-dihydroxyindole (**7**), and 5,6-indoloquinone (**8**), which are utilized in the polymerization process to give a eumelanin-type polymer (**9**).

The formation of phaeomelanins is initiated by the condensation of tyrosine (**1**) with cysteine [**Sch. 1C-2**], resulting in the formation of 5-cystein-*S*-yldopa (**11**) and other isomers of lesser importance [5, 6, 11–13]. 5-Cystein-*S*-yldopa (**11**) is then oxidized enzymatically by tyrosinase in the presence of **3** and oxygen to cyclodopaquinone (**12**) which undergoes a cyclization reaction to form, presumably, either the dihydrobenzothiazine derivative (**14**) via the cyclodopa-ortho-quinoneimine (**13**) which is unstable, and/or the 2*H*-1,4-benzothiazine derivatives **15** and **16** via a partial decarboxylation reaction. The ensuing instant polymerization process results in the formation of the phaeomelanins polymer (**17**) containing these components [5,11,12].

The initial steps in the formation of phaeomelanins may also involve reaction of tyrosine (**1**) with glutathione (GSH), analogous to the reaction with cysteine [**Sch. 1C-1**], resulting in the formation of glutathionedopa (**10**), which, however, is rapidly converted into cysteinyldopa (**11**), by the enzymatic reaction mediated by γ-glutamyltranspeptidase [4, 5]. In contrast to the phaeomelanin compounds **14–16**, structures have been proposed that contain the benzothiazole rings (**21**) [5, 9]. However, there is some uncertainty about whether this type of ring structure was present in the original native polymer or was obtained by the harsh degradation procedures [5].

The polymerization processes of all melanins can be envisaged to occur by either an ionic or a radical mechanism, or both. Since the polymerizations occur in aerated environments, often in the presence of transition-metal cations, radical processes would be favored in many steps of the polymerization sequence [3].

At this juncture, no attempt will be made to expand and critically analyze the structural and mechanistic details of the formation of melanins. Instead, the emphasis will be on the photophysical, photochemical, and chemical reactions of melanins, resulting in the formation of reactive oxygen species and their transformation. This area is of paramount importance in connection with the preservation, prevention, and protection of human skin against harmful endogeneous and exogeneous agents.

All melanins and their intermediates, which have been encountered in the formation of melanins, have several well-defined unifying structural elements, the so-called chromophores, which are of decisive importance in the absorption of solar energy and subsequent reactions. The chromophores **22** and **23** [**Fig. 1C-2**] are part of the quinhydrone systems (**19**) in melanins. The chromophores **24**–**26** are conjugated to aromatic and heteroaromatic ring structures, which have also chromophoric properties. In addition, melanins have an abundance of hydroxyl groups, which act as auxochromes causing the "red shift", i.e., to absorbances at longer wavelengths. In the ground state of these chromophores, there are π-bonding electrons on unsaturated functions and nonbonding n electrons on the heteroatoms. Irradiation with ultraviolet and visible lights causes π,π^* and n,π^* transitions to excited singlet and triplet states. (For additional details, see **Chapter 3**.)

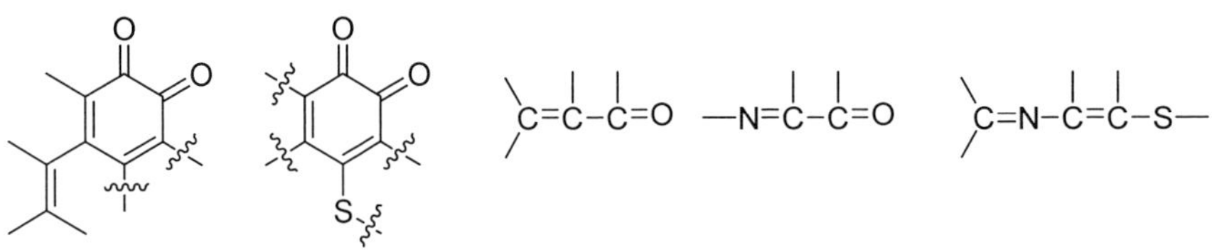

22 **23** **24** **25** **26**

Fig. 1C-2. Chromophores of melanins.

Thus, based on these chromophores, it can be expected that melanins should be excellent absorbers of ultraviolet and visible light energies. In instances where the absorbed energies would be efficiently dissipated as heat and/or scattered, the melanins could be regarded as ideal natural sunscreen agents. However, melanins seem to have only low scatter and heat dissipation properties in the visible part of the spectrum [7, 9, 23, 26]. Hence, the absorbed energies of light are utilized in the elevation of the melanins from the ground state to the excited diamagnetic singlet state and via intersystem crossing (ISC) to the paramagnetic triplet state [**Sch. 1C-4**].

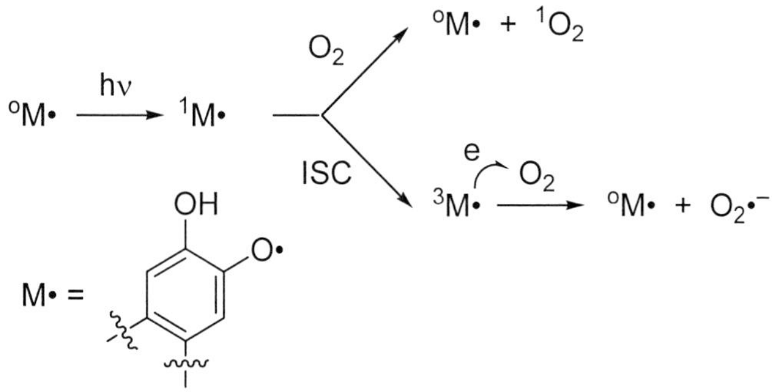

Sch. 1C-4. Photochemistry of melanins. Generation of singlet oxygen ($^1O_2$) and superoxide anion radical ($O_2\cdot^-$). $^oM\cdot$ = ground state melanin, $^1M\cdot$ = singlet state, $^3M\cdot$ = triplet state, ISC = intersystem crossing, $^oM\cdot$ = melanin in equilibrium with semiquinone.

These species readily interact with molecular oxygen, which is a diradical in the ground state, to give reactive oxygen species (ROS), such as singlet oxygen ($^1O_2$), superoxide anion radical ($O_2\cdot^-$), hydroxyl radicals (HO·), and hydrogen peroxide [**Sch. 1C-4** and **Sch. 1C-5**]. The hydrogen peroxide, hydroxyl radical, and superoxide anion radicals can also be generated by a variety of secondary reactions, including the ground state components of melanins and transition-metal cations bound to the melanins [**Sch. 1C-6**] [7, 9, 10, 21–32].

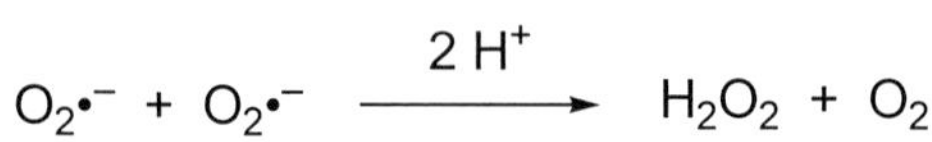

Sch. 1C-5. Formation of hydrogen peroxide and molecular oxygen by dismutation of superoxide anion radical.

$$M{-}Fe^{2+} + O_2{\bullet}^- \xrightleftharpoons{2\,H^+} M{-}Fe^{3+} + H_2O_2$$

$$M{-}Fe^{2+} + H_2O_2 \longrightarrow M{-}Fe^{3+} + HO{\bullet} + HO^-$$

$$M{-}Fe^{3+} + H_2O_2 \rightleftharpoons M{-}Fe^{2+} + HOO{\bullet} + H^+$$

$$M{-}Fe^{2+} + O_2 \rightleftharpoons M{-}Fe^{3+} + O_2{\bullet}^-$$

Sch. 1C-6. Reactions of iron cation–melanin complexes with reactive oxygen species, generated by photochemical reactions with melanins.

The energy of the singlet state melanin species can be transferred to molecular oxygen, resulting in the inversion of one electron spin on oxygen to give a singlet oxygen with an electron pair located in the same orbital. This species, denoted as delta (Δ) singlet oxygen, can undergo reactions both as an electrophile and as a nucleophile. In the case where the excited electron is located unpaired in a different orbital, the species is a sigma (Σ) singlet oxygen species. However, this species is very unstable and decays before reacting with substrates, such as lipids and DNA [30].

$$\uparrow O_2 \uparrow \;\rightarrow\; \uparrow O_2 \downarrow {}^1\Sigma_g \;\rightarrow\; \uparrow\downarrow O_2 \; {}^1\Delta_g$$

All ROS, including singlet oxygen, have much longer half-lives than the 0.3 ns of the hydroxyl radical. The hydroxyl radical is also the most electrophilic of all ROS. It would be expected that, besides the reactions with molecular oxygen, the triplet species of melanins could also undergo reactions with various hydrogen donor compounds of biological origin [**Sch. 1C-7**]. Indeed, it was shown [8] that the reactions of melanins with nicotinamide adenine dinucleotide (NADH) and the phosphate NADPH in the presence of oxygen resulted in oxidations of these compounds. The oxidations were increased when the reactants were irradiated with a broad-spectrum light source, while the oxidations were decreased in the presence of the hydrogen donor phenothiazine [8]. Similarly, the irradiation of NADH, NADPH, and ascorbic acid with visible light resulted in oxidations of the compounds [7]. It is most likely that these reactions occurred by hydrogen-transfer reactions [22]. This type of reaction has been extensively studied over the years with 1,4-benzoquinones and various donor compounds, such as NADH, glutathione, ascorbic acid, α-tocopherol, phenothiazines, and other compounds to give semiquinones and donor compound radicals or anion radicals [33]. The results and mechanistic interpretations of these studies [33] can be applied, no doubt, to the 1,2-indoquinone systems of eumelanins [22]. When a mixture of two hydrogen donor compounds is used, a competition reaction ensues [8]. The semiquinone imine type radical (**18**) of phaeomelanins, which was detected by EPR spectroscopy [11, 12], could also be formed by a hydrogen-transfer process involving the melanin triplet species [22]. The photolysis of the phaeomelanin component 5-cystein-*S*-yldopa (**11**) with ultraviolet light of 290 nm produces the sulfur- and carbon-centered radicals [**Sch. 1C-8**] [6]. The free radical species that are generated by various reactions of melanins could accumulate in the solid-state type melanin matrixes as is frequently implied in the literature. It has also been found that melanins can function as pseudodismutases, i.e., as superoxide dismutase mimics [24, 26, 27, 29, 30, 32]. In the redox reactions [**Sch. 1C-9**], the melanins could function either in the formation or elimination of reactive oxygen species.

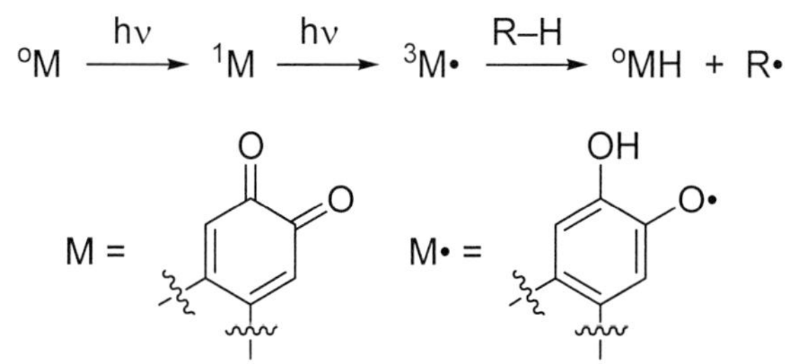

Sch. 1C-7. Photochemistry of melanins with hydrogen donors. R–H = hydrogen donors, e.g., NADH, NADPH, ascorbic acid. R· = radicals derived from donor compound, e.g., ascorbyl radical.

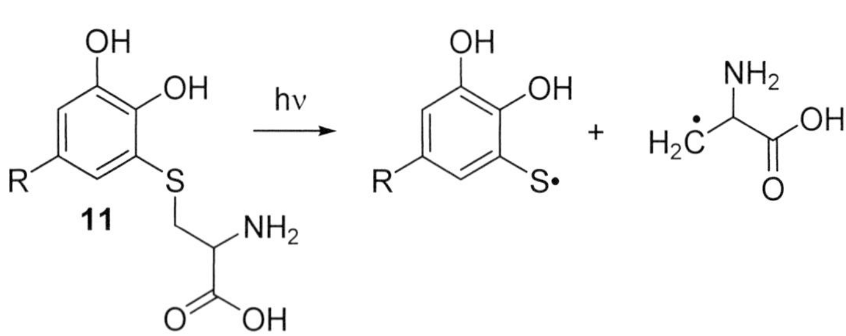

Sch. 1C-8. Photolysis of phaeomelanin component 5-cystein-S-yldopa with UV light (290 nm) resulting in sulfur- and carbon-centered radicals.

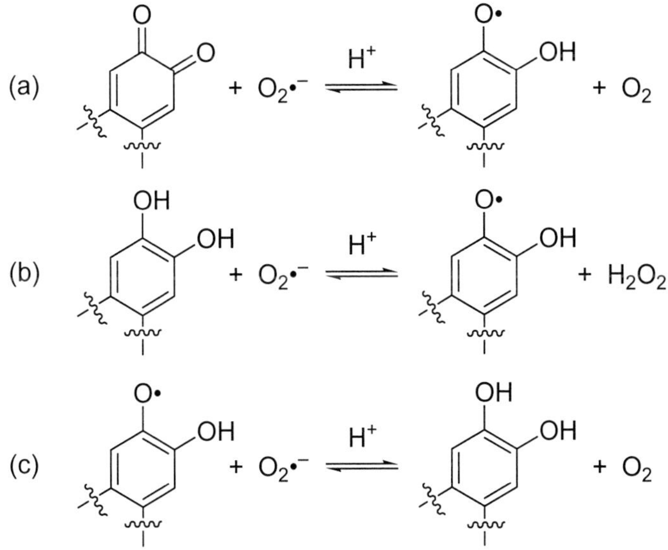

Sch. 1C-9. Eumelanins as possible pseudodismutases; (a) oxidizing form of melanins, (b) reducing form of melanins, and (c) semiquinone radical form of melanins.

In conjunction with the elucidation of mechanisms of action of nitroxyl (aminoxyl)-labeled drugs against melanomas, studies have been conducted [31] to probe the nature of melanin components by using spin-labeled compounds, such as the nitroxyl radical, 4-oxo-2,2,6,6-tetramethylpiperidine-1-oxyl. (See **Section 2G**.) It was known that aminoxyls can mimic superoxide dismutase [**Sch. 1C-10**] [34, 35]. Hence, reactions of aminoxyl radicals with the superoxide anion radicals, which are generated by the photochemical and other reactions of melanins could occur in accordance with **Sch. 1C-11**. Aminoxyl radicals have been found [36–40] to "trap" carbon-centered radicals. Since it was shown [31] that the aminoxyl radicals bind to synthetic melanins, it is possible that reactions occur between nitroxyl radicals and the "trapped" radicals to give O-substituted hydroxylamine derivatives [**Sch. 1C-12**], although there is some doubt concerning this proposition [31]. Aminoxyl radicals also facilitate the activity of tyrosinase in the synthesis of eumelanins, probably by trapping those free radical species which function as inhibitors of the enzymatic process [31].

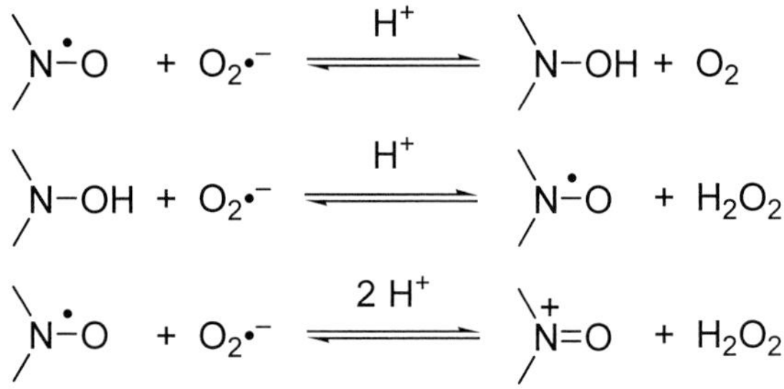

Sch. 1C-10. Reactions of aminoxyl radical as superoxide dismutase mimic.

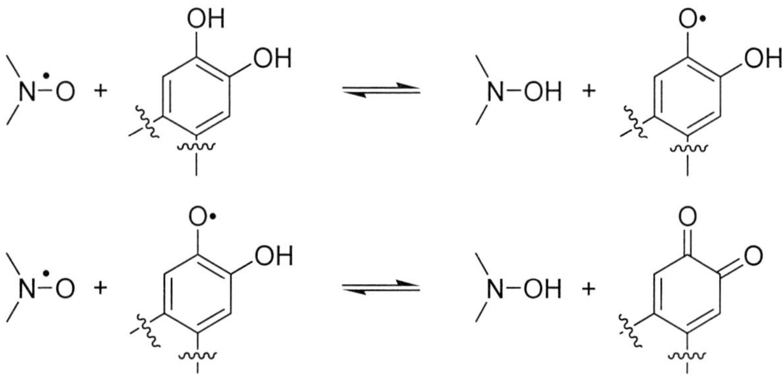

Sch. 1C-11. Possible reactions of eumelanins with aminoxyl radicals.

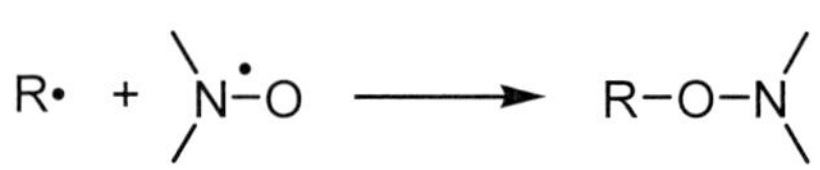

Sch. 1C-12. "Trapping" reactions of carbon-centered radicals by aminoxyl radicals.

In general, melanins have been considered to have benign properties in protecting the human skin against the harmful effects of solar radiations [6, 8, 9, 21–30, 32]. However, the phenolic and quinoid components of melanins were found to be toxic to cells [4, 8, 18, 28]. Irradiations with gamma rays and UVC light of DNA samples in the presence of eumelanins, which were prepared by autoxidations of D,L-dopa (**2**) [**Sch. 1C-1**], resulted in significant strand breaks and formations of thymine glycols. These products were also obtained in the absence of radiations after incubations at 4 °C and 37 °C [41–43].

Irradiation of a phage DNA sample together with 5,6-dihydroxy-2-indolecarboxylic acid (**6**) [**Sch. 1C-1**] with ultraviolet light of 313 nm resulted in single-strand breaks, whereby hydroxyl radicals, superoxide anion radicals, and probably singlet oxygen species were involved in causing this degradation [44].

The formation of reactive oxygen species (ROS) derived from melanins by photophysical and photochemical processes has been well documented throughout this section. However, a question remains as to whether the redox reactions of melanins in the absence of irradiations can also produce ROS. Such reactions have been known to occur with the antibiotic anticancer drugs containing the para-quinone and para-hydroquinone moieties [31, 45], such as rubomycin [31], for the treatment of melanoma, involving the reaction of a para-semiquinone intermediate with molecular oxygen [46]. In numerous studies with these clinically used drugs, it was found that increases in the anticancer activity and the undesirable cardiotoxicity occurred either on reductions of para-quinones or on oxidations of para-hydroquinones to para-semiquinones [46]. The reductions in a cellular environment are mediated by various enzymes, such as NADPH cytochrome P450 reductase [30, 31]. During this process, the toxic superoxide anion radicals and hydroxyl radicals are always formed. Therefore, this process is also always accompanied by peroxidation reactions of lipids [30, 31]. The formation of ROS seems to point to reactions of the para-semiquinone groups of the drugs with molecular oxygen, whereby the para-semiquinone moiety is reoxidized to the para-quinone moiety with the formation of superoxide anion radicals ($O_2^{\bullet -}$). The latter are converted, by a dismutation process, to molecular oxygen and hydrogen peroxide, which is the source of hydroxyl radicals [**Sch. 1C-13**, and, by analogy, **Sch. 1C-5**, **Sch. 1C-6**, and **Sch. 1C-8**].

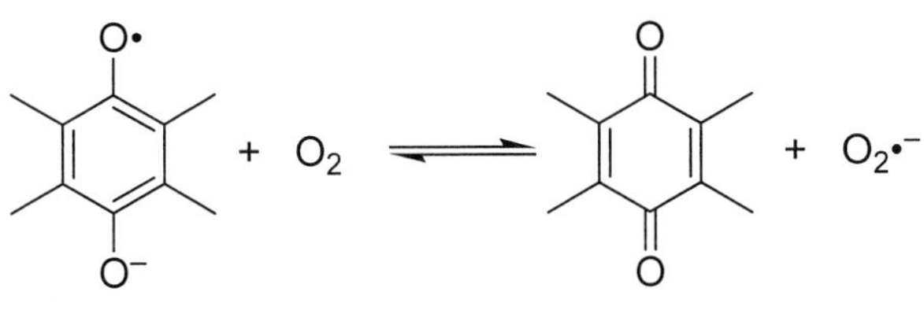

Sch. 1C-13. Oxidation of para-semiquinones of anticancer drugs.

This idea is supported by the fact that the para-semiquinones derived from the one-electron reductions of the para-quinone-containing anticancer drugs undergo reactions with molecular oxygen at the very rapid rates of K = 10^7–10^9 $M^{-1}s^{-1}$ [46]. Therefore, it is tempting to speculate that analogous processes occur with the ortho-quinone, ortho-hydroquinone, and ortho-semiquinone moieties of melanins [**Sch. 1C-3**], derived from such precursors as dopa (**2**) and 5-cystein-*S*-yldopa (**11**) [**Sch. 1C-1** and **Sch. 1C-2**] and molecular oxygen to give superoxide anion radicals, and subsequently hydroxyl radicals [**Sch. 1C-5**, **Sch. 1C-6**, and **Sch. 1C-8**]. Indeed, mechanisms for such interactions have been proposed on several occasions. However, it was shown, using EPR spectroscopy, that such reactions are insignificant since they proceed, in the case of dopa (**2**) and 5-cystein-*S*-yldopa (**11**) at the very slow rates of ≤ 10^5 $M^{-1}s^{-1}$ [46]. Consequently, the observed consumption of molecular oxygen during the redox reactions of melanin components probably proceeds by different mechanisms. Thus, the tyrosinase-mediated oxidations of dopa (**2**) to dopaquinone (**3**) and 5-cystein-*S*-yldopa (**11**) to cyclodopaquinone (**12**) [**Sch. 1C-1** and **Sch. 1C-2**] via the corresponding ortho-semiquinone intermediates [**Sch. 1C-3**] cannot proceed by direct interactions with molecular oxygen, but are, most likely, formed by catalytic oxidations with cupric cations that are continuously regenerated by molecular oxygen, resulting in the formation of superoxide anion radicals as byproducts [**Sch. 1C-14**]. This type of cupric-catalyzed oxidations have a precedent in the conversion of the hydroxyl groups in ascorbic acid to the 1,2-dione group via the ascorbyl anion radical. (See **Section 5B** on antioxidants.) Recapitulating, the UV light induced reactions of melanins with molecular oxygen initially produce the singlet oxygen species and superoxide anion radicals. These peroxides and the derived peroxides from superoxide anion radicals can readily undergo photochemical reactions with melanins; in the case of eumelanins, primarily with the hydroquinone groups [**Sch. 1C-4** to **Sch. 1C-7**, **Sch. 1C-9**, **Sch. 1C-12**, **Sch. 1C-13**, and **Sch. 1C-15**]. The severity of these often-damaging processes was shown [47, 48] to depend on the degree of aggregations of small oligo units of eumelanins into larger units. This coalescence results in a decrease of the hydroquinone units at the surfaces of eumelanins, and, consequently, in a reduced formation of photoproducts and an alleviation of oxidative stress [47, 48]. Thus, solar energy causes the melanins to generate self-inflicting damages. However, at the same time, these reactions of melanins in the skin can be viewed as benign effects for the prevention of free radical reactions by ROS with other biological systems [49, 50].

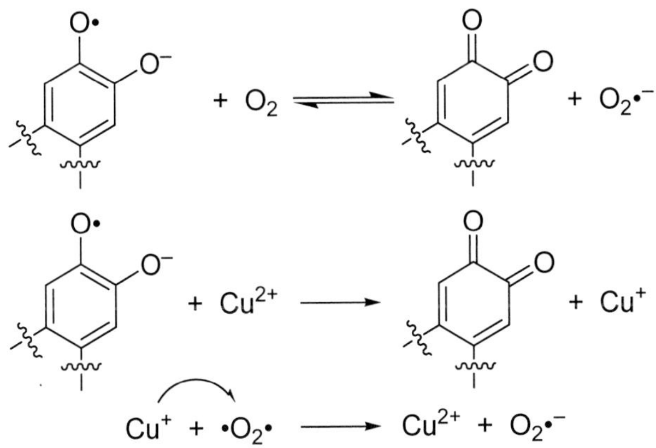

Sch. 1C-14. Proposed oxidations of ortho-semiquinones of melanins by molecular oxygen in the presence of copper cations as catalysts.

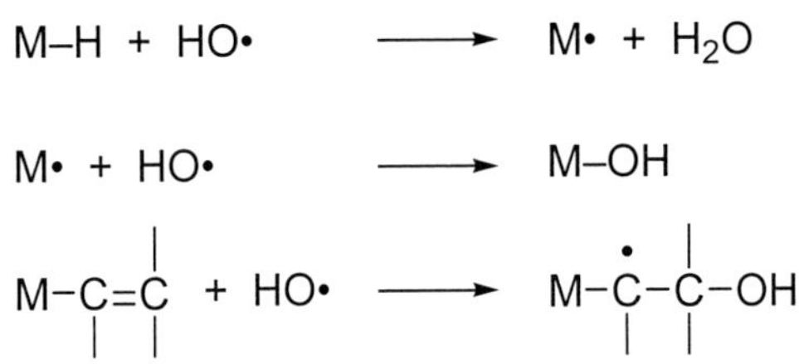

Sch. 1C-15. Reactions of the hydroxyl radical with various melanin functions.

In conclusion, melanins have been destined by evolutionary processes to have only partially protecting qualities in human skin. Prolonged and intense exposures to solar radiations can result in melanin-mediated damages to the skin and other biological entities.

Various aspects of their biology, physiology, and biochemistry have been intensely investigated and reviewed in recent years [48, 51–53].

References

1. Blois M. S., Zahlan A. B. and Mailing J. E. (1964) Electron spin resonance studies on melanin. *Biophys. J.* **4**: 471–490.
2. Nicolaus R. A. (1968) Melanins. In: *Chemistry of natural products,* pp 9–305, Lederer E. (ed.), Hermann, Paris, and references therein.
3. Swan G. A. (1973) Current knowledge of melanin structure. *Pigm. Cell* **1**: 151–157.

4. Pawelek J. M. and Korner A. M. (1982) The biosynthesis of mammalian melanin. *Am. Sci.* **70**: 136–145.
5. Prota G. (1988) Progress in the chemistry of melanins and related metabolites. *Med. Res. Rev.* **8**: 525–556, and references therein.
6. Chedekel M. R. and Zeisel L. (1988) Sunlight, melanogenesis and radicals in the skin. *Lipids* **23**: 587–591.
7. Glickman R. D., Gallas J. M., Jacques S. L., Rockwell B. A. and Sardar D. K. (2000) *The physical and photochemical properties of ocular melanin.* Internet presentation for Saratov Fall Conf. 3–6 Oct. 2000, and references therein.
8. Menon I. A. and Haberman H. F. (1977) Mechanisms of action of melanins. *Br. J. Dermatol.* **97**: 109–112.
9. Chedekel M. R. (1982) Photochemistry and photobiology of epidermal melanins. Yearly review. *Photochem. Photobiol.* **33**: 881–885.
10. Arnoud R., Perbet G., Deflandre A. and Lang G. (1983) Electron spin resonance of melanin from hair. Effects of temperature, pH and light irradiation. *Photochem. Photobiol.* **38**: 161–168.
11. Sealy R. C. (1984) Radicals in melanin biochemistry. *Meth. Enz.* **105**: 479–483.
12. Sealy R. C., Hyde J. S., Felix C. C., Menon I. A., Prota G., Swartz H. M., Persad S. and Haberman H. F. (1982) Novel free radicals in synthetic and natural phaeomelanins: distinction between dopa melanins and cysteinyl dopa melanins by ESR spectroscopy. *Proc. Natl. Acad. Sci. U. S. A.* **79**: 2885–2889.
13. Sealy R. C., Hyde J. S., Felix C. C., Menon I. A. and Prota G. (1982) Eumelanins and phaeomelanins: characterization by electron spin resonance spectroscopy. *Science* **217**: 545–547.
14. Sarna T., Froncisz W. and Hyde J. S. (1980) Cu^{2+} probe of metal-ion binding sites in melanin using electron paramagnetic resonance spectroscopy. II. Natural melanins. *Arch. Biochem. Biophys.* **202**: 304–313.
15. Sarna T., Hyde J. S. and Swartz H. M. (1976) Ion-exchange in melanin: an electron spin resonance study with lanthanide probes. *Science* **192**: 1132–1134.
16. Felix C. C., Hyde J. S., Sarna T. and Sealy, R. C. (1978) Interactions of melanin with metal ions. Electron spin resonance evidence for chelate complexes of metal ions with free radicals. *J. Am. Chem. Soc.* **100**: 3922–3926.
17. Froncisz W., Sarna T. and Hyde J. S. (1980) Cu^{2+} probe of metal-ion binding sites in melanin using electron paramagnetic resonance spec-

troscopy. I. Synthetic melanins. *Arch. Biochem. Biophys.* **202**: 289–303.

18. Felix C. C. and Sealy R. C. (1981) Electron spin resonance characterization of radicals from 3,4-dihydroxyphenylalanine: semiquinone anions and their metal chelates. *J. Am. Chem. Soc.* **103**: 2831–2836.
19. Kalyanaraman B., Felix C. C. and Sealy R. C. (1985) Semiquinone anion radicals of catechol(amine)s, catechol estrogens and their metal ion complexes. *Environ. Health Perspect.* **64**: 185–198.
20. Commoner B., Townsend J. and Pake G. E. (1954) Free radicals in biological materials. *Nature* **174**: 689–691.
21. Felix C. C., Hyde J. S., Sarna T. and Sealy R. C. (1978) Melanin photoreaction in aerated media: electron spin resonance evidence for production of superoxide and hydrogen peroxide. *Biochem. Biophys. Res. Commun.* **84**: 335–341.
22. Felix C. C., Hyde J. S. and Sealy R. C. (1979) Photoreactions of melanin: a new transient species and evidence for triplet state involvement. *Biochem. Biophys. Res. Commun.* **88**: 456–461.
23. Chio S. S., Hyde J. S. and Sealy R. C. (1980) Temperature-dependent paramagnetism in melanin polymers. *Arch. Biochem. Biophys.* **199**: 133–139.
24. Sarna T. and Sealy R. C. (1984) Free radicals from eumelanins: quantum yields and wavelength dependence. *Arch. Biochem. Biophys.* **232**: 574–578.
25. Sarna T. and Sealy R. C. (1984) Photoinduced oxygen consumption in melanin systems. Action spectra and quantum yields for melanin and synthetic melanin. *Photochem. Photobiol.* **39**: 69–74.
26. Korytowski W., Kalyanaraman B., Menon I. A., Sarna T. and Sealy R. C. (1986) Reaction of superoxide anions with melanins: electron spin resonance and spin trapping studies. *Biochim. Biophys. Acta* **882**: 145–153.
27. Sarna T., Pilas B., Land E. J. and Truscott T. G. (1986) Interaction of radicals from water radiolysis with melanin. *Biochim. Biophys. Acta* **883**: 162–167.
28. Korytowski W., Sarna T., Kalyanaraman B. and Sealy R. C. (1987) Tyrosinase-catalyzed oxidation of dopa and related catechol(amine)s: a kinetic electron spin resonance investigation using spin-stabilization and spin label oximetry. *Biochim. Biophys. Acta* **924**: 383–392.
29. Korytowski W., Pilas B., Sarna T. and Kalyanaraman B. (1987) Photoinduced generation of hydrogen peroxide and hydroxyl radicals in melanins. *Biochem. Biophys.* **45**: 185–190.

30. Fuchs J. (1992) *Oxidative injury in dermatopatology*, Springer-Verlag, Berlin.
31. Raikov Z. D. (2000) *Spin-labeled antitumor compounds*, Robev S. K. (ed.), Bulgaria. ISBN 954-9736-02-5, and references therein.
32. Goodchild N. T., Kwock L. and Lin P-S. (1981) Melanin: a possible cellular superoxide scavenger. In: *Oxygen and oxy-radicals in chemistry and biology*, pp 645–649, Rodgers M. A. J. and Powers E. L. (eds.), Academic Press, New York.
33. Biondi C., Galeazzi R., Littarru G. and Greci L. (2002) Reduction of 1,4-quinone and ubiquinones by hydrogen atom transfer and UVA irradiation. *Free Radical Res.* **36**: 399–404.
34. Carloni P., Damiani E., Greci L., Stipa P., Marrosu G., Petrucci R. and Trazza A. (1996) Chemical and electrochemical study on the interactions of aminoxyls with superoxide anion. *Tetrahedron* **52**: 11257–11264.
35. Greci L., Damiani E., Carloni P. and Stipa P. (1997) Indolinic and quinolinic aminoxyls as biological antioxidants. In: *Free radicals in biology and environment*, pp 223–232, Minisci F. (ed.), Kluwer Academic Publishers, The Netherlands.
36. Gerlock J. L., Zacmanidis P. J., Bauer D. R., Simpson D. J., Blough N. V. and Salmeen I. T. (1990) Fluorescence detection of free radicals by nitroxide scavenging. *Free Radical Commun.* **10**: 119–121.
37. Damiani E., Greci L., Parsons R. and Knowland J. (1999) Nitroxide radicals protect DNA from damage when illuminated in vitro in the presence of dibenzoylmethane and a common sunscreen ingredient. *Free Radical Biol. Med.* **26**: 809–816.
38. Damiani E., Carloni P., Stipa P. and Greci L. (1999) Reactivity of an indolinic aminoxyl with superoxide anion and hydroxyl radicals. *Free Radical Res.* **31**: 113–121.
39. Damiani E., Kalinska B., Canapa A., Canestrari S., Wozniak M., Olmo E. and Greci L. (2002) Effects of nitroxide radicals on oxidative DNA damage. *Free Radical Biol. Med.* **28**: 1257–1265.
40. Scalia, S., Simeoni S., Barbieri A. and Sostero S. (2002) Influence of hydroxypropyl-beta-cyclodextrin on photo-induced free radical production by the sunscreen agent butyl-methoxydibenzoylmethane. *J. Pharm. Pharmacol.* **54**: 1553–1558.
41. Hill H. Z. and Hill G. F. (1987) Eumelanin causes DNA strand breaks and kills cells. *Pigm. Cell Res.* **1**: 163–170.
42. Hubbard-Smith K., Hill H. Z. and Hill G. J. (1992) Melanin both causes and prevents oxidative base damage in DNA: quantification by anti-thymine glycol antibody. *Radiat. Res.* **130**: 160–165.

43. Huselton C. A. and Hill H. Z. (1990) Melanin photosensitizes ultraviolet light (UVC) DNA damage in pigment cells. *Environ. Mol. Mutat.* **16**: 37–43.
44. Routaboul C., Serpentini C. L., Msika P., Cesarini J. P. and Paillous N. (1985) Photosensitization of supercoiled DNA damage by 5,6-dihydroxyindole-2-carboxylic acid, a precursor of eumelanin. *Photochem. Photobiol.* **62**: 469–475.
45. Gnewuch C. T. and Sosnovsky G. (2002) Critical appraisals of approaches for predictive designs in anticancer drugs. *Cell. Mol. Life Sci.* **59**: 959–1023.
46. Kalyanaraman B., Korytowski W., Pilas B., Sarna T., Land E. J. and Truscott T. G. (1988) Reaction between ortho-semiquinones and oxygen: pulse radiolysis, electron spin resonance and oxygen uptake studies. *Arch. Biochem. Biophys.* **266**: 277–284.
47. Nofsinger J. B., Liu Y. and Simon J. D. (2002) Aggregation of eumelanin mitigates photogeneration of reactive oxygen species. *Free Radical Biol. Med.* **32**: 720–730.
48. Liu Y. and Simon J. D. (2003) Isolation and Biophysical Studies of Natural Eumelanins: Applications of Imaging Technologies and Ultrafast Spectroscopy. *Pigm. Cell Res.* **16**: 606–618.
49. Herrling T., Jung K. and Fuchs J. (2008) The role of melanin as protector against free radicals in skin and its role as free radical indicator in hair. *Spectrochim. Acta, Part A* **69**: 1429–1435.
50. Brenner M. and Hearing V. J. (2008) The protective role of melanin against UV damage in human skin. *Photochem. Photobiol.* **84**: 539–549.
51. Young A. R. and Sheehan J. M. (2001) UV-induced Pigmentation in Human Skin. In: *Sun Protection in Man*, pp 357–375, Giacomoni, P. U. (ed.), Elsevier, Amsterdam.
52. Calzavara-Pinton P. G. and Ortel B. (2007) Pigmentation after Solar Radiation. In: *Biophysical and Physiological Effects of Solar Radiation on Human Skin*, pp 65–97, Giacomoni P. U. (ed.), The Royal Society of Chemistry, Cambridge.
53. Beer J. Z. and Hearing V. J. (2007) Skin Color, Melanin, Race/Ethnicity and UV-Induced DNA Damage. In: *Biophysical and Physiological Effects of Solar Radiation on Human Skin*, pp 99–125, Giacomoni P. U. (ed.), The Royal Society of Chemistry, Cambridge.

CHAPTER TWO

DAMAGES TO THE HUMAN SKIN BY SOLAR RADIATION: NONCANCEROUS AND PRECANCEROUS CHANGES

A. Allergic and Photoallergic Properties of Sunscreens

The photosensitivity of humans to sunscreens that cause allergic and/or photoallergic responses has been extensively studied over the past fifty years [1–15]. Several excellent review articles covering specific aspects of this topic have been published during this period [4–7]. Therefore, there is no need in the present review for another critical assemblage of all data on this topic. Instead, several examples may suffice to emphasize the health problems that have been encountered by a large number of individuals upon using the freely available "over the counter" commercial sunscreen products. Thus, in studies involving 305 patients using a number of commercial UVA and UVB sunscreen filters, it was shown that 239 allergic and/or 150 photoallergic responses occurred, whereby many individuals developed allergies to more than one sunscreen product. In other studies with 402 patients using commercial sunscreen agents, 80 patients (20%) developed clinically observed sensitivity, i.e., allergic and/or photoallergic dermatitis, whereby 102 allergies were attributable to the UVA radiation absorbing agents and 73 allergies to the UVB radiation absorbing filters. Furthermore, the use of UVA agents elicited more allergic (48) and photoallergic (54) responses than the UVB absorbing agents with 43 allergic and 30 photoallergic reactions, and patients were afflicted with allergies caused by more than one kind of sunscreen agent [5,6]. The commercial sunscreen formulations are composed of a multitude of different, often unrelated, ingredients. Usually, one formulation contains about 30–50 different ingredients (excipients), including such preservatives as parabens, i.e., methyl, ethyl, *n*-propyl, and *n*-butyl hydroxybenzoates, phenoxylethanol, dehydroacetic acid, 2-bromo-2-nitro-1,3-propanediol (bromopol), benzyl alcohol, benzoic acid, sorbic acid, triclosan, chlorohexidine, DMDM hydantoin, diazolidinyl urea, and imidazolidinyl urea. All of these compounds were found to cause allergic reactions in some users of sunscreen products. Several of these preservatives, such as bromopol, DMDM hydantoin, diazolidinyl urea, and imidazolidinyl urea can undergo decompositions with the formation of formaldehyde, which is a chemical hazard, a primary irritant of the human skin, and a possible carcinogen [1]. In many sunscreen formulations, specific compounds are included for fragrance effects, often without adequate structural information, although this type of compound is known to cause allergic reactions [1–13]. Thus, for example, in 47 patients exposed to fragrance compounds, 178 allergic and 15 photoallergic reactions were observed [6, 7]. Also, it is generally not realized that various prescription and nonprescription medications that are taken orally, inadvertently, can surface either unchanged or as metabolites at the human skin and cause allergic and photoallergic reactions [13–15]. (See **Section 3D**.)

Sunscreen agents are often included in skin care cosmetics, such as creams, moisturizers, conditioners, lipsticks, anti-aging creams, and other cosmetic products. Routinely included in those formulations are various parabens, which have been shown to have acute and toxic effects on fish and algae, and have been detected in cancerous breast tissues of women [3]. The recently used sunscreen agent 2-hydroxy-4-methoxybenzophenone (oxybenzone), which has been shown to have allergic and photoallergic properties, readily penetrates the human skin, and can be detected in urine.

Other frequently used UV filters such as 4-*tert*-butyl-4-methoxydibenzoylmethane, 2-ethylhexyl 4-methoxycinnamate and isoamyl 4-methoxydibenzoylmethane cause photoallergic contact dermatitis [1]. Furthermore, the photodegradation of 4-*tert*-butyl-4-methoxydibenzoylmethane produces cytotoxic benzils and photocontact allergies by arylglyoxals [2].

These enlightening, but rather troubling, results convey a serious but apparently somewhat minimized problem [9] caused by the prevailing casual use of prescription-free sunscreen preparations in order to prevent reddening and inflammation of the skin without suspecting more serious but latent health problems.

B. Sunburn Effect, Erythema, and Photoaging

The skin of humans is the ultimate defense against the biological, chemical, and physical malfeasances that originate from internal and external stimuli and agents [16–25]. The human skin consists of two major layers, i.e., the outer epidermis and the inner dermis. The epidermis has been divided into four or five sublayers consisting mainly of keratinocytes, which are continually undergoing renewal processes. The keratinocytes contain, through the evolutionary process, various reactive oxygen species (ROS) and a number of diverse classes of detoxifying agents such as the enzymes superoxide dismutase, catalase, glutathione peroxidase and reductase; the antioxidant β-carotene and vitamins C and E; the proteins for metal cation binding transferrin, albumin, haptoglobin; and compounds with radical scavenging properties such as bilirubin and urates [22–26]. Thus, in a healthy body, a balance is maintained between the oxidant and antioxidant species. This homeostasis can be easily upset by various exogenous agents and intracellular and extracellular endogeneous metabolic processes, such as the generation of radical species from inflammations involving xenobiotics, gamma rays, ultraviolet radiations, and visible and infrared light stimuli [22–38]. Hence, this imbalance of oxidants and antioxidants results in the so-called oxidative stress leading to cellular reactions, such as oxidations of proteins, with a loss of normal cell functions, inflammations, photoaging, many other maladies, and ultimately to cancers [15, 22–37]. By the way, oxidative stress is not restricted to mammals, but is also found in plant tissues when irradiated with 400–700 nm light resulting in the formation of singlet oxygen species. (See **Section 4A.**)

Exposures of the human skin to sun rays even for short periods of time can result in erythema, an abnormal reddening of the skin caused by capillary congestion [33–38]. In extreme cases, prolonged exposures to radiation will inevitably produce severe inflammation, blistering, and peeling of the skin. The inflammation initially is a local response to cellular injury marked by capillary dilation, leukocytic infiltration, reddening, heat and pain and serves as a mechanism for initiating the elimination of noxious agents and damaged tissue, such as reactive oxygen species, arachidonic acid, prostaglandin metabolites, and DNA pyrimidine dimers. Thus, the degree of inflammation and damage to the skin components will depend on a number of factors, but also on the types of person who were subjected to the radiation [36–45]. Thus, persons with a light-colored skin may always experience erythema, but not tanning, while people with a dark skin may not be susceptible to erythema, and enjoy excellent tanning. The tanning of human skin involves pigmentation of melanins, primarily the brown-black eumelanin and the less common red pheomelanin. Tanning can occur either immediately on exposure, i.e., immediate pigment tanning (IPO), or by delayed pigment darkening. The IPO usually fades within minutes, while the persistent pigment darkening (PPO) may remain for hours and days. The darkening of melanin is accompanied by oxidative processes of melanin, an increase of melanocytes, an increase of the tyrosinase activity, and a transfer of melanosomes to keratinocytes. Melanin is an antioxidant, a natural filter of solar energy radiation, and a photosensitizer for the formation of ROS. Thus, melanin has benign and malign qualities. (See **Section 1C** on melanins.) An exposure of human skin to solar radiations either of prolonged duration or frequently recurring radiation, i.e., chronic exposure, will result in some visible changes on the skin, such as yellowing, dryness, thickness, leathery property, freckles, wrinkles, loss of elasticity, and invisible, latent changes such as a severe damage of dermal connective tissues, epidermal thickening, dermal inflammation, collagen damage, increase of glucosamineglycans, and a possible formation of premalignant neoplasms.

It is often incorrectly assumed that photoaging is simply an accelerated, otherwise "normal" aging process of the skin. However, it was shown that these phenomena are distinctly different. Thus, while the "normally" aged skin, which has not been subjected to excessive solar exposure, may show loss of elasticity, it can be, nevertheless, unblemished and smooth, unlike the photodamaged skin [17–21, 29, 36–39, 44, 46–55].

C. Penetration of the Human Skin by UVA and UVB Radiations and Sunscreen Agents. Endogenous Production of Hydroxyl Radicals in Various Layers of the Human Skin

The penetration of human skin by the UVB radiation will affect the components of the epidermis and some components of the dermis, while the UVA radiation, with longer wavelengths, will penetrate the dermis down to the junction of dermis and the subcutaneous tissue [**Fig. 1B-1**].

It was initially assumed that only the UVB radiation of the ultraviolet spectrum was causing the troublesome reddening and inflammation of the skin, since the required UVA doses for such an effect were expected to be 1000 times greater than those of the UVB radiation. However, in sunrays, the UVA radiation is present in levels 1000 times greater than those of the UVB radiation. Hence, it is obvious that the UVA radiation could cause such an erythema effect [34–38, 45, 46]. Unfortunately, many sunscreen formulations have been initially developed based on the premise that the UVB radiation should be prevented from reaching the skin, while neglecting the "deep seated" damages caused by the UVA radiation.

Hydroxyl radicals can be formed in the human skin by various endogenous and exogenous processes. The endogenous processes involve oxygen metabolisms in the cellular environment, whereas the exogenous processes are induced by various radiation stimuli. Thus, the components of the human skin, such as melanin, can undergo photosensitization reactions by solar radiations to give excited singlet and triplet species which are effectively quenched by molecular oxygen, resulting in the formation of reactive oxygen species (ROS) that are the source of hydroxyl radicals. (See **Section 4**.) Water in the human skin is also a source of hydroxyl radicals when irradiated with ultraviolet light. The radicals are produced by homolysis of the water molecules [56]. This reaction is facilitated by the presence of transition metal cations, in particular, the ubiquitous iron cations [**Sch. 2C-1**] [56, 57].

$$H_2O + Fe^{3+} \xrightarrow{h\nu} H_2O^{\bullet +} + Fe^{2+}$$

$$H_2O^{\bullet +} \longrightarrow HO^{\bullet} + H^+ \qquad (k = 10^{12}\ s^{-1}\ [34])$$

$$HO^{\bullet} + Fe^{2+} + H^+ \longrightarrow H_2O + Fe^{3+}$$

Sch. 2C-1. The formation of hydroxyl radicals by ultraviolet radiation of human skin in the presence of iron cations.

Another source of hydroxyl radicals in biological environments could also be considered, whereby the hydroxyl radicals are formed by the Fenton-type decomposition of hydrogen peroxide in the presence of ferrous cations. (See **Section 4**.) However, it appears that an accumulation of hydrogen peroxide in biological systems, including the skin, caused by pathological processes is low, i.e., 10^{-10} to 10^{-8} M [57, 58]. Instead, it is possible that because of high molecular oxygen content in biological systems, reactions can ensue between molecular oxygen and ferrous cations to produce superoxide anion radicals ($O_2{\cdot}^-$), followed by conversion of $O_2{\cdot}^-$ to hydrogen peroxide and a subsequent Fenton-type reaction to give hydroxyl radicals [**Sch. 2C-2**] [57, 58].

$$Fe^{2+} + O_2 \longrightarrow Fe^{3+} + O_2^{\bullet -}$$

$$Fe^{2+} + O_2^{\bullet -} \xrightarrow{2H^+} Fe^{3+} + H_2O_2$$

$$Fe^{2+} + H_2O_2 \longrightarrow Fe^{3+} + HO^{\bullet} + HO^{-}$$

Sch. 2C-2. Formation of hydroxyl radicals via molecular oxygen and ferrous cations.

The various layers of the human skin contain different amounts of water. Thus, the stratum corneum contains about 15%, the epidermis about 35%, and the dermis about 70% of water. Consequently, if it is assumed that UV radiation has an equal effect on the cleavage of water in all layers, the dermis should contain the largest quantity of hydroxyl radicals. However, the UVA and UVB radiations have different penetration potentials. Thus, 15–35% of the UVB light and 60–80% of the UVA light penetrates the metabolically active epidermis, whereas 60% of the UVA and none of the UVB radiation can reach the upper dermis [52, 53, 56]. Thus, the generation of hydroxyl radicals and of other reactive oxygen species will depend on the wavelength and intensity of the UV light and on the water content of the layers. Consequently, the UVB radiation will have an influence on the stratum corneum and epidermis with low water content, while the UVA radiation will exert its full effect in the dermis with a 70% water content.

The erythema and inflammation of the skin, the so-called sunburn effect will be caused, therefore, primarily by the UVB radiation in the epidermis, while the deeper penetrating UVA radiation with longer wavelengths will have a more lasting effect in the dermis. Although the UVA radiation is about 1000 times energetically less effective than the UVB radiation, it contains about 90–95% of the solar energy which is reaching the earth's inhabitants.

The permeation of the human skin by the UV light induced excited sunscreen species could be expected to readily occur since the UV filters and their possible degradation products and metabolites have mostly lipophilic properties with molecular weights below 500. (See **Section 3D**.) These properties enable the species to penetrate the stratum corneum, the epidermis, and transdermal layers [59–63]. Therefore, it is not surprising that various widely used commercial UV filters, when applied topically to the human skin of volunteers, have been detected in the plasma and urine of the volunteers [63–65].

Thus, benzophenone-3 was found in the urine of about 97% of human volunteers. Oxybenzone tested on human volunteers in topical applications with and without UV radiation was excreted in 3–5 hours after application, and it was detected in the urine of 98% of six-to-eight-year old girls. The levels of oxybenzone were higher in girls and women than in boys and men. The estrogenic sunscreens, 4-methylbenzylidene camphor and 3-benzylidene camphor, which are part of various skin care cosmetics, were tested for the transdermal passage from mothers to offsprings through breast milk. It was found that 79% of women regularly used skin cosmetics and 76% of their milk samples contained these filters [66].

Exposure of the frequently used sunscreens 4-*tert*-butyl-4-methoxydibenzoylmethane, 4-methylbenzylidene camphor, 2-ethylhexyl 4-methoxycinnamate, and benzophenone-3 to UV radiations facilitates the systemic absorption and permeation of these compounds through the human skin into deeper nucleated layers of the dermis, where living cells are encountered. These compounds are then detected in human plasma and urine [63–65, 67, 68].

Furthermore, it was found that the sunscreens 2-ethylhexyl 4-methoxycinnamate, 2-ethylhexyl salicylate, 3,3,5-trimethylcyclohexyl salicylate (homosalate), 2-ethylhexyl 4-di-ethylaminobenzoate, benzophenone-3, and benzophenone-4 can function as skin permeation enhancers of insecticides, herbicides, and other xenobiotics [63, 69]. The UV light induced photoreactions of most sunscreen molecules with molecular oxygen species produce a cascade of reactive oxygen species (ROS). In nucleated layers of the epidermis is maintained a certain level of ROS that are formed naturally by photoreactions of epidermal chromophores upon irradiation with UV light. The permeation of photoexcited sunscreen species into the nucleated epidermis causes an enhancement of the natural level of ROS, in particular upon illumination with the deeply penetrating UVA light [70, 71].

It was also shown that when all three sunscreens octocrylene, 2-ethylhexyl 4-methoxycinnamate, and benzophenone-3 penetrate the nucleated layers of the human skin on UV irradiation, the levels of the generated ROS increase above the levels that normally are formed by irradiation of epidermal chromophores in the absence of sunscreens [71]. Hence, the sunscreens have only a limited capacity for protecting the skin against the highly reactive ROS.

In conclusion, and based on such results, it is surprising to find that the harmlessness of photoexcited sunscreens to humans is a widely held opinion.

References

1. Collaris E. J. and Frank J. (2008) Photoallergic contact dermatitis caused by ultraviolet filters in different sunscreens. *Int. J. Dermatol.* **47** (Suppl. 1): 35–37.
2. Karlsson I., Hillerström L., Stenfeldt A. L., Mårtensson J. and Börje A. (2009) Photodegradation of dibenzoylmethanes: potential cause of photocontact allergy to sunscreens. *Chem. Res. Toxicol.* **22**: 1881–1892.
3. Reisch M. S. (2010) Preservatives under fire. Concerns over the cancer-causing potential of commonly used skin and hair care components dog cosmetic ingredient makers. *Chem. Eng. News* **88**: 13–16.
4. Schauder S. and Ippen H. (1986) Photoallergic and allergic contact dermatitis from dibenzoylmethanes. *Photodermatol.* **3**: 40–147.
5. Schauder S. (1990) Survey of the literature on adverse reactions to preparations containing UV filters (1947–1989). *Z. Hautkrankh.* **65**: 982–998.
6. Schauder S. and Ippen H. (1997) Contact and photocontact sensitivity to sunscreens. Review of a 15-year experience and of the literature. *Contact Derm.* **37**: 221–232, and references therein.
7. Schauder S. (2001) Dermatologische Verträglichkeit von UV-Filter, Duftstoffen und Konservierungsmitteln in Sonnenschutz Präparaten. *Bundesgesundheitsblatt-Gesundheits-forschung-Gesundheitsschutz* **44**: 471–479.
8. Vainio H. and Bianchi F. (eds.) (2001) *IARC Handbooks of Cancer Prevention Sunscreens*. Vol. 5, Chapter 1, International Agency on Cancer, Lyon.
9. Nohynek G. J. and Schaefer H. (2001) Benefit and risk of organic ultraviolet filters. *Regul. Toxicol. Pharmacol.* **33**: 285–299.
10. Molière P., Hüppe G., Averbeck D., Young A. R., Santus R. and Dubertret L. (1990) In vitro photostability and photosensitizing of bergamot oil. Effects of a cinnamate sunscreen. *J. Photochem. Photobiol., B* **7**: 199–208.
11. Dubertret L., Serraf-Tircazes D., Jeanmougin M., Molière P., Averbeck D. and Young A. R. (1990) Phototoxic properties of perfumes

containing bergamot oil on human skin: photoprotective effect of UVA and UVB sunscreens. *J. Photochem. Photobiol., B* 7: 251–259.
12. Young A. R., Walker S. L., Kinley J. S., Plastow S. R., Averbeck D., Molière P. and Dubertret L. (1990) Phototumorigenesis studies of 5-methoxypsoralen in bergamot oil: evaluation and modification of risk on human use in an albino mouse skin model. *J. Photochem. Photobiol., B* 7: 231–250.
13. Orentreich D., Leone A.- S., Arpino G. and Burack H. (2001) Sunscreens: practical application. In: *Sun Protection in Man*, pp 535–559, Giacomoni, P. U. (ed.), Elsevier, Amsterdam.
14. Moore D. E. (2002) Drug-induced cutaneous photosensitivity. Incidence, mechanism, prevention and management. *Drug Safety* **25**: 345–372.
15. Marrot L. and Meunier J.-R. (2008) Skin DNA photodamage and its biological consequences. *J. Am. Acad. Dermatol.* **58** (5 Suppl. 2): S139–S148.
16. Anderson R. R. and Parrish J. A. (1981) The optics of human skin. *J. Invest. Dermatol.* **7**: 13–19.
17. Hawk J. L. M. and Parrish J. A. (1982) Responses of normal skin to ultraviolet radiation. In: *The Science of Photomedicine*, pp 219–260, Regan J. D. and Parrish J. A. (eds.), Plenum Press, New York.
18. Goldberg L. H. and Altman A. (1984) Benign skin changes associated with chronic sunlight exposure. *Cutis* **34**: 33–39.
19. Kollias N., Sayre R. M., Zeise L. and Chedekel M. R. (1991). Photoprotection by melanin. *J. Photochem. Photobiol., B* **9**: 135–160.
20. Sarna, T. (1992) Properties and function of ocular melanin–A photobiophysical view. *J. Photochem. Photobiol., B* **12**: 215–258.
21. Tyrrell R. M. (1994). The molecular and cellular pathology of solar ultraviolet radiation. *Mol. Aspects Med.* **15**: 1–77.
22. Fuchs J. (1992) *Oxidative Injury in Dermatopathology*, Springer Verlag, Berlin.
23. Halliwell B. (1993) Reactive oxygen species in pathology with special reference to the skin. In: *Oxidative Stress in Dermatology*, pp 3–11, Fuchs J. and Packer L. (eds.), Marcel Dekker, New York.
24. Tyrell R. M. (1991) UVA (320–380 nm) radiation as oxidative stress. In: *Oxidative Stress: Oxidants and Antioxidants*, pp 57–84, Sies H. (ed.), Academic Press, New York.
25. Vessey D. (1993) Cutaneous antioxidant system. In: *Oxidative Stress in Dermatology*, pp 81–103, Fuchs J. and Packer L. (eds.), Marcel Dekker, New York.

26. Young A. R. (1997) Chromophores in human skin. *Phys. Med. Biol.* **42**: 789–802.
27. Kasai H. and Nishimura S. (1991) Formation of 8-hydroxydeoxyguanosine in DNA by oxygen radicals and its biological significance. In: *Oxidative Stress: Oxidants and Antioxidants*, pp 99–118, Sies H (ed.), Academic Press, New York.
28. McCord J. M. (1997) Oxygen-derived radicals: a link between reperfusion injury and inflammation. *Fed. Proceed.* **46**: 2402–2406, and references therein.
29. Pinnels R. (2003) Cutaneous photodamage, oxidative stress, and topical antioxidative stress. *J. Am. Dermatol.* **48**: 1–19.
30. Herrling T., Jung K. and Fuchs J. (2006) Measurements of UV-generated free radicals/reactive oxygen species (ROS) in skin. *Spectrochim. Acta, Part A* **63**: 840–845.
31. Grether-Beck S., Wiaschek M., Krutmann J. and Scharffetter-Kochanek K. (2005) Photodamage and photoaging-prevention and treatment. *J. Dtsch. Dermatol Ges.* (Suppl 2): S19–25.
32. Stege H., Roza L., Vink A. A., Grewe M., Ruzicka T., Grether-Beck S. and Krutmann J. (2000) Enzyme plus light therapy to repair DNA damage in ultraviolet-B-irradiated human skin. *Proc. Natl. Acad. Sci. U. S. A.* **97**: 1790–1795.
33. Parrish J. A., Jaenike K. F. and Anderson R. R. (1982). Erythema and melanogenesis action spectra of normal human skin. *Photochem. Photobiol.* **36**: 187–191.
34. Farr P. M. and Diffey B. L. (1985) The erythemal response of human skin to ultraviolet radiation. *Br. J. Dermatol.* **113**: 65–76.
35. Auletta M., Granges R. W., Tan O. T. and Matzinger E. (1986) Effect of cutaneous hypoxia upon erythema and pigment responses to UVA, UVB and PUVA (8-MOP±UVA) in human skin. *J. Invest. Dermatol.* **86**: 649–652.
36. Kligman L. H. (1987) Full spectrum solar radiation as a cause of dermal photodamage: UVB to infrared. *Acta Derm.-Venereol.* **134** (Suppl.): 53–61.
37. Kligman L. H. (1989) Photoaging. Manifestations, prevention and treatment. *Clin. Geriatr. Med.* **5**: 235–251.
38. Kitazawa M., Ishitsuka Y., Kobayashi M., Nakano T., Iwasaki K., Sakamoto K., Arakane K., Suzuki T. and Kligman L. H. (2005) Protective effects of an antioxidant derived from serine and vitamin B6 on skin photoaging in hairless mice. *Photochem. Photobiol.* **81**: 970–974.

39. Wlaschek M., Tantcheva-Poor I., Naderi L., Ma W., Schneider L. A., Razi-Wolf Z., Schuller J. and Scharffetter-Kochanek K. (2001) Solar UV irradiation and dermal photoaging. *J. Photochem. Photobiol., B* **63**: 41–51.
40. Plummer W. A., Greaves M. W., Hensby C. N. and Black A. K. (1977) Inflammation in human skin induced by ultraviolet radiation. *Postgrad. Med. J.* **53**: 656–657.
41. Greaves M. W., Hensby C. N., Black A. K., Plummer N. A., Fincham N., Warin A. P. and Camp R. (1978) Inflammatory reactions induced by ultraviolet radiation. *Bull. Cancer* **65**: 299–304.
42. Gallagher R. P., McLean D. I., Young C. P., Coldman A. J., Silver H. K. B., Spinelli J. J. and Beagric M. (1990) Suntan, sunburn and pigmentation factors and the frequency of acquired melanocytic nevi in children. Similarities to melanoma; the Vancouver mole study. *Arch. Dermatol.* **126**: 770–776.
43. Gilchrest B. A. (1996) A review of skin ageing and its medical therapy. *Br. J. Dermatol.* **135**: 867–875.
44. Scharffeter-Kochanek K., Wlaschek M., Brenneisen P., Schauen M., Blaudschun R. and Wenk J. (1997) UV-induced reactive oxygen species in photocarcinogenesis and photoaging. *Biol. Chem.* **378**: 1247–1257, and references therein.
45. Scharffeter-Kochanek K., Brenneisen P., Wenk J., Herrmann G., Ma W., Kuhr L., Meewes C. and Wlaschek M. (2000) Photoaging of the skin from phenotype to mechanisms. *Exp. Gerontol.* **35**: 307–316, and references therein.
46. Wlaschek M., Tantcheva-Poor I., Brenneisen P., Kuhr L., Razi-Wolf Z., Hellweg C., Schneider L.-A., Meewes C. and Scharffetter-Kochanek K. (2001) The negative effects of solar and artificial irradiation: photoaging of the skin, its clinical appearance and underlying mechanisms. In: *Sun Protection in Man*, pp 115–130, Giacomoni, P. U. (ed.), Elsevier, Amsterdam.
47. Pillai S., Oresajo C., and Hayward J. (2005) Ultraviolet radiation and skin aging: roles of reactive oxygen species, inflammation and protease activation, and strategies for prevention of inflammation-induced matrix degradation – a review. *Int. J. Cosmet. Sci.* **27**: 17–34.
48. Svobodova A., Walterova D. and Vostalova J. (2006) Ultraviolet light induced alteration to the skin. *Biomed. Pap. Med. Fac. Univ. Palacky Olomouc Czech Repub.* **150**: 25–38.
49. Wondrak G. T. (2007) Let the sun shine in: mechanism and potential for therapeutics in skin photodamage. *Curr. Opin. Invest. Drugs* **8**: 390–400.

50. Lübeck R. P., Berneburg M., Trelles M., Friquet B., Ogden S., Esrefoglu M., Kaya G., Goldberg D. J., Mordon S., Calderhead R. G., Griffiths C. E., Saurat J. H. and Thappa D. M. (2008) How best to half and/or revert UV-induced skin ageing: strategies, facts and fiction. *Exp. Dermatol.* **17**: 228–240.
51. Wang S. Q., Setlow R., Berwick M., Polsky D., Marghoob A. A., Kopf A. W. and Bart R. S. (2001) Ultraviolet A and melanoma: a review. *J. Am. Acad. Dermatol.* **44**: 837–846.
52. Roberts J. E. (2007) The effects of visible and near infrared light in humans. In: *Biophysical and Physiological Effects of Solar Radiation on Human Skin*, pp 211–224, Giacomoni P. U. (ed.), The Royal Society of Chemistry, Cambridge.
53. Wlaschek M., Schneider L. A., Kohn M., Nüßeler E., Treiber N. and Scharffetter-Kochanek K. (2007) Aging after solar radiation. In: *Biophysical and Physiological Effects of Solar Radiation on Human Skin*, pp 191–210, Giacomoni P. U. (ed.), The Royal Society of Chemistry, Cambridge.
54. Young A. R. (2007) Damage from acute vs. chronic solar exposure. In: *Biophysical and Physiological Effects of Solar Radiation on Human Skin*, pp 3–23, Giacomoni P. U. (ed.), The Royal Society of Chemistry, Cambridge.
55. Foster K. W., Katiyar S. K., Yusuf N. and Elmets C. A. (2007) Inflammation after solar radiation. In: *Biophysical and Physiological Effects of Solar Radiation on Human Skin*, pp 25–63, Giacomoni P. U. (ed.), The Royal Society of Chemistry, Cambridge.
56. Herrling Th., Groth N., Golz K. and Zastrow L. (2000) The role of aggressive •OH free radicals in skin – their generation, detection and prevention. *SÖFW-J.* **126**: 20–27.
57. Kruszewski M. (2003) Labile iron pool: the main determinant of cellular response to oxidative stress. *Mutat. Res.* **53**: 81–92.
58. Qian S. Y. and Buettner G. R. (1999) Iron and dioxygen chemistry is an important route to initiation of biological free radical oxidations: an electron paramagnetic resonance spin trapping study. *Free Radical Biol. Med.* **26**: 1447–1456.
59. Fernandez C., Nielloud F., Fortunè R., Vian L. and Marti-Mastres G. (2002) Benzophenone-3: rapid prediction and evaluation using non-invasive methods of in vivo human penetration. *J. Pharm. Biomed. Anal.* **28**: 57–63.
60. Zastrow L., Ferrero L., Herrling T. and Groth N. (2004) Integrated sun protective factor: a new sun protection factor based on free radi-

cals generated by UV radiation. *Skin Pharmacol. Physiol.* **17**: 219–231.

61. Haywood R. (2006) Relevance of sunscreen application method, visible light and sunlight intensity to free-radical protection: A study of ex vivo human skin. *Photochem. Photobiol.* **82**: 1123–1131.
62. Klinubol P., Asawanonda P. and Wanichwecharungruang S. P. (2008) Transdermal penetration of UV filters. *Skin Pharmacol. Physiol.* **21**: 23–29.
63. Bens G. (2008) Sunscreens. In: *Sunlight, Vitamin D and Skin Cancer*, pp 137–161, Reichrath J. (ed.), Springer Science + Business Media, LLC, New York, and Landes Bioscience, Austin, TX.
64. Janjua N. R., Morgensen B., Anderson A. M., Petersen J. H., Henriksen M., Skakkebaek N. E. and Wulf H. C. (2004) Systemic absorption of sunscreens benzophenone-3, octyl methoxycinnamate and 3-(4-methylbenzylidene)camphor after whole-body topical application and reproductive hormone levels in human. *J. Invest. Dermatol.* **123**: 56–57.
65. Sarveiya V., Risk S. and Benson H. A. E. (2004) Liquid chromatography assay for common sunscreen agents: application to in vivo assessment of skin penetration and systemic absorption in human volunteers. *J. Chromatogr. B* **803**: 225–231.
66. Schlumpf M., Kypke K., Vökt C. C., Birchler M., Durrer S., Faass O., Ehnes, C., Fuetsch, M., Gaille, C., Henseler, M., Hofkamp, L., Maerkel, K., Reolon, S., Zenker, A., Timms, B., Tresguerres, J. A. F. and Lichtensteiger, W. (2008) Endocrine active UV filters: developmental toxicity and exposure through breast milk. *Chimia, Int. J. Chem.* **62**: 345–351.
67. Gonzalez H., Farbrot A., Larko O. and Wennberg A. M. (2006) Percutaneous absorption of the sunscreen benzophenone-3 after repeated whole body applications, with and without ultraviolet irradiation. *Br. J. Dermatol.* **154**: 337–340.
68. Hayden C. G., Roberts M. S. and Benson H. A. (1997) Systemic absorption of sunscreen after topical application. *Lancet* **350** (9081): 863–864.
69. Pont A. R., Charron A. R. and Brand R. M. (2004) Active ingredients in sunscreens act as topical penetration enhancers for the herbicide 2,4-dichlorophenoxyacetic acid. *Toxicol. Appl. Pharmacol.* **195**: 348–354.
70. Haywood R., Wardman P., Sanders R. and Linge C. (2003) Sunscreens inadequately protect against ultraviolet-A-induced free radi-

cals in skin: implications for skin aging and melanoma. *J. Invest. Dermatol.* **121**: 862–868.
71. Hanson K. M., Gratton E. and Bardeen C. J. (2006) Sunscreen enhancement of UV-induced reactive oxygen species in the skin. *Free Radical Biol. Med.* **41**: 1205–1212.

D. DNA Damage Mediated by Ultraviolet Radiation. Formation of Photoproducts of Heterobases by Photoadditions and Reactions with Hydroxyl Radicals and Singlet Oxygen Species

An extensive literature has been generated over the past fifty years on the UV light induced changes in the heterobases of deoxyribonucleic acid (DNA). Hence, the cited selection of literature references was restricted to roughly the preceeding two decades, and it is not exhaustive. During this process, some publications of merit may have been inadvertently omitted from the following discourse. However, a supplemental collection of relevant topics is assembled at the end of this discourse.

The present discussion contains the UV light induced photophysical and photochemical transformations of the DNA heterobases and mechanisms of reactions of heterobases with reactive oxygen species to give oxygenated derivatives and degradation products, and comments concerning efforts to prevent those changes of the DNA by the use of sunscreen agents. Nucleic acids have an absorption maximum at about 260 nm, i.e., in the region of the non-solar UVC radiation. Since the UVC radiation is almost entirely absorbed by the ozone layer, only a tiny amount of UVC energy might be reaching the earth surface, and, hence, it is unlikely that it has a noticeable effect on the photosensitization of the DNA. However, nucleic acids absorb, in part, the solar UVB radiation ranging from 280 to 320 nm and even the UVA radiation covering the 320–380 nm range.

In aqueous media, under physiological conditions, the absorption of solar energy by the DNA results in the photosensitization of the DNA followed by subsequent reactions. The DNA has been considered a chromophore, although it is unlikely that the whole DNA molecule can be involved in this function. Therefore, instead of such an indistinct term for a chromophore, the following rationale may clarify this matter somewhat. Thus, the double helix of the DNA is composed of carbohydrate groups, phosphoric acid, and four heterobases, i.e., the pyrimidines cytosine (**1**) and thymine (**2**) and the purines adenine (**3**) and guanine (**4**). The polynucleotide strands are held together by hydrogen bonds between pairs of complementary purines and pyrimidines. The adenine amino group is always hydrogen bonded to the keto group of thymine and the keto group of guanine is hydrogen bonded to the amino group of cytosine. In addition, virtually all of the sugar molecules and phosphate groups are bonded to water molecules. These well-defined chromophores are functioning as endogenous photosensitizers of heterobases, and, ultimately of the DNA. The absorption of ultraviolet light by these chromophores results in the promotion of electrons from π and n orbitals of molecules in the ground state to higher energy levels, whereby the unsaturated functions, such as double bonds with π orbitals, are elevated to the antibonding π* orbitals by the π,π* transitions, while the nonbonding n electrons on oxygen and nitrogen atoms undergo the n,π* transitions. The heterobase guanine, containing four chromophores and the amino group as the auxochrome, would be the most susceptible to UV light sensitized processes of Type I and II [1–5, 17–20, 27–29, 42, 43]. In addition, the guanine base has the lowest oxidation potential of all heterobases of the DNA [15, 41]. Consequently, the reactions of guanine with reactive oxygen species, such as hydroxyl radicals (HO·) and singlet oxygen ($^1O_2$), proceed with the highest rate constants [15].

The photosensitized heterobases in the singlet and triplet states are very efficiently quenched by molecular oxygen to give initially the reactive oxygen species superoxide anion radical $O_2^{\cdot -}$ and singlet oxygen $^1O_2$. The superoxide anion radical is formed by an electron transfer from the excited triplet state of the UV light induced heterobase to molecular oxygen $^3O_2$ which is triplet in the ground state. The superoxide anion radical undergoes dismutation to hydrogen peroxide and molecular oxygen, followed by a cascade of reactive oxygen species, including hydroxyl radicals formed by the Fenton reaction. Singlet oxygen is formed by energy transfer from the excited triplet state of a heterobase to molecular oxygen. The minimum energy requirement for this process is 22 kcal/mol. Of all reactive oxygen species, the hydroxyl radicals would be expected to inflict the most damage to nucleic acids, because the hydroxyl radical is the most electronegative and the strongest thermodynamically stable one-electron oxidant, whereby the heterobases are the most favorable target for reactions with hydroxyl radicals. Indeed, it was found that more than 80% of hydroxyl radicals react with the heterocyclic ring systems by addition reactions rather than by hydrogen abstraction from the carbohydrate moieties. The reactions of cytosine (**1**) and thymine (**2**) with hydroxyl radicals occur by additions at the 5-carbon and 6-carbon positions of the double bonds to give the resulting radicals [**Sch. 2D-1**] [36–40]. The reactions of these radicals with hydrogen donor compounds result in the formation of 5-hydroxy-6-hydropyrimidines (**5**) and 6-hydroxy-5-hydropyrimidines (**6**)

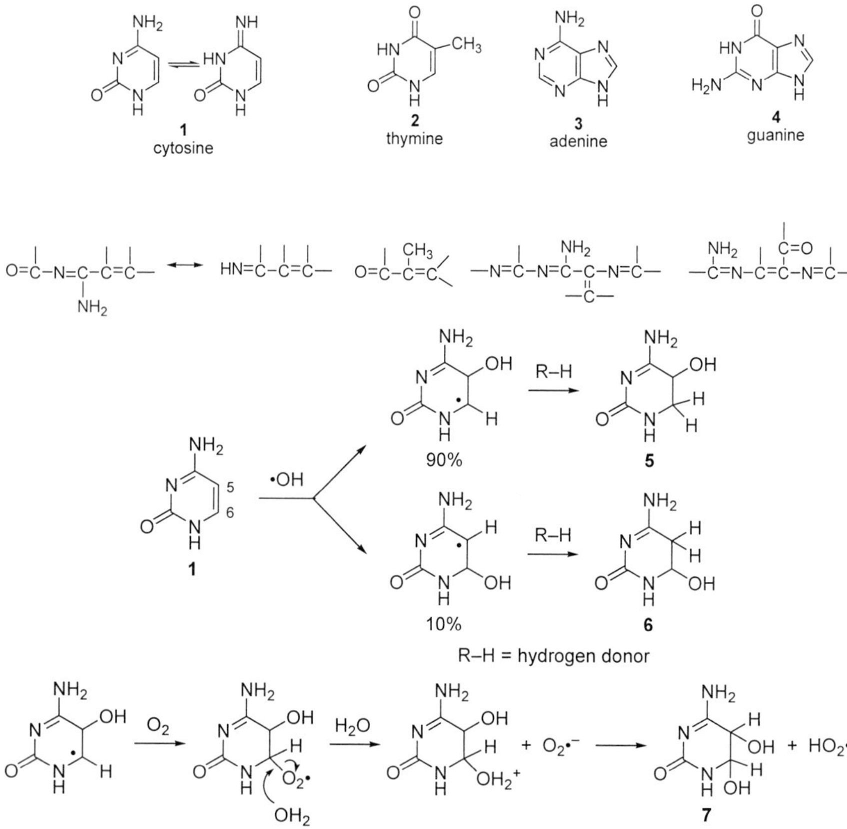

Sch. 2D-1. Reaction of cytosine with hydroxyl radical.

with the former derivative in excess of the latter derivative [**Sch. 2D-1**]. Such reactions tend to be very site-specific [4, 15, 28]. Thus, the reactions of the hydroxyl radicals with cytosine occur preferentially at position 5 of the olefinic double bond, since this position has the highest electron density. Addition of the hydroxyl radicals to the nitrogen–carbon double bond of cytosine could not be substantiated. The radical formed is an alkylamino-type radical, and was shown to have good one-electron-donor properties [**Sch. 2D-1**]. Molecular oxygen is a diradical and is known to readily react with carbon radicals by addition reactions. Hence, the reactions of radicals derived from such additions with molecular oxygen result in the formation of the corresponding cytosine peroxy radicals. These peroxy radicals in aqueous media can undergo elimination reactions to give the corresponding cis and trans glycols (**7**) and superoxide anion radical ($O_2 \cdot^-$) or the more stable hydroperoxy radical ($HO_2 \cdot$). Analogous reactions of thymine radicals result in the formation of the corresponding hydroxy derivatives **8** and **9** and cis and trans glycols (**10**) of thymine (**2**). In the schemes, the stereochemistry is not indicated; i.e., four cis and trans diastereoisomers are formed [1–5, 15].

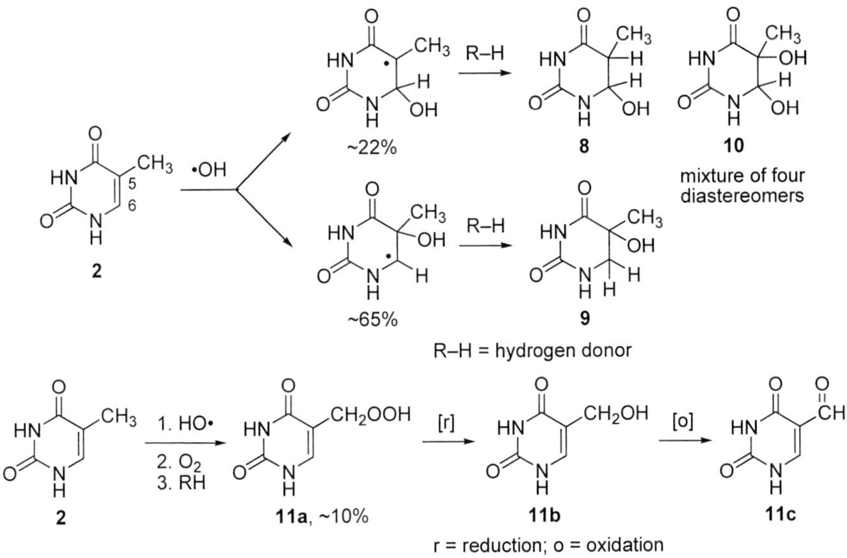

Sch. 2D-2. Reaction of thymine with hydroxyl radical.

In the case of thymine (**2, Sch. 2D-2**), the outcome of the addition of the hydroxyl radicals to the double bond is less predictable than in the case of cytosine because of the methyl group at the 5 position. Since the methyl group is an electron-donating substituent, the electron density at position 5 should be enhanced and, thus, reaction with the hydroxyl radical should be facilitated at this position. The formation of a radical at position 5 would give a tertiary radical, i.e., a more stable radical than that at position 6, which would be a secondary radical. However, the steric requirement of the methyl group is another factor, which could be important. It would be expected that approach of the hydroxyl radical to position 5 would be somewhat hindered, as compared to that in the reaction with cytosine [4]. Based on the product distribution of **8** and **9**, it is evident that the steric factor was somewhat important, but not decisive. The methyl group in **2** is also vulnerable to hydrogen abstraction by the hydroxyl radicals to give a resonance-stabilized allylic radical, and, as a result, the hydroperoxide derivative **11a** is formed, albeit in a low yield [3], followed by reduction to the corresponding allylic alcohol **11b**, which is oxidized to the corresponding aldehyde **11c** [4, 28]. The photosensitized heterobases can undergo [2 + 2] cycloadditions and [4 + 2] Diels–Alder-type condensations [13, 16, 20, 22, 27, 28, 31, 32, 34, 35, 38, 40]. The photoinduced condensations of two thymine molecules involve the π,π^* transitions of the carbon–carbon double bond. The excited singlet-state species produced undergo intersystem crossing (ISC) to the more stable, lower energy triplet species that produce, by a [2 + 2] cycloaddition, the cyclobutane derivatives **12**. The [2 + 2] cycloaddition reaction of thymine to give oxetane derivative **13** involves the carbon–carbon double bond π,π^* transition and the n,π^* transition of the carbonyl group [**Sch. 2D-3**, **Sch. 2D-4**, and **Sch. 2D-5**]. An analogous [2 + 2] cycloaddition reaction of cytosine (**1**) with the tautomer of thymine (**2**) involves the π,π^* transition of the carbon–carbon double bond and the n,π^* transition of the C=NH group to give azetidine derivative **17** [**Sch. 2D-3** and **Sch. 2D-6**]. As expected, the oxetane (**13**) and the azetidine (**17**) derivatives are unstable and undergo rearrangements to the (6-4) compounds **14** and **18**, respectively, in equilibrium with the corresponding pyridone isomers, the so-called "Dewar compounds" **15** and **19**, respectively [**Sch. 2D-5** and **Sch. 2D-6**] [13, 16, 20, 27, 28, 42,]. Under acidic conditions, compounds **14** and **18** lose water and ammonia molecules, respectively, to give compounds **16** and **20** [**Sch. 2D-5** and **Sch. 2D-6**].

It is important to be aware that the reactions involving the movements of odd electrons are shown in the schemes by "half-arrows", in contrast to the use of regular arrows for ionic mechanisms. The photosensitized condensation of thymine (**2**) with adenine (**3**), involving the π,π^* transitions, results in the formation of the cyclobutane derivative **21**, which undergoes rearrangement to give the eight-membered-ring valence isomer **22** [**Sch. 2D-7**] [26, 28]. The reaction of guanine (**4**) with the hydroxyl radicals was shown to give, as expected, the 8-oxoguanine derivative **25** [**Sch. 2D-8**] [21, 26, 41, 43]. The reaction in a biological environment of the hydroxyl radical with guanine (**4**) results in a resonance-stabilized radical, whereby the odd electron can be located either on the oxygen, carbon, or nitrogen atoms. The selection of radical **23**, with the electron on the nitrogen atom, represents an oxidizing radical [15], i.e., a hydrogen-atom-abstracting radical from the prevailing substrate to give the 8-hydroxy derivative **24.** The oxidation of **24** results in the formation of 8-oxoguanidine (8-oxo-Gua, **25**), probably as a tautomer [20, 21, 28]. The intermediate, **24**, can suffer a degradation to 2,6-diamino-5-formamidopyrimidine, the so-called Fapy Gua (**26**). Analogous transformations, as exemplified in **Sch. 2D-8**, occur also with the adenine heterobase to 8-oxoadenine (8-oxo-Ade, **27**) and 4,6-diamino-5-formamidopyrimidine (Fapy Ade, **28**) [28, 45–48]. However, as expected, the radiation-mediated formations of **27** and **28** are less effective, resulting in much lower yields than those obtained with **25** and **26** [28, 45–47]. The excision and repair of the mutant 8-oxoguanine in human DNA, mediated by the human 8-oxoguanine DNA glycosylase, has been extensively studied [28, 43, 44]. The [4 + 2] Diels–Alder-type cycloaddition reaction of guanine (**4**) with singlet oxygen proceeds by a convoluted but well-understood mechanism to give **25** [26, 28] [**Sch. 2D-9**]. In addition, the oxidative reactions of **4** with the hydroxyl radicals and singlet oxygen result in a number of degradations products, such as the guanidinohydantoin **29**, two stereoisomers of spiroiminohydantoins (**30**), the imidazolone derivative **31**, oxazolone derivative **32**, imidazolidinetrione (oxalylurea) (**33**), and guanidine (**34**) [26, 28, 41], just to mention a few. In the end, one comes to the realization that even such a vital and benign substance as the DNA can become, under the influence of solar radiation, the source of self-inflicting damaging species. Over the years, many experimental attempts have been made in the hope to firmly establish a complete effectiveness of commercial sunscreens in the prevention of UV-light induced damages to the DNA heterobases and other biological entities, albeit with inconclusive results [6–9, 39]. (See **Sections 2F** and **3E**.) The inconsistencies are, in part, attributable to the experimental design, such as the choice and number of human volunteers used in the experiments, the mode of application of sunscreens to the human skin, the choice of sunscreens, their stabilities, penetration through the skin, and the choice of light sources for irradiations [6–12, 32, 39, 45]. However, the main reason can probably be attributed to the fact that it has been assumed that the onset of the UV light induced damages to biological systems coincides with the onsets of erythema at the human skin, and that these onsets could be either delayed or prevented on the basis of knowing the skin protection factor (SPF) of the sunscreen in use. This assumption is incorrect, since it was recently found [8, 45, 49] that the suberythemogenic doses of UV irradiations can initiate, for example, the onsets of immunosuppression and sertain skin cancers, and, hence, knowing the sun protection factor of the sunscreen cannot be used for the prevention of those onsets [49]. (See **Sections 1A** and **2B**.)

Supplemental Collection of Relevant Sources

These sources contain a variety of topics, such as formation of photoproducts [1, 5, 12, 17, 19, 22, 27, 28, 34, 35, 38–40, 46], photoproducts in the human skin [14, 16, 17, 30–36], structures of photoproducts [16, 21, 22, 27, 28], cytotoxicity of photoproducts [13, 42], genotoxic effects of solar radiation [42], single-strand breaks [6], replication errors [41], photolesions in the human skin [41, 42, 48], repair of photoproducts in the human skin [24, 30, 34, 37–40, 43–45], involvement of reactive oxygen species [1–5, 15, 20, 21, 23, 26–29], possible sunscreen protection against photolesions [7–12, 39, 49], and mechanisms of formation of photoproducts [1–5, 15, 18, 25–28, 42, 43, 47, 48].

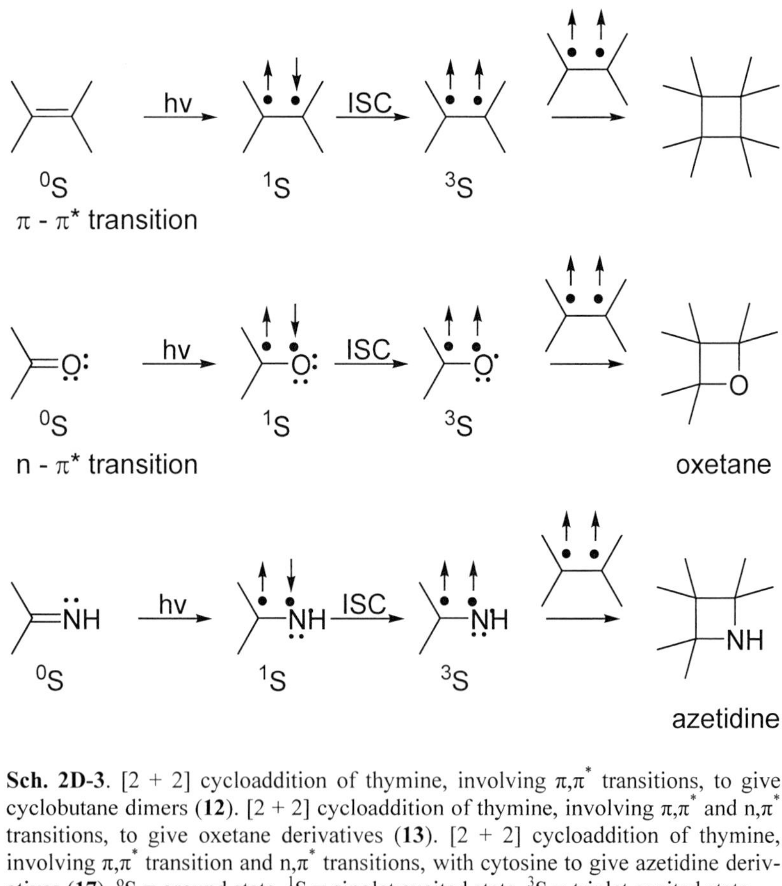

Sch. 2D-3. [2 + 2] cycloaddition of thymine, involving π,π^* transitions, to give cyclobutane dimers (**12**). [2 + 2] cycloaddition of thymine, involving π,π^* and n,π^* transitions, to give oxetane derivatives (**13**). [2 + 2] cycloaddition of thymine, involving π,π^* transition and n,π^* transitions, with cytosine to give azetidine derivatives (**17**). ^{0}S = ground state, ^{1}S = singlet excited state, ^{3}S = triplet excited state.

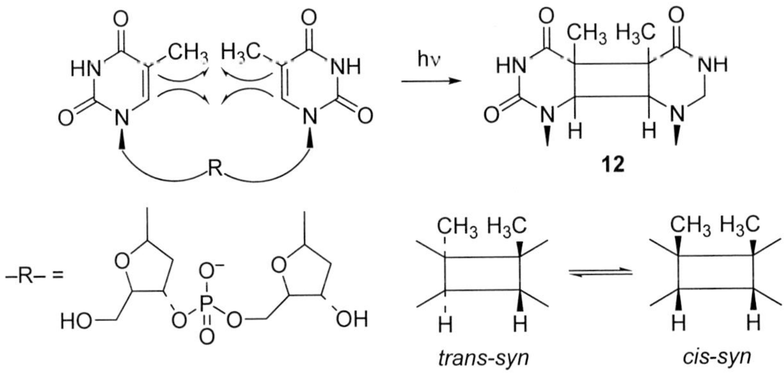

Sch. 2D-4. Photosensitized [2 + 2] cycloaddition of pyrimidine heterobases to give cyclobutane derivatives.

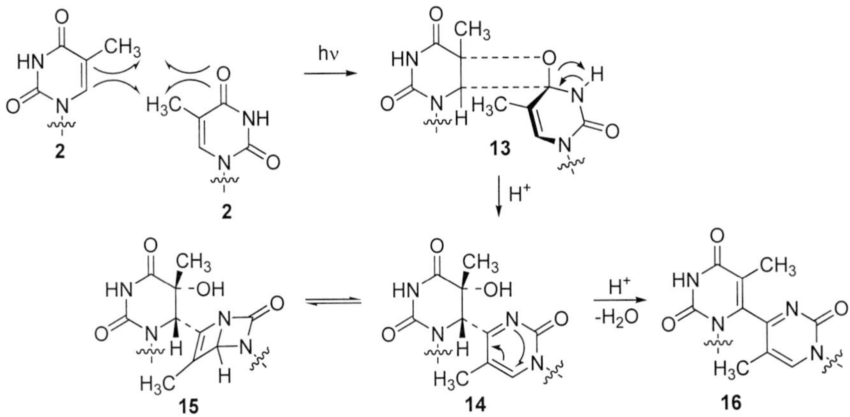

Sch. 2D-5. Photosensitized [2 + 2] cycloaddition of pyrimidine heterobases to give oxetane intermediates, which rearrange to pyrimidine in equilibrium with a "Dewar component". Dehydration of isomer **14** results in product **16**.

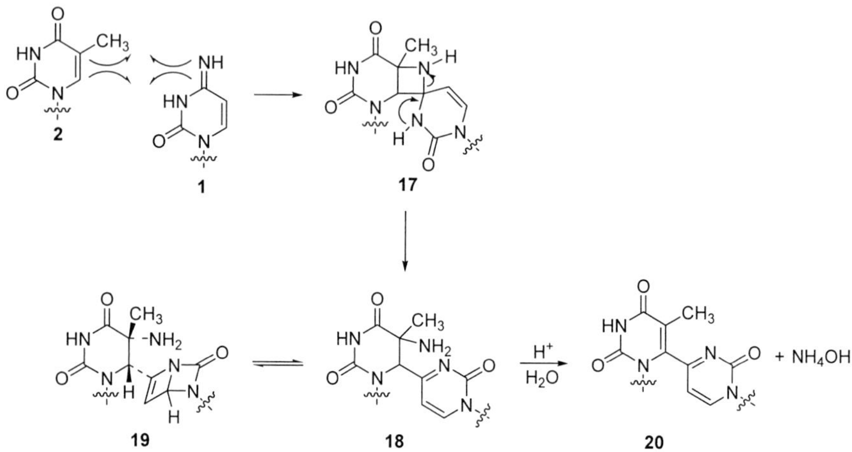

Sch. 2D-6. Photosensitized [2 + 2] cycloaddition of pyrimidine heterobases to give an azetidine intermediate, which rearranges to (6-4) pyrimidine–pyridine photoproduct in equilibrium with a “Dewar” isomer. Deamination of **18** results in compound **20**.

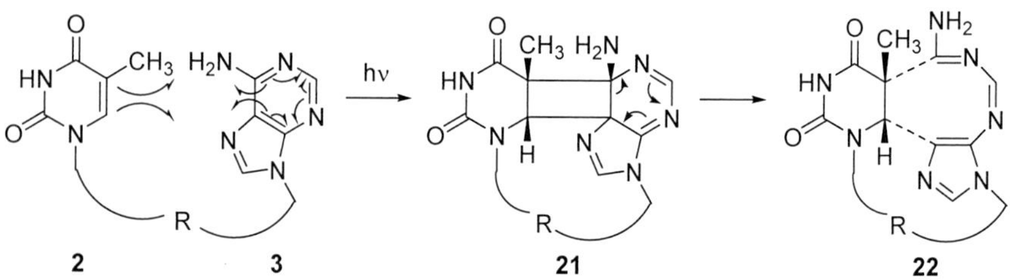

Sch. 2D-7. Photosensitized [2 + 2] condensation of thymine with adenine.

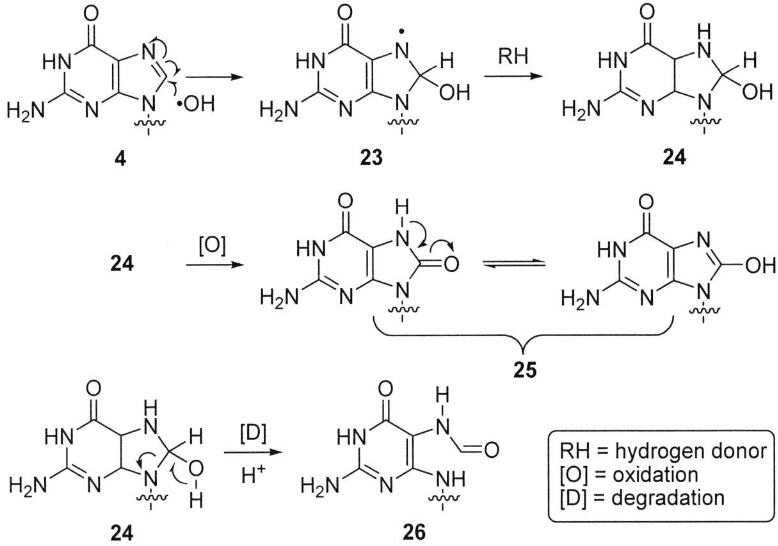

Sch. 2D-8. The reaction of guanine with singlet oxygen and the hydroxyl radicals.

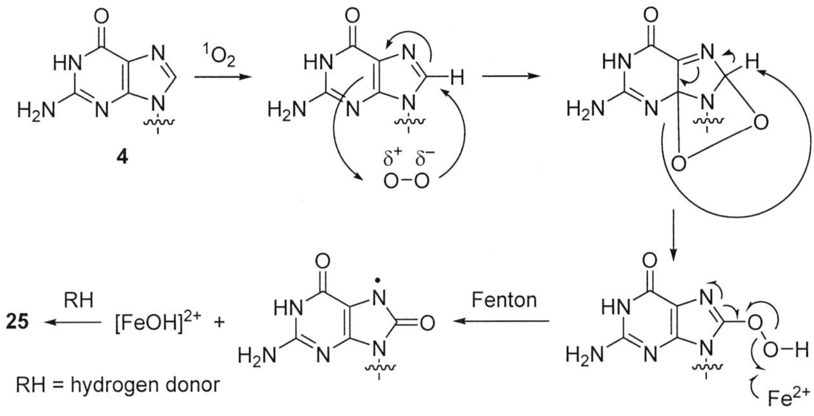

Sch. 2D-9. Diels–Alder-type [4 + 2] cycloaddition reaction of guanine with singlet oxygen.

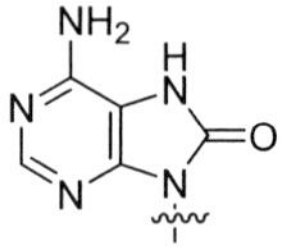

27
8-oxo Ade

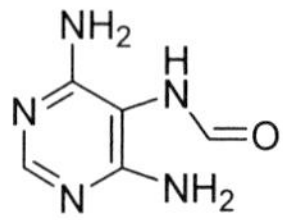

28
Fapy Ade

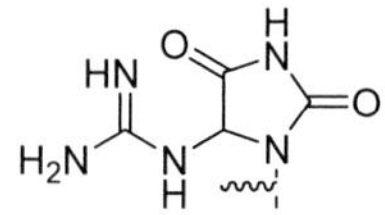

29
guanidino-hydantoin

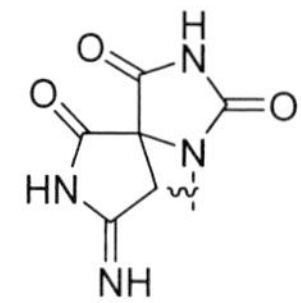

30
spiroiminohydantoins
two stereoisomers

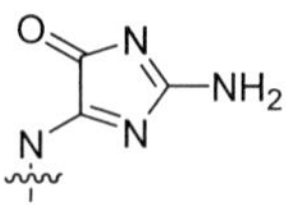

31
imidazolidone derivative

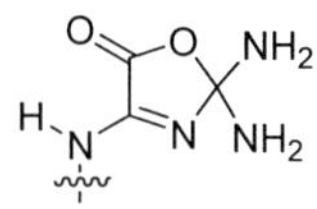

32
oxazolone derivative

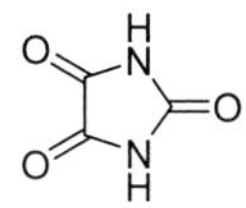

33
trioxoimidazole

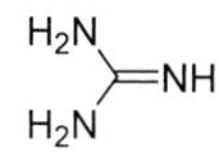

34
guanidine

Fig. 2D-1. Radiation-mediated formation of heterocyclic bases.

References

1. Fisher G. J. and Johns H. E. (1976) Pyrimidine photohydrates. In: *Photochemistry and Photobiology of Nucleic Acids*, Vol. 1, pp 169–224, Wang, S. (ed.), Academic Press, New York.
2. Hariharan P. V. and Cerutti P. A. (1977) Formation of products of the 5,6-dihydroxydihydrothymine type by ultraviolet light in HeLa cells. *Biochemistry* **16**: 2391–2395.
3. Fujita S. and Steenken S. (1981) Pattern of OH radical addition to uracil and methyl- and carboxyl-substituted uracils. Electron transfer of OH adducts with *N,N,N',N'*-tetramethyl-*p*-phenylenediamine and tetranitromethane. *J. Am. Chem. Soc.* **103**: 2540–2545.
4. Steenken S. (1989) One-electron redox reactions between radicals and molecules. Dominance of inner-sphere mechanisms. In: *Free Radicals in Synthesis and Biology*, pp 213–231, Minisci F. (ed.), Klluwert Academic Publishers, Dordrecht.
5. Hazra D. K. and Steenken S. (1983) Pattern of OH radical addition to cytosine and 1-, 3-, 5-, and 6-substituted cytosines. Electron transfer and dehydration reactions of the OH adducts. *J. Am. Chem. Soc.* **105**: 4380–4386.
6. Gulston M. and Knowland J. (1999) Illumination of human keratocytes in the presence of the sunscreen ingredient Padimate-O and through an SPF-15 sunscreen reduces direct photodamage to DNA but increases strand breaks. *Mutat. Res.* **444**: 49–60.

7. Freeman S. E., Ley R. D. and Ley, K. D. (1988) Sunscreen protection against UV-induced pyrimidine dimers in DNA of human skin in situ. *Photodermatology* **5**: 243–247.
8. Liardet S., Scaletta C., Panizzon R., Hohlfeld P. and Laurent-Applegate L. (2001) Protection against pyrimidine dimers, p53, and 8-hydroxy-2'-deoxyguanosine expression in ultraviolet-irradiated human skin by sunscreens: difference between UVB + UVA and UVB alone sunscreens. *J. Invest. Dermat.* **117**: 1437–1441.
9. Al Mahroos M., Yaar M., Phillips T. J., Bhawan J. and Gilchrest B. A. (2002) Effect of sunscreen application on UV-induced thymine dimers. *Arch. Dermatol.* **138**: 1480–1485.
10. Bykov V. J., Marcusson J. A. and Hemminki K. (1998) Ultraviolet B-induced DNA damage in human skin and its modulation by a sunscreen. *Cancer Res.* **58**: 2961–2964.
11. Young A. R., Sheehan J. M., Chadwick C. A. and Potten C. S. (2000) Protection by UVA and UVB sunscreens against in situ dipyrimidine photolesions in human epidermis is comparable to protection against sunburn. *J. Invest. Dermatol.* **115**: 37–41.
12. Vainio H. and Bianchini (eds.) (2001) IARC Handbooks of Cancer Prevention. *Sunscreens*, Vol. **5**, International Agency for Research on Cancer, Lyon.
13. Mitchell D. L. (1988) The relative cytoxicity of (6-4) photoproducts and cyclobutane dimers in mammalian cells. *Photochem. Photobiol.* **48**: 51–57.
14. Freeman S. E., Hacham H., Gange R. W., Maytum D. J., Sutherland C. and Sutherland B. M. (1989) Wavelength dependence of pyrimidine dimer formation in DNA of human skin irradiated in situ with ultraviolet light. *Proc. Natl. Acad. Sci. U. S. A.* **86**: 5605–5609.
15. Steenken S. (1989) Purine bases, nucleosides and nucleotides: aqueous solution redox chemistry and transformation reactions of their radical cations and e- and OH adducts. *Chem. Rev.* **89**: 503–520.
16. Mitchell D. L. and Nairm R. S. (1989) The biology of the (6-4) photoproduct. *Photochem. Photobiol.* **49**: 805–819.
17. Gallagher P. E. and Duker N. J. (1989) Formation of purine photoproducts in a defined human DNA sequence. *Photochem. Photobiol.* **49**: 599–605.
18. Cadet J. and Vigny P. (1990) Bioorganic photochemistry. In: *The Photochemistry and Photobiology of Nucleic Acids*, Vol. **1**, pp 1–273, Morrison, H. (ed.), John Wiley & Sons, New York.
19. Mitchell D. L., Jen J. and Cleaver J. E. (1991) Relative induction of cyclobutane dimers and cytosine photohydrates in DNA irradiated in

vitro and in vivo with ultraviolet-C and ultraviolet-B light. *Photochem. Photobiol.* **54**: 741–746.
20. Sies H. (ed.) (1991) Oxidative Stress: Oxidants and Antioxidants, Academic Press, New York.
21. Kasai H. and Nishimura S. (1991) Formation of 8-hydroxydesoxyguanosine in DNA by oxygen radicals and its biological significance. In: *Oxidative Stress: Oxidants and Antioxidants*, pp 99–119, Sies H. (ed.), Academic Press, New York.
22. Mitchel D. L., Jen J. and Cleaver J. E. (1992) Sequence specificity of cyclobutane pyrimidine dimers in DNA treated with solar (ultraviolet B) radiation. *Nucl. Acids Res.* **20**: 225–229.
23. Fuchs J. (1992) The skin and oxidative stress. In: *Oxidative Injury in Dermatopathology*, Springer-Verlag, Berlin.
24. Sage E. (1993) Distribution and repair of photolesions in DNA: Genetic consequences and the role of sequence context. *Photochem. Photobiol.* **57**: 163–174.
25. Tyrell R. M. (1994) The molecular and cellular pathology of solar, ultraviolet radiation. *Mol. Aspects Med.* **15**: 1–77.
26. Cadet J., Berger M., Douki T., Morin B., Raoul, S., Ravanat J. L. and Spinelli S. (1997) Effects of UV and visible radiation on DNA-final base damage. *Biol. Chem.* **378**: 1275–1286.
27. Ravanat J.-L., Douki T. and Cadet J. (2001) UV damage to nucleic acid Components. In: *Sun Protection in Man*, pp 207–230, Giacomoni, P. U. (ed.), Elsevier, Amsterdam.
28. Douki T. (2007) UV-induced DNA damage. In: *Biophysical and Physiological Effects of Solar Radiation on Human Skin*, pp 227–269, Giacomoni P. U. (ed.), The Royal Society of Chemistry, Cambridge.
29. Marrot L. and Meunier J.-R. (2008) Skin DNA photodamage and its biological consequences. *J. Am. Acad. Dermatol.* **58** (5 Suppl. 2): S139–S148.
30. Bykov. V. J., Jansen C. T. and Hemminki K. (1998) High levels of dipyrimidine dimers are induced in human skin by solar-simulating UV radiation. *Cancer Epidemiol. Biomarkers Prev.* **7**: 199–202.
31. Bykov V. J., Marcusson J. A. and Hemminki K. (2000) Effect of constitutional pigmentation on ultraviolet B-induced DNA damage in fair-skinned people. *J. Invest. Dermat.* **114**: 40–43.
32. Hemminki K., Xu G., Kause L., Koulu L. M., Zhao C. and Jansen C. T. (2002) Demonstration of UV-dimers in human skin DNA in situ 3 weeks after exposure. *Carcinogenesis* **23**: 605–609.

33. Young A. R., Potten C. S., Nikaido O., Parsons P. G., Boenders J., Ramsden J. M. and Chadwick C. A. (1998) Human melanocytes and keratinocytes exposed to UVB or UVA in vivo show comparable levels of thymine dimers. *J. Invest. Dermatol.* **111**: 936–940.
34. Wilms L. C., Zhao C., Snellman E., Segerbäck D. and Hemminki K. (2002) Measurements of cyclobutane dimers in melanocytic nevi and surrounding epidermis in human skin in situ. *Mutagenesis* **17**: 181–191.
35. Zhao C., Snellman E., Jansen C. T. and Hemminki K. (2002) Ultraviolet photoproduct levels in melanocytic nevi and surrounding epidermis in human skin in situ. *J. Invest. Dermatol.* **118**: 180–184.
36. Young A. R., Chadwick C. A., Harrison G. I., Nikaido O., Ramsden J. and Potten C. S. (1998) The similarity of action spectra for thymine dimers in human epidermis and erythema suggests that DNA is the chromophore for erythema. *J. Invest. Dermatol.* **111**: 982–988.
37. Bykov V. J., Sheehan, J. M., Hemminki, K. and Young A. R. (1999) In situ repair of cyclobutane pyrimidine dimers and 6-4 photoproducts in human skin exposed to solar simulating radiation. *J. Invest. Dermatol.* **112**: 326–331.
38. Xu G., Snellman E., Jansen C. T. and Hemminki K. (2000) Levels and repair of cyclobutane pyrimidine dimers and 6-4 photoproducts in skin and sporadic basal cell carcinoma patients. *J. Invest. Dermatol.* **115**: 95–99.
39. Hemminki K., Xu G. and Le Curieux F. (2001) Ultraviolet radiation-induced photoproducts in human skin DNA as biomarkers of damage and its repair. In: *Biomarkers in Cancer Chemoprevention*, Miller A. B., Bartsch H., Boffetta P., Dragsted L. and Vainio H. (eds.), IARC Scientific Publications No. 154, International Agency for Research on Cancer, Lyon.
40. Zhao C., Snellman E., Jansen C. T. and Hemminki K. (2002) In situ repair of cyclobutane pyrimidine dimers and in skin and melanocytic nevi of cutaneous melanoma patients. *Int. J. Cancer* **98**: 331–334.
41. Henderson P. T., Delaney J., Muller J. G., Neeley W. L., Tannenbaum S. R., Burrows C. J. and Essigmann J. M. (2003) The hydration lesions formed from oxidation of 7,8-dihydro-8-oxoguanine are potent sources of replication errors in vivo. *Biochemistry* **42**: 9257–9263.
42. Douki T., Reynaud-Angelin A., Cadet J. and Sage E. (2003) Bipyrimidine photoproducts rather than oxidative lesions are the main type of DNA damage involved in the genotoxic effect of solar UVA radiation. *Biochemistry* **42**: 9221–9226.

43. Bruner S. D., Norman D. P. G. and Verdine G. L. (2000) Structural basis for recognition and repair of the endogeneous mutagen 8-oxoguanine in DNA. *Nature* **403**: 859–866.
44. Fromme J. C., Bruner S. D., Yang W., Karplus M. and Verdine G. L. (2003) Product-assisted catalysis in base-excision DNA repair. *Nature* **10**: 204–211.
45. Yarosh D. B. and Smiles K. A. (2009) DNA Repair and Photoprotection. In: *Clinical Guide to Sunscreens and Photoprotection*, pp 169–179, Lim H. W. and Draelos Z. D. (eds.), Informa Healthcare, New York.
46. Pouget J.-P., Frelon S., Ravanat J.-L., Testard I., Odin F. and Cadet J. (2002) Formation of modified DNA bases in cells exposed either to gamma radiation or to high-LET particles. *Radical Res.* **157**: 589–595.
47. Bodepudi V., Shibutani S. and Johnson F. (1992) Synthesis of 2′-deoxy-7,8-dihydro-8-oxoguanosine and 2′-deoxy-7,8-dihydro-8-oxoadenosine and their incorporation into oligomeric DNA. *Chem. Res. Toxicol.* **5**: 608–617.
48. Haraguchi K., Delaney M. O., Wiederholt C. J., Samabandam A., Hantosi Z. and Greenberg M. M. (2002) Synthesis and characterization of oligodeoxynucleotides containing formamidopyrimidine lesions and nonhydrolyzable analogues. *J. Am. Chem. Soc.* **124**: 3263–3269.
49. Halliday G. M. and Hönigsmann G. M. (2009) Sunscreens, photoimmunosuppression, and photoaging. In: *Clinical Guide to Sunscreens and Photoprotection*, pp 101–116, Lim H. W. and Draelos Z. D. (eds.), Informa Healthcare, New York.

E. Glycation. Maillard Reaction and Amadori–Heyns Rearrangement Reactions Resulting in Protein Damage by Reducing Carbohydrates and Other Carbonyl Compounds. UV Photodamage of DNA. Photoaging, Photocarcinogenesis, and Various Diseases Derived from Advanced Glycation Endproducts (AGE)

Glycoproteins, derived from the Maillard reaction and Amadori–Heyns rearrangements, are widely distributed in the human body, and they possess very important biological functions, e.g., as components of blood groups, antigens, and antibodies, just to mention a few areas. The nonenzymatic condensation process of various reducing carbohydrates and amino acids, proteins, and peptides is known as the Maillard Reaction [1–4]. The products of this reaction and Amadori and Heyns rearrangements have been detected in the so-called long-lived human proteins, such as collagen, eye lens crystallins, and membranes of arteries, nerves, and connective tissues, and it is believed that these products are the manifestation of the aging processes. Thus, the Maillard reaction and its subsequent reactions are very common in nature, and furthermore, they occur always in food processing when carbohydrates and amino acids or proteins are present.

The chemistry of the Maillard and Amadori–Heyns reactions is very complex, often resulting in a multitude of products with chemically unrelated structures. Thus, a possible mutagenic and carcinogenic acrylamide was discovered in high-temperature processed food, such as French fries, potato chips, and even bread [5, 6]. A study of the thermal degradation of the fructose–methionine Amadori intermediate by GC/MS revealed that the major product (70%) was methional with an additional 82 minor compounds, of which 70 were identified [7]. The minor compounds were composed of aliphatics and alicyclics, pyrans and furans, pyrazines, pyridines, and pyrroles [7]. Free radicals have been detected by ESR spectroscopy in early stages of the Maillard reaction between glycolaldehyde or glyceraldehyde and *N,N'*-dialkylethylenediamines [8]. Two series of cyclic cation radicals are formed. The first involves one ethylenediamine molecule bridged by a sugar molecule and the second, and more stable, involves a dihydropyrazine cation radical, formed by the reaction of the two amines with two sugars [8]. Details were reported about the formation of the pyrazinium radical cation in the Maillard reaction between glycine and glucose using ESR spectroscopy [**Sch. 2E-1**] [9].

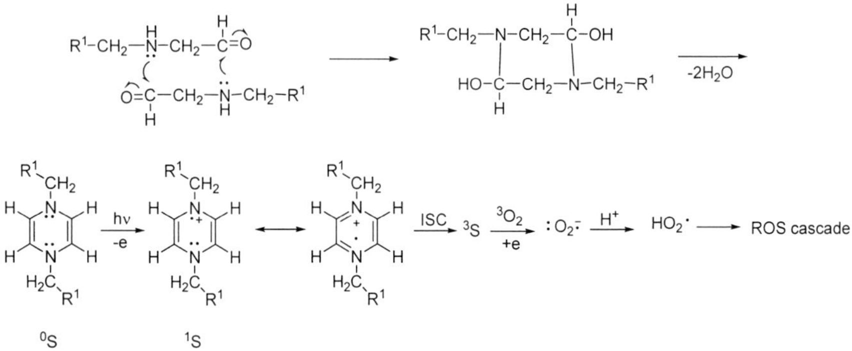

Sch. 2E-1. Proposed mechanism of the formation of pyrazinium cation radicals and their reactions with molecular oxygen ($^3O_2$). R^1 = various moieties, derived from condensations of proteins with sugar fragmentation products. ^0S = singlet ground state, ^1S excited singlet state, ^3S excited triplet state. ISC = intersystem crossing. $O_2{\cdot}^-$ = superoxide anion radical, $HO_2\cdot$ = hydroperoxide radical.

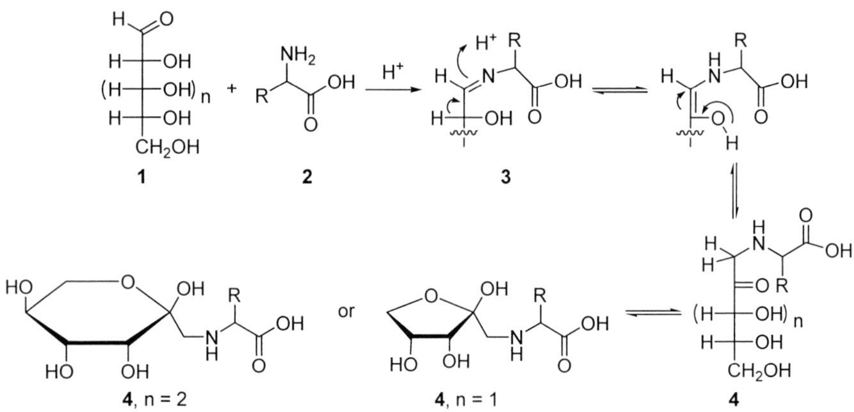

Sch. 2E-2. Products (**4**) of the Amadori rearrangement of the Maillard reaction condensation products (**3**) of pentoses (**1**, n = 1) and hexoses (**1**, n = 2) with α-amino acids (**2**). R = alkyl and aryl groups. Reactions with compounds containing several amino groups, such as lysine, proceed analogously, but the products have complex structures, e.g., **6** [**Sch. 2E-3**].

In some cases, the reactions of monomeric starting materials can be mechanistically readily explained. Thus, in the first step, the Maillard reaction between D-glucose and other carbohydrates (**1**) with L-amino acids (**2**) yields Schiff base intermediates **3**, which then undergo cyclizations to give, in the case of D-glucose, *N*-glucosyl amino acid derivatives. Analogous condensations with D-fructose result in *N*-fructosyl amino acid derivatives. These condensation products readily undergo further well-defined reactions. Thus, glucose derivatives on protonation are converted into 1-amino-1-desoxy ketoses (**4**) by the Amadori Rearrangement [**Sch. 2E-2**], while the fructose derivatives undergo an analogous Heyns Rearrangement to give a product with an aldehyde group (**6**) [**Sch. 2E-3**] [10]. This type of reaction also occurs in biological environments with many metabolites containing carbonyl groups (C=O), such as glyoxal, methylglyoxal, 3-deoxyglucosone, and malondialdehyde.

The Maillard–Amadori-type reactions are also involved in the glycation (glycosylation) of proteins, i.e., in the spontaneous amino–carbonyl reaction between reducing carbohydrates, other carbonyl compounds, and long-lived proteins [11–13]. The initial glycation products are further converted by oxidative and nonoxidative pathways into reactive carbonyl species (RCS) [1, 11, 14–16], leading to the formation of the so-called advanced glycation end products (AGE) [17–19], which accumulate on long-lived skin proteins, such as collagen and elastin, in the process of skin aging [1–4, 12]. The RCS are mainly composed of α-dicarbonyl compounds, such as glyoxal, methylglyoxal, 3-deoxyosones, and malondialdehyde [14], that originate from pathways such as glycation [14], carbohydrate degradations via retroaldol condensations [20], lipid peroxidations [21], and UV-induced photodamage [22]. The AGE products include protein–protein aldimino crosslinks (–N=C<), proteins containing ε-(carboxymethyl)lysine groups (HO_2CCH_2-εNH$(CH_2)_4CH(NH_2)CO_2H$) derived from the initial Maillard–Amadori reactions, and other heterogeneous modifications, such as products derived from proteins and from ubiquitous entities like heme, hematin, hemoglobin, bilirubin, protoporphyrin, and chlorophyll. A model reaction for protein–DNA interaction was investigated between 2-deoxyguanosine, L-lysine and different carbohydrates [23]. The reaction between the sugar degradation products dihydroxyacetone (DHA) and D,L-glyceraldehyde and lysine led to the formation of two new cross-link products, the two diastereomers of N^6-[2-(N^2-deoxyguanosyl)propionyl]lysine [23]. Further interactions of DHA and DHA phosphate with various biological systems have been intensively investigated [24–32].

DHA is commercially used as the active browning ingredient in the so-called sunless self-tanning agents. The reactions in the human skin of DHA with amino acids, followed by a Heyns rearrangement, produce AGE products [**Sch. 2E-3**]. During exposure to the sun, these products undergo reactions with molecular oxygen to produce ROS in quantities that are much larger than those obtained with untanned skin [25]. Hence, it is important to avoid prolonged exposures to the sun shortly after application of the DHA agent to the skin, in order to permit completion of the browning process.

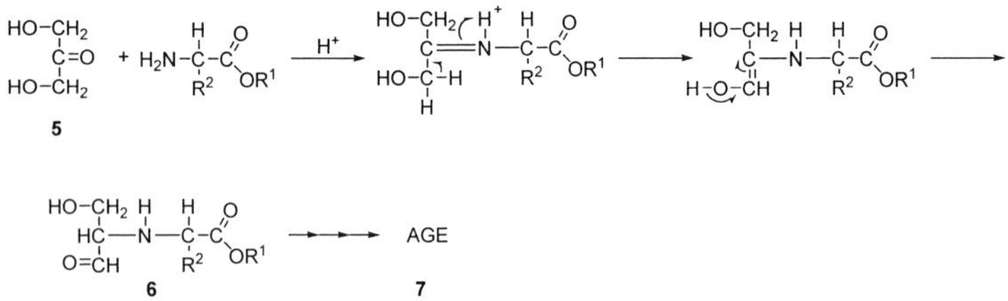

R^1, R^2 = various groups

Sch. 2E-3. Proposed mechanism for the Maillard Reaction and Heyns Rearrangement with dihydroxyacetone (DHA).

Various model reactions have been studied to determine the mechanism of AGE formation [19, 31–36]. DHA phosphate undergoes a nonenzymatic glycation reaction with the nucleotide guanosine triphosphate (GTP) [31, 32]. This reaction occurs by the classical Heyns pathway [31, 32]. The concentration of DHA is elevated in the erythrocytes of diabetic patients [31, 32]. AGEs are formed intracellularly at a much faster rate from fructose, trioses, and dicarbonyl compounds than from glucose [33]. While the concentration of glucose is much higher extracellularly than that of fructose, the concentration of intracellular fructose is elevated in diabetic patients, and its seven-fold greater reactivity than that of glucose could represent a significant pathway for the formation of intracellular AGEs [33].

The reaction of glyceraldehyde and the lysine residue of proteins produced glyceraldehyde-derived pyridinium compounds (GLAP) [34]. The reaction of bovine serum albumin (BSA) with various carbonyl compounds, at 37 °C and pH 7.4 for one week, resulted in the formation of GLAP only in the glyceraldehyde modified BSA. Apparently, GLAP is a specific AGE derived from glyceraldehydes. GLAP induced the formation of reactive oxygen species in HL-60 cells and caused oxidative stress [34]. Thus, GLAP could be a biomarker for AGE-related diseases, such as diabetes and chronic renal failure [34].

The reaction of lens proteins with oxidation products of ascorbic acid produced AGEs. These AGEs can readily undergo UV light induced reactions with molecular oxygen to give reactive oxygen species (ROS) and other oxidation products [19]. Reaction of the most active of these oxidation products, L-threonine, with *N*-acetyllysine, produced a mixture of six AGEs, which were isolated by HPLC and recognized by their fluorescent spectra. The UV light induced reactions of AGEs with molecular oxygen produced the superoxide anion radical ($O_2\cdot^-$) by the Type I mechanism and singlet oxygen ($^1O_2$) by the Type II mechanism [**Sch. 2E-4** and **Sch. 2E-5**]. After purification, the UV light induced reaction of these AGEs generated 20–60 times more singlet oxygen on a weight basis than either crude ascorbic glycated proteins or a mixture of water-soluble proteins from aged normal human lenses [19]. The AGE could account for the sensitizer activity of these reaction products, if they represent less than 1% of the total amino acids [19]. Polycationic, basic proteins, such as histones with their lysine, glycine, arginine, and cysteine amino acids, are potential targets for protein carbonylation processes involved in the nuclear chromatin structure and functions [35–39]. A possible pathway for histone glycation was obtained from studies on isolated PC12 (rat) cell nuclei [37]. In this case, the condensation reaction of the nucleotide adenosine diphosphate ribose (ADP-ribose, **8**) with H1 histone yielded an ADP-ribose-H1 conjugate [14, 40, 41] [**Fig. 2E-1**]. In order to have some idea about the product, which may be formed between ADP-ribose and histone, a reaction was carried out between ADP-ribose and N^{α}-acetyl-L-lysine [35]. The main product was the acyclic ketoamine **9**, presumably formed by the Maillard–Amadori reaction, according to **Sch. 2E-2** [35]. In a biological environment, the acyclic aminoketose could also be formed from the metabolic precursor of ADP-ribose, i.e., the nicotinamide–adenine dinucleotide (NAD, **10**).

The use of ADP-ribose and histone H1 was based on the following facts. ADP-ribose contains a reducing pentose sugar, which is formed in the nucleus in proportion to DNA-strand breaks following genotoxic stress [42, 43]. This stress can be produced by alkylating agents, such as *N*-methyl-*N*′-nitro-*N*-nitrosoguanidine (MNNG), which are potent inducers of DNA strand breaks that activate the nuclear enzymes, such as poly(ADP-ribose) polymerase and poly(ADP-ribose) glycohydrolase [35]. These two enzymes convert a large portion of the NAD (**10**), which is a metabolic precursor of ADP-ribose, to free ADP-ribose in close proximity to H1 histones [35, 42]. Histone H1 was investigated because it is a lysine-rich subtype and a linker histone with a greater accessibility and a higher level of protein carbonylation than the core histones [44, 45]. The photosensitization of the histone–ADP-ribose conjugate with UV radiations is facilitated by the adenine heterobases of ADP-ribose containing a conjugated chromophore. The pyrazinium free radical cation was identified on histone H1 glycated by glycolaldehyde or ADP-ribose [46].

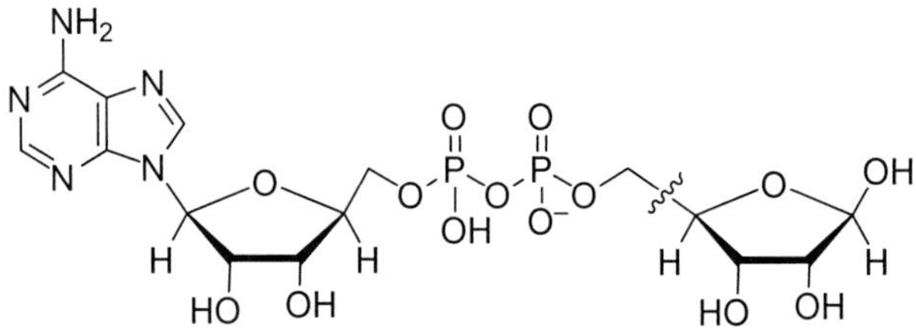

8

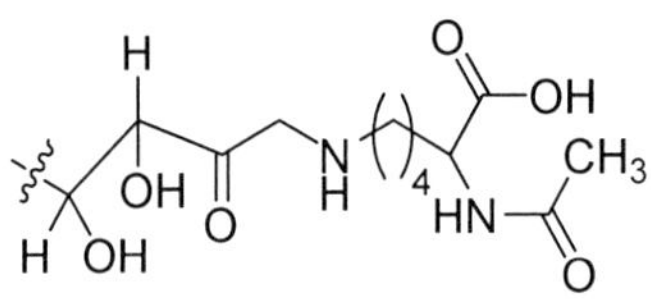

9

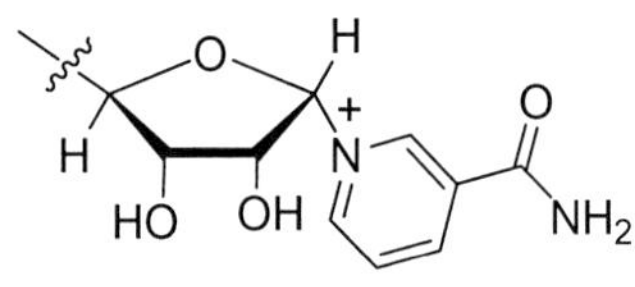

10

Fig. 2E-1. Structures of ADP-ribose (**8**) and product (**9**) derived from the Maillard condensation and Amadori rearrangement using N^{α}-acetyl-L-lysine and ADP-ribose according to **Sch. 2E-1**. An analogous reaction is possible with nicotinamide–adenine dinucleotide (NAD, **10**).

Many AGE products contain chromophores that absorb UV radiations resulting in photosensitization and fluorescence processes [11–19] and, subsequently, in the production of reactive oxygen species (ROS) which are damaging to the DNA [11–13]. (See **Section 2D**.) The advanced glycation end products (AGEs), their intermediates and related entities in human biosystems contain a variety of "simple" and conjugated chromophores and the auxochromes amino (NH_2), hydroxyl (OH), and sulfhydryl (SH) groups. The chromophores readily absorb the energies of UVA and UVB radiations, and the auxochromes cause a shift of absorptions to longer wavelengths. The radiation-induced species ^0S undergo either n,π^* or π,π^* transitions to excited singlet state species (^1S), followed by intersystem crossing (ISC) to excited triplet state species (^3S) [**Sch. 2E-4** and **Sch. 2E-5**].

The reactions of the excited species, in particular the triplet state species, are very efficiently quenched by molecular oxygen which is a triplet in the ground state ($^3O_2$). (See **Sections 2D**, **3**, and **4**.) The photoinduced reactions with molecular oxygen can proceed either by the Type I mechanism or by the Type II mechanism. In the Type I mechanism, a transfer of an electron occurs from the excited triplet state species to the oxygen with formation of superoxide anion radical ($O_2\cdot^-$). The dismutation of the superoxide anion radical produces hydrogen peroxide and molecular oxygen, and a cascade of various reactive oxygen species, such as the Fenton reaction of hydrogen peroxide with iron cations to give the very reactive hydroxyl radical (HO·). The formation of singlet oxygen ($^1O_2$) depends on the transfer of energy from the triplet species to molecular oxygen. The minimum energy requirements are 22.7 kcal.mol^{-1}. Singlet oxygen is a very reactive species, and its reactions are well documented with most biological systems. (See **Sch. 2E-4** and **Sch. 2E-5**, **Sections 2D**, **3**, and **4**.)

A multistep mechanism was proposed for the AGE photosensitization in human skin under UVA radiations [11–13]. First, an accumulation of AGEs in the skin cell nuclei occurs as a result of RCS-mediated glycation. Second, the nuclear AGEs are photoexcited by solar radiation. Third, DNA damage occurs as a result of direct electron transfer between the excited chromophores of AGEs and DNA. Fourth, DNA damage occurs by ROS that are generated from AGE sensitization [11] [**Sch. 2E-5**]. Extracellular accumulations of AGE-modified proteins may also cause damage to cellular membranes, proteins, and DNA as a result of extracellular generation of hydrogen peroxide followed by intracellular Fenton-type chemistry [11].

The chemistry of AGE-photosensitized ROS production can involve both Type I and Type II photoreactions [see **Sch. 2E-5**] [12, 47]. UVA irradiation of human dermal fibroblasts in the presence of AGE-BSA resulted in decreased cell viability, increased photoaging, and an increase in ROS [48, 49]. The reactive oxygen species were identified as singlet oxygen, hydrogen peroxide, and hydroxyl radicals using EPR spin-trapping experiments [**Sch. 2E-5**] [11, 12, 48, 49]. The formation of hydrogen peroxide observed in cellular assays [9] is derived from a superoxide anion radical, formed by a Type I photosensitization process. This radical undergoes spontaneous dismutation with the formation of molecular oxygen and hydrogen peroxide, which is converted by a Fenton-type ferrous cation catalyzed reaction into highly reactive and toxic hydroxyl radicals [50]. The AGE-photosensitized production of ROS not only results in cellular toxicity, but also in the further generation of RCS derived from peroxidations of lipids and/or autoxidations of carbohydrates. Hence, a cycle between RCS and ROS formation, mediated by solar radiation, is maintained [12].

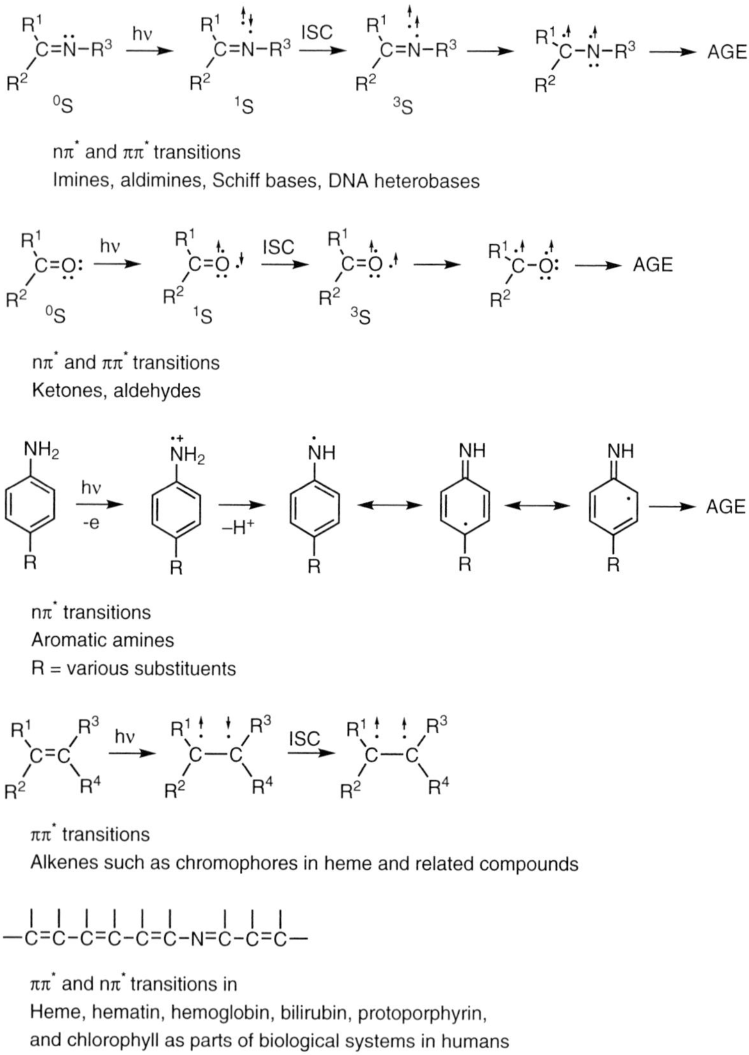

Sch. 2E-4. Chromophores in AGE aggregates. Simple chromophores are often in conjugation with chromophores of various biological entities. The UV light induced n,π^* and π,π^* transitions of chromophores proceed from the ground singlet state, ^0S, to the excited singlet state, ^1S, and by intersystem crossing (ISC) to the excited triplet state, ^3S, that can undergo reactions with molecular oxygen. $R^1 - R^4$ = various groups.

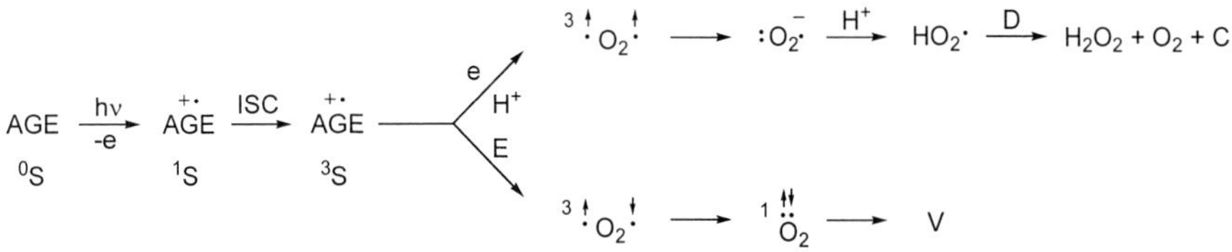

Sch. 2E-5. Formation of reactive oxygen species (ROS) by UV light induced reactions of advanced glycation end product (AGE) aggregates. ISC = intersystem crossing. E = energy of the excited triplet species. Minimum required 22.7 kcal.mol^{-1}. $\cdot{}^{\uparrow}O_2\cdot^{\uparrow}$ = molecular oxygen in the ground state triplet. $^1{:}O_2$ = singlet oxygen with paired electrons. D = dismutation. C = cascade of other oxygen species. V = reactions of $^1O_2$ with entities of various classes, such as lipids, proteins, carbohydrates, heterobases of DNA, steroids, and AGEs.

The third step of the proposed mechanism involves UV photosensitization of AGE-conjugates in close proximity to DNA resulting in DNA damages [11]. Thus, irradiation of supercoiled XΦ174 DNA with simulated solar light in the presence of either an AGE derived from the proteins BSA, or an AGE derived from ribonuclease (RNAse) induced DNA single strand breaks [11]. The increased photosensitization of the glycated proteins could be correlated with the increase of AGE modification, whereas the nonglycated proteins could not undergo photosensitization [11]. The biologicals BSA and RNAse contain chromophores, which can undergo, on absorption of UV radiation, elevations to excited state species that can react with molecular oxygen to give ROS [**Sch. 2E-5**].

A growth inhibition of skin cells as a result of AGE photosensitization with UVA radiation and solar-simulated light radiations was demonstrated in human keratinocytes and fibroblasts, using the AGE species derived from BSA and from collagen as photosensitizers [12]. The UVA radiation of these conjugates induced the formation of hydrogen peroxide that was recognized as a key mediator of skin cell growth inhibition, since a prior catalase treatment completely negated the inhibition. A similar growth inhibition was found with non-irradiated cells when treated with pre-irradiated BSA-AGE conjugate [12]. In contrast to the BSA-AGE conjugate, the non-glycated Type I calfskin collagen was photosensitized by solar-simulated light irradiation in CFE fibroblasts, resulting in the formation of hydrogen peroxide [12, 51]. This somewhat surprising result could be explained by several factors. The native collagen contains some tyrosine and is cross-linked with elastin, which contains phenylalanine units. The Type I calfskin collagen is also cross-linked with malondialdehyde by aldimine chromophores, which can undergo oxidative changes during the aging processes in human epidermis. These cross-links together with tyrosine and phenylalanine are chromophores, which can contribute to photosensitization processes [**Sch. 2E-4**]. The UVA irradiation of elastin induces ROS formation and cell growth inhibition [48], attributed either to tryptophan residues [12, 53, 54] or to native collagen and elastin cross-links [12].

The cysteine derivative 3,3-dimethyl-D-cysteine (D-penicillamine) is a potent inhibitor of the non-oxidative glycation processes [13]. The addition of D-penicillamine protected against the AGE-photosensitized growth inhibition even when added after the irradiation, since the reaction of D-penicillamine with α-dicarbonyl compounds (RCSs), such as glyoxal and methylglyoxal, results in the formation of thiazolidine derivatives [13]. The addition of D-penicillamine to human skin keratinocytes and fibroblasts protected against glyoxal- and methylglyoxal induced carbonyl toxicity. Based on these results, it was proposed that a further search of D-penicillamine analogs could generate suitable therapeutic agents for the protection against UVA radiation damages to human skin [13].

The AGE-photosensitized production of significant amounts of hydrogen peroxide in human skin [48, 49] also has important implications for the photocarcinogenesis of human skin [12]. Thus, it is conceivable that an interference could occur between the AGE-mediated photoproduction of hydrogen peroxide and the hydrogen peroxide induced mitogenic redox signaling processes [55], since various human cancer cells spontaneously produce substantial amounts of hydrogen peroxide as an autocrine stimulant for the maintenance of proliferative signaling in melanoma cells [55]. The mitogenic signaling in fibroblasts through both the Ras and Rac genes is mediated by superoxide anion radical production with spontaneous formation of molecular oxygen and hydrogen peroxide. The endogenous production of ROS could be responsible for an essential activation of the transcription factor NF-kβ in malignant melanoma cells [56]. Therefore, scavengers of ROS, especially the catalase enzyme, are inhibitors of melanoma cell proliferation.

In recent years, much attention has been devoted to the role of AGEs and the receptor for AGE (RAGE) in various diseases, including diabetes [17, 18, 33, 34], oxidative stress and aging [57], smoking and dental disease [58], cardiovascular disease [59], lens disease and macular degeneration [60–63], Alzheimer's disease (AD) [64–71], Parkinson's disease [72], Creutzfeldt–Jacob disease [73], amyotrophic lateral sclerosis (Lou Gehrig's disease) [74,75], cardiovascular disease [76, 77], and polycystic ovarian syndrome [78]. The level of RAGE may be associated with periodontal disease linked to smoking [62]. Immunolocalization of RAGE in retinal pigment epithelium (RPE) and photoreceptors coincided with AGE deposits and macular disease in aged and early-age-related macular degeneration (AMD) and geographic atrophy (GA) retinas [62]. AGE accumulation during normal aging and in disease may induce receptor-mediated activation of RPE/photoreceptor cells, contributing to disease progression in the aging human retinas [62].

RAGEs have been shown to play a central role in the pathology of important neurological diseases, including AD and stroke [64–75]. It was hypothesized that serum or cerebrospinal fluid (CSF) levels of glyceraldehyde-derived AGE could become a biomarker for early detection of AD [65]. The glyceraldehyde-AGE has a toxic effect on primary cultured rat cortical neurons in vitro [66] and is a toxic moiety for neuronal cells in AD in vivo [66, 67]. In the brains of AD patients, glyceraldehyde-AGE was mainly present in the cytosol of neurons in the hippocampus and parahippocampal gyrus but not in the senile plaques and astrocytes [66, 67].

There are two functional types of RAGE associated with neurological diseases: cell membrane-bound full length (fl) and soluble (s) [64]. Ligand binding to fl-RAGE initiates sustained cellular activation and receptor-dependent signaling, resulting in inflammation and cellular stress and increased RAGE expression. The cell surface RAGE receptor and ligand interaction provides a positive feedback mechanism that can rapidly accelerate disease progression [64]. The s-RAGE significantly inhibits these positive feedback mechanisms, because they contain functional ligand-binding domains but lack the cellular signaling domains. Thus, the s-RAGE can reduce the severe outcomes of ligand–membrane interactions by binding to RAGE ligands and preventing their interaction with fl-RAGE. The soluble forms of RAGE can serve a protective role against various neurological diseases and as potential therapeutic targets [64].

In conclusion, it appears that the protein glycoxidation products, the so-called advanced glycosylation end products (AGE), are the endogenous photosensitizers. The reactions of the photoexcited singlet and triplet species with molecular oxygen generate the reactive oxygen species (ROS), which cause the oxidative cell damages in human skin and other organs of the human body, and, thus, probably contribute to photoaging and photocarcinogenesis processes.

References

1. Walter G. R. and Feather M. S. (eds.) (1983) *The Maillard Reaction in Foods and Nutrition*, ACS Symposium Series 215, American Chemical Society, Washington, DC.

2. Vernin G. and Parkanyi C. (1982) Mechanisms of formation of heterocyclic compounds in Maillard reaction. In: *Chemistry of Heterocyclic Compounds in Flavors and Aromas*, pp 151–207, Vernin G. (ed.), Halsted Press, New York; Ellis Horwood, Chichester, West Sussex, England.
3. Sosnovsky G., Gnewuch, C. T. and Ryoo E. S. (1993) In the search for new anticancer drugs. XXV: Role of N-nitrosated Amadori compounds derived from glucose-amino acid conjugates in cancer promotion or inhibition. *J. Pharm. Sci.* **82**: 649–656.
4. Sosnovsky G. and Gnewuch C. T. (1994) In the search for new anticancer drugs. 27. Synthesis and comparison of anticancer activity in vivo of amino acids, carbohydrates and carbohydrate-amino acid conjugates containing the [*N*'-(2-chloroethyl)-*N*'-nitrosoamino]-carbonyl group. *J. Pharm. Sci.* **83**: 989–998.
5. Rothweiler B., Kuhn E. and Prest H. (2004) GC-MS approaches to the analysis of acrylamide in foods. *Am. Lab.* (June), pp 35–38.
6. Hogervorst J. G., Schouten L. J., Konings E. J., Goldbohm R. A. and van den Brandt P. A. (2007) A prospective study of dietary acrylamide intake and the risk of endometrial, ovarian, and breast cancer. *Cancer Epidemiol. Biomarkers Prev.* **11**: 2304–2313.
7. Vernin G., Metzger J., Boniface C., Murello M.-H., Siouffi A., Larice J.-L. and Parkanyi C. (1992) Kinetics and thermal degradation of the fructose-methionine Amadori intermediates. GC-MS/SPECMA data bank identification of volatile aroma compounds. *Carbohydr. Res.* **230**: 15–29.
8. Roberts R. L. and Lloyd R. V. (1997) Free radical formation from secondary amines in the Maillard reaction. *J. Agric. Food Chem.* **45**: 2413–2418.
9. Stoesser R., Klein J., Peschke S., Zehl A., Cammerer B. and Kroh L. W. (2007) On the time behaviour of the concentration of pyrazinium radical cations in the early stage of the Maillard reaction. *Spectrochim. Acta, Part A* **67**: 1161–1168.
10. Shipar M. A. H. (2006) Formation of the Heyns Rearrangement products in dihydroxyacetone and glycine Maillard reaction: A computational study. *Food Chem.* **97**: 231–243.
11. Wondrak G. T., Jacobson E. L. and Jacobson M. K. (2002) Photosensitization of DNA damage by glycated proteins. *Photochem. Photobiol. Sci.* **1**: 355–363.
12. Wondrak G. T., Roberts M. J., Jacobson M. K. and Jacobson E. L. (2002) Photosensitized growth inhibition of cultured human skin

cells: mechanism and suppression of oxidative stress from solar irradiation of glycated proteins. *J. Invest. Dermatol.* **119**: 489–498.
13. Wondrak G. T., Cervantes-Laurean D., Roberts M. J., Qasem J. G., Kim M., Jacobson E. L. and Jacobson M. K. (2002) Identification of α-dicarbonyl scavengers for cellular protection against carbonyl stress. *Biochem. Pharmacol.* **63**: 361–373.
14. Thornalley P. J., Langborg A. and Minhas H. S. (1999) Formation of glyoxal, methylglyoxal and 3-deoxyglucosone in the glycation of proteins by glucose. *Biochem. J.* **344**: 109–116.
15. Glomb M. A. and Monnier V. M. (1995) Mechanism of protein modification by glyoxal and glycolaldehyde, reactive intermediates of the Maillard reaction. *J. Biol. Chem.* **270**: 10017–10026.
16. Wondrak G. T., Varadarajan S., Butterfield D. A. and Jacobson M. K. (2000) Formation of a protein-bound pyrazinium free radical cation during glycation of histone H1. *Free Radical Biol. Med.* **29**: 557–567.
17. Brownlee M. (1995) Advanced protein glycosylation in diabetes and aging. *Annu. Rev. Med.* **46**: 233–234.
18. Monnier V. M., Sell D. R., Nagaraj R. H., Miyata S., Grandhee S., Odetti P. and Ibrahim S. A. (1992) Maillard reaction-mediated molecular damage to extracellular matrix and other tissue proteins in diabetes, aging, and uremia. *Diabetes* **41** (Suppl. 2) 36–41.
19. Ortwerth B. J., Prabhakaram M., Nagaraj R. H. and Linetsky M. (2008) The relative UV sensitizer activity of purified advanced glycation endproducts. *Photochem. Photobiol.* **65**: 666–672.
20. Wolff S. P., Bascal Z. A. and Hunt J. V. (1989) Autoxidative glycosylation: free radicals and glycation theory. *Prog. Clin. Biol. Res.* **304**: 259–275.
21. Fu M.-X., Requena J. R., Jenkins A. J., Lyons T. J., Baynes J. W. and Thorpe S. R. (1996) The advanced glycation end product, N^{ε}-(carboxymethyl)lysine, is a product of both lipid peroxidation and glycoxidation reactions. *J. Biol. Chem.* **271**: 9982–9986.
22. Mizutari K., Ono T., Ikeda K., Kayashima K. and Horiuchi S. (1997) Photoenhanced modification of human skin elastin in actinic elastosis by N^{ε}-(carboxymethyl)lysine, one of the glycoxidation products of the Maillard reaction. *J. Invest. Dermatol.* **108**: 797–802.
23. Peich C. C., Seidel W., Hanak N., Waibel R., Schneider M. and Pischetsrieder M. (2005) Potential DNA-protein cross-link products formed by sugar degradation products: identification of N^6-[2-(N^2-deoxyguanosyl)propionyl]lysine. *Eur. Food Res. Tech.* **221**: 1438–2377.

24. Steenken S., Jaenicke-Zauner W. and Schulte-Frohlinde D. (2008) Photofragmentation of hydroxyacetone, 1,3-dihydroxyacetone, and 1,3-dicarboxyacetone in aqueous solution. An EPR study. *Photochem. Photobiol.* **21**: 21–26.
25. Jung K., Seifert M., Herrling T. and Fuchs J. (2008) UV-generated free radicals (FR) in skin: their prevention by sunscreens and their induction by self-tanning agents. *Spectrochim. Acta, Part A* **69**: 1423–1428.
26. Lloyd R. V., Fong A. J. and Sayre R. M. (2001) *In vivo* formation of Maillard reaction free radicals in mouse skin. *J. Invest. Dermatol.* **117**: 740–742.
27. Molin M., Pilon M. and Blomberg A. (2007) Dihydroxyacetone-induced death is accompanied by advanced glycation endproduct formation in selected proteins of *Saccharomyces cerevisiae* and *Caenorhabditis elegans*. *Proteomics* **7**: 3764–3774.
28. Wondrak G. T., Jacobson M. K. and Jacobson E. L. (2006) Endogenous UVA-photosensitizers: mediators of skin photodamage and novel targets for skin photoprotection. *Photochem. Photobiol. Sci.* **5**: 215–237.
29. Petersen A. B., Wulf H. C., Gniadecki R. and Gajkowska B. (2004) Dihydroxyacetone, the active browning ingredient in sunless tanning lotions, induces DNA damage, cell-cycle block and apoptosis in cultured HaCaT keratinocytes. *Mutat. Res.* **560**: 173–186.
30. Okano Y., Masaki H. and Sakurai H. (2001) Pentosidine in advanced glycation end-products (AGEs) during UVA irradiation generates active oxygen species and impairs human dermal fibroblasts. *J. Dermatol. Sci.* (Suppl 1): S11–18.
31. Li Y., Cohenford M. A., Udayan D. and Dain J. A. (2008) Nonenzymatic glycation of guanosine 5'-triphosphate (GTP) by dihydroxyacetone phosphate (DHAP): an in vitro study of AGE formation. *FASEB J.* **22**: 1056.3.
32. Li Y., Cohenford M. A., Dutta U. and Dain J. A. (2008) In vitro nonenzymatic glycation of guanosine 5'-triphosphate by dihydroxyacetone phosphate. *Anal. Bioanal. Chem.* **392**: 1189–1196.
33. Schalkwijk C. G., Stehouwer C. D. A. and van Hinsbergh V. W. M. (2004) Fructose-mediated non-enzymatic glycation: sweet coupling or bad modification. *Diabetes/Metab. Res. Rev.* **20**: 369–382.
34. Usui T., Shimohira K., Watanabe H. and Hayase F. (2008) Detection and determination of glyceraldehyde-derived advanced glycation endproduct. *Biofactors* **21**: 391–394.

35. Wondrak G. T., Cervantes-Laurent D., Jacobson E. L. and Jacobson M. K. (2000) Histone carbonylation in vivo and in vitro. *Biochem. J.* **351**: 769–777.
36. Halliwell B. and Gutteridge J. M. C. (1989) Free radicals, aging, and disease. In: *Free radicals in biology and medicine*, pp 279–313, Clarendon press, Oxford.
37. Berlett B. S. and Stadtman E. R. (1997) Protein oxidation in aging, disease, and oxidative stress. *J. Biol. Chem.* **272**: 20313–20316.
38. Dean R. T., Fu S., Stocker R. and Davies M. J. (1997) Biochemistry and pathology of radical-mediated protein oxidation. *Biochem. J.* **324**: 1–18.
39. Stadtman E. R. (1992) Protein oxidation and aging. *Science* **257**: 1220–1224.
40. Kreimeyer A., Wielkens P., Adamletz P. and Hilz H. (1984) DNA repair-associated ADP-ribosylation in vivo. Modification of histone H1 differs from that of the principal acceptor proteins. *J. Biol. Chem.* **259**: 890–896.
41. Cervantes-Laurean D., Minter D. E., Jacobson E. L. and Jacobson M. K. (1993) Protein glycation by ADP-ribose: studies of model conjugates. *Biochemistry* **32**: 1528–1534.
42. Jacobson E. L., Antol K. M., Juarez-Salinas H. and Jacobson M. K. (1983) Poly(ADP-ribose) metabolism in UV irradiated human fibroblasts. *J. Biol. Chem.* **258**: 103–107.
43. Jacobson E. L., Cervantes-Laurean D. and Jacobson M. K. (1997) ADP-ribose in glycation and glycoxidation reactions. *Adv. Exp. Med. Biol.* **419**: 371–379.
44. Strahl B. D. and Allis C. D. (2000) The language of covalent histone modifications. *Nature (London)* **403**: 41–45.
45. Wolffe A. P. (1992) Chromatin structure. In: *Chromatin structure and function*, pp 4–67, Academic Press, London.
46. Wondrak G. T., Varadarajan S., Butterfield D. A. and Jacobson M. K. (2000) Formation of a protein-bound pyrazinium free radical cation during glycation of histone H1. *Free Radical Biol. Med.* **29**: 557–567.
47. Foote C. S. (1991) Definition of type I and type II photosensitized oxidation. *Photochem. Photobiol.* **54**: 659.
48. Masaki H., Okano Y. and Sakurai H. (1997) Generation of active oxygen species from advanced glycation end-products (AGE) under ultraviolet light A (UVA) irradiation. *Biochem. Biophys. Res. Commun.* **235**: 306–310.

49. Masaki H., Okano Y. and Sakurai H. (1999) Generation of active oxygen species from advanced glycation end-products (AGEs) during ultraviolet light A (UVA) irradiation and a possible mechanism for cell damaging. *Biochem. Biophys. Acta* **1428**: 45–56.
50. Scharffetter-Kochanek K., Wlaschek M., Brenneisen P., Schauen M., Blaudschun R. and Wenk J. (1997) UV-induced reactive oxygen species in photocarcinogenesis and photoaging. *Biol. Chem.* **378**: 1247–1257.
51. Kollias N., Gilles R., Moran M., Kochevar I. E. and Anderson R. R. (1998) Endogenous skin fluorescence includes bands that may serve as quantitative markers of aging and photoaging. *J. Invest. Dermatol.* **111**: 776–780.
52. Petruska J. A. and Sandberg L. B. (1968) The amino acid composition of elastin in its soluble and insoluble state. *Biochem. Biophys. Res. Commun.* **33**: 222–228.
53. McCormick J. P., Fischer J. R., Pachlatko J. P. and Eisenstark A. (1976) Characterization of a cell-lethal product from the photooxidation of tryptophan: hydrogen peroxide. *Science* **191**: 468–469.
54. Grossweiner L. I. (1984) Photochemistry of proteins: a review. *Curr. Eye Res.* **3**: 137–144.
55. Schmidt K. N., Amstad P., Cerutti P. and Baeuerle P. A. (1996) Identification of hydrogen peroxide as the relevant messenger in the activation pathway of transcription factor NF-kappaβ. *Adv. Exp. Med. Biol.* **387**: 63–68.
56. Brar S. S., Kennedy T. P., Whorton A. R., Sturrock A. B., Huercksteadt T. P., Ghio A. J. and Hoidal J. R. (2001) Reactive oxygen species from NAD(P)H, quinone oxidoreductase constitutively activate NF-kappaβ in malignant melanoma cells. *Am. J. Physiol. Cell Physiol.* **280**: C659–C676.
57. Uribarri J., Cai W., Peppa M., Goodman S., Ferrucci L., Striker G. and Vlassara H. (2007) Circulating glycotoxins and dietary advanced glycation endproducts: two links to inflammatory response, oxidative stress, and aging. *J. Gerontol., Ser. A* **62**: 427–433.
58. Katz J., Yoon T. Y. H., Mao S., Lamont R. J. and Caudle R. M. (2007) Expression of the receptor of advanced glycation end products in the gingival tissue of smokers with generalized periodontal disease and after nornicotine induction in primary gingival epithelial cells. *J. Periodontol.* **78**: 736–741.
59. Yamagishi S., Matsui T. and Nakamura K. (2009) Possible involvement of tobacco-derived advanced glycation end products (AGEs) in

an increased risk for developing cancers and cardiovascular disease in former smokers. *Med. Hypotheses* **71**: 259–261.
60. De La Rochette A., Birlouez-Aragon I., Silva E. and Morliere P. (2003) Advanced glycation endproducts as UVA photosensitizers of tryptophan and ascorbic acid: consequence for the lens. *Biochem. Biophys. Acta* **1621**: 235–241.
61. Glenn J. V. and Stitt A. W. (2009) The role of advanced glycation end products in retinal ageing and disease. *Biochim. Biophys. Acta* **1790**: 1109–1116.
62. Howes K. A., Liu Y., Dunaief J. L., Milam A., Frederick J. M., Marks A. and Baehr W. (2004) Receptor for advanced glycation end products and age-related macular degeneration. *Invest. Ophthalmol. Visual Sci.* **45**: 3713–3720.
63. Gottsch. J. D., Pou S., Bynoe L. A. and Rosen G. M. (1990) Hematogenous photosensitization. A mechanism for the development of age-related macular degeneration. *Invest. Ophthalmol. Visual Sci.* **31**: 1674–1682.
64. Lue L-F., Walker D. G., Jacobson S. and Sabbagh M. (2009) Receptor for advanced glycation end products: its role in Alzheimer's disease and other neurological diseases. *Future Neurol.* **4**: 167–177.
65. Yamagishi S., Nakamura K., Inoue H., Kikuchi S. and Takeuchi M. (2005) Serum or cerebrospinal fluid levels of glyceraldehyde-derived advanced glycation end products (AGEs) may be a promising biomarker for early detection of Alzheimer's disease. *Med. Hypotheses* **64**: 1205–1207.
66. Choei H., Sasaki N., Takeuchi M., Yoshida T., Ukai W., Yamagishi S., Kikuchi S. and Saito T. (2004) Glyceraldehyde-derived glycation end products in Alzheimer's disease. *Acta Neuropathol.* **108**: 189–193.
67. Takeuchi M., Kikuchi S., Sasaki N., Suzuki T., Watai T., Iwaki M., Bucala R. and Yamagishi S. (2004) Involvement of advanced glycation end-products (AGEs) in Alzheimer's disease. *Curr. Alzheimer Res.* **1**: 39–46.
68. Smith M. A., Taneda S., Richey P. L., Miyata T., Yan S. D., Stern D., Sayre L. M., Monnier V. M. and Perry G. (1994) Advanced Maillard reaction end products are associated with Alzheimer disease pathology. *Proc. Natl. Acad. Sci. U. S. A.* **91**: 5710–5714.
69. Vitek M. P., Bhattacharya K., Glendening J. M., Stopa E., Vlassara H., Bucala R., Manogue K. and Cerami A. (1994) Advanced glycation end products contribute to amyloidosis in Alzheimer disease. *Proc. Natl. Acad. Sci. U. S. A.* **91**: 4766–4770.

70. Yan S. D., Chen X., Schmidt A. M., Brett J., Godman G., Zou Y. S., Scott C. W., Caputo C., Frappier T. and Smith M. A. (1994) Glycated tau protein in Alzheimer disease: a mechanism for induction of oxidant stress. *Proc. Natl. Acad. Sci. U. S. A.* **91**: 7787–7791.
71. Sasaki N., Toki S., Choei H., Saito T., Nakano N., Hayashi Y., Takeuchi M. and Makita Z. (2001) Immunohistochemical distribution of the receptor for advanced glycation end products in neurons and astrocytes in Alzheimer's disease. *Brain Res.* **888**: 256–262.
72. Castellani R., Smith M. A., Richey P. J. and Petty G. (1996) Glycoxidation and oxidative stress in Parkinson disease and diffuse Lewy body disease. *Brain Res.* **737**: 195–200.
73. Sasaki N., Takeuchi M., Chowei H., Kikuchi S., Hayashi Y., Nakano N., Ikeda H., Yamagishi S., Kitamoto T., Saito T. and Makita Z. (2002) Advanced glycation end products (AGE) and their receptor (RAGE) in the brain of patients with Creutzfeldt-Jacob disease with prion plaques. *Neurosci. Lett.* **326**: 117–120.
74. Kikuchi S., Shinpo K., Ogata A., Tsuji S., Takeuchi M., Makita Z. and Toshiro K. (2002) Detection of *N*-epsilon-(carboxymethyl)lysine (CML) and non-CML advanced glycation end products in the anterior horn of amyotrophic lateral sclerosis spinal cord. *Amyotrophic Lateral Scler. Other Mot. Neuron Disord.* **3**: 63–68.
75. Choi S. M., Wang H. S., Taniguchi A. and Bucala R. (1998) Advanced glycation end products in neurofilament conglomeration of motoneurons in familial and sporadic amyotrophic lateral sclerosis. *Mol. Med.* **4**: 324–332.
76. Peppa M. and Raptis S. A. (2008) Advanced glycation end products and cardiovascular disease. *Curr. Diabetes Rev.* **4**: 92–100.
77. Robinet A., Alouane L., Hozey G. and Millart H. (2007) Advanced glycation end products (AGEs) derived from glycate albumin suppress early β1-adrenergic preconditioning. *Fund. Clin. Pharmacol.* **21**: 35–43.
78. Diamanti-Kandarakis E., Piperi C. and Nicolopoulou-Stamati P. (2007) Advanced glycation end products in polycystic ovarian syndrome. In *Environmental Science and Technology Library*, Vol. 22, pp 119–140, Reproductive Health and the Environment, Springer, The Netherlands.

F. The Ultraviolet Light Induced Impairments of Nucleic Acids, Immunity, Cancer Suppressor Gene P53, and Other Cell Protective Systems in the Human Skin. Possible Alleviating Properties of Sunscreen Agents

The process of immunosuppression begins with the interaction of UVB and UVA radiations with various chromophores such as DNA, *trans*-urocanic acid, and porphyrins in the epidermis, resulting in the formation of reactive oxygen species (ROS). It also activates the enzymes cyclooxygenase-2 (COX-2) and nitric oxide synthase (NOS), leading to the production of prostaglandins (PG) such as PGE-2 and nitric oxide, respectively. These events are followed by the release of various cytokines, mutations in the cell signaling events, and mutations of the p53 tumor suppressor gene and other genes, leading to cancer [1–6]. The application of sunscreen agents would be expected to either ameliorate or even protect against all these adverse events and, in particular, against the all-important event, the induction of DNA damage.

i. The Interaction of UV Radiation with Chromophores in DNA and Urocanic Acid

a. DNA Damage

UV radiations, especially the UVB radiations, cause the formation of a number of DNA photoproducts, such as cyclobutane pyrimidine dimers (CPD), (6-4) pyrimidine-pyrimidone and other photoproducts [7–12]. (See **Section 2D**.) These lesions are formed mainly at sites of adjacent pyrimidine moieties where the UVR-induced DNA damages and mutations occur. The regions of high mutation occurrence for the p53 gene in skin cancers are also the regions of low occurrence for DNA repair [1]. The UVA and visible light radiations are known to cause DNA damage indirectly by producing first the reactive oxygen species (ROS), which then cause single-strand breaks, DNA-protein cross-links and altered bases, such as 8-hydroxyguanine [1]. (See **Section 2D**.) Recently, it was discovered that UVB radiation induced DNA damages can be repaired by the application of the DNA repair enzyme photolyase that specifically converts the cyclobutane dimers into their original DNA structure after exposure to photoactivating light [13–15]. Thus, the topical application of photolyase-containing liposomes to UVB-irradiated skin and subsequent exposure to photoreactivating light decreased the number of UVB radiation induced dimers by 40 to 45%. The enzyme application can also prevent the hypersensitivity reactions as well as erythema and sunburn-cell formations [13]. The protection rendered by the use of sunscreen agents against the UVR-induced DNA damage was investigated in a number of studies [15–25]. DNA damage is considered to be a transient, causal, and an early biomarker in the pathway of photocarcinogenesis. Protection by sunscreens against DNA damage was found in several cases, but only in one study [22] was solar-simulated UVR used and information was provided based on a dose-response relationship.

The application of the broad spectrum UVA absorber terephthalylidene-3,3'-dicamphor-10,10'-sulfonic acid (Mexoryl® SX) was significantly more effective than that of the UVBR absorber 2-ethylhexyl 4-methoxycinnamate (OMC) in preventing the induction of pyrimidine dimers [22]. The DNA protection factors (11.5 and 6.6, respectively) were greater than the sun protection factor, SPF = 4, for both sunscreens, whereby the DNA protection factor is defined as the ratio of the UVR dose needed to inhibit 50% of DNA synthesis with sunscreens, to the UVR dose needed to inhibit 50% DNA synthesis without sunscreens. The application of sunscreens containing either 1% *para*-aminobenzoic acid (PABA) or 1% urocanic acid resulted in low protection against the UVB-induced suppression of epidermal DNA synthesis, whereas the use of a sunscreen containing 10% titanium dioxide gave complete protection [23].

b. Urocanic Acid (UCA)

As one of the major chromophores in skin, UCA undergoes a conversion from the trans form to the cis form upon absorption of UV light [26–29]. This isomerization has been shown to produce reactive oxygen species (ROS) [30, 31]. (See **Section 1A.**) *cis*-UCA is responsible for initiating some of the processes causing UV-induced immunosuppression in humans and mice [2, 4, 26–28, 32, 33]. The prevention of the urocanic acid (UCA) mediated immunosuppression [34, 35] and its effect on photoaging processes have been studied [36, 37]. Thus, it was found that inclusion of *N*-acetylcysteine (NAC) inhibited the UVB radiation induced suppression of contact hypersensitivity (CHS) in mice [34, 35]. The inhibitory effect on CHS was attributed, in part, to interference by NAC in the function of *cis*-UCA in UVBR-induced suppression of CHS [34]. Support for this conclusion was obtained from an experiment with mice that were kept in the dark where no photoisomerization of *cis*-urocanic acid (*cis*-UCA) could occur. The oral administration to mice of *N*-acetylcysteine (NAC) together with *cis*-UCA resulted in a complete inhibition of the CHS suppression, whereas the administration independently of either NAC or *cis*-UCA produced no effect [34]. A control experiment revealed that topical application of NAC to mice 20 minutes prior to irradiation did not influence the photoisomerization of *trans*- to *cis*-UCA.

ii. Chemical Mediators of Skin Immunosuppression

a. ROS and Nitric Oxide (NO)

ROS and NO can interact to form peroxy nitrite, a powerful oxidant. In addition, these two species at high doses can cause oxidative damage to lipids, proteins, and DNA, resulting in stress or damage to the cell, and, at higher doses, they can kill the cells [33]. ROS and NO contribute to immunosuppression in both humans and mice [38, 39, 40–43].

Reactive oxygen- and nitrogen-centered species, such as ROS and NO, produced in response to UV radiations, constitute important factors in processes of erythema, immunosuppression, and carcinogenesis [40, 41]. Thus, it was found that the administration to mice of a mixture consisting of the UVB radiation absorbing sunscreen agent OMC and the oxygen radical inhibitors (ORI) 2,2'-dipyridyl and N(G)-monomethyl-L-arginine acetate (L-NMMA), followed by irradiation of the mice with simulated solar (ss) radiation containing UVA and UVB wavelengths, resulted in prevention of the UVA-induced suppression of CHS [40, 44]. The use of ORI in conjunction with ssUV radiation of mice lowers the levels of the erythema and improves the effectiveness of sunscreens in the prevention of carcinogenesis, but fails to improve the immune protection by sunscreen agents [40].

b. Prostaglandins and Histamine

Prostaglandin levels, especially PGE-2, are elevated after exposure to UV irradiation. This lipoid compound is produced by the action of the enzyme cyclooxygenase-2 (COX-2) on arachidonic acid. PGE-2 production is effected indirectly by the mediators histamine and platelet activating factor (PAF) [45]. PGE-2 affects immunosuppression by increasing the serum levels of the cytokines IL-4 and IL-10 [46, 47].

c. Neuropeptides

UV-induced calcitonin gene-related peptide (CGRP) modulates Langerhans cells (LC) by stimulating TNF release by mast cells, and producing premature LC migration out of the skin [48, 49].

d. LC Loss and Dysfunctional APC Activity

UV light causes damaged LC to migrate from the epidermis to draining lymph nodes, where they have an impaired ability to induce immunity [2, 3, 50–52]. The UV radiations suppress the immunity directly by modifying the antigen presentation by cutaneous antigen presenting cells (APC) [53]. The defect in the CHS response is mediated, in part, by a direct damage to APCs in the epidermis resulting in a reduction of $ATPase^{+}$ and Ia^{+} Langerhans cells and alterations in the morphology and functions of the remaining Langerhans cells [1, 54, 55].

e. Regulatory Cells

UV irradiation induces the generation of a unique population of suppressor cells that actively inhibit immunity and induce tolerance in an antigen-specific manner [56]. This unique population of cells includes regulatory T cells [57], suppressor B cells [58], and suppressor NKT cells [59]. These cells produce IL-10 and IL-4, which mediate the immunosuppression. Thus, IL-10 inhibits the production of Il-12 by dendritic (DC) cells and the production of interferon gamma (IFN-γ) by T cells [2].

The immunological impairment caused by UV radiation can be divided into local and systemic effects. The local immune suppression is a Tcell mediated response, e.g., a diminished contact hypersensitivity response (CHR) [3, 60–65], evoked by topically applied antigens that occur at UV-irradiated sites, while the systemic immune suppression occurs when the exposure to UVR results in a diminished CHR to haptens at a distant, not irradiated site [66]. A delayed-type hypersensitivity (DTH) response is a T cell mediated response evoked by internally administered antigen, e.g., injected into the skin [67].

Chronic exposure of mice to UVB radiations induces systemic changes in the immune system that result in an inability to reject highly antigenic transplanted UVBR-induced cancers, and in an inability to develop DTH skin responses to xenobiotics, such as dinitrochlorobenzene (DNCB) and dinitrofluorobenzene (DNFB) [30, 50, 53, 54, 60, 68]. These changes appear to be associated with the development of suppressor T cells [63–65]. A hypothesis was proposed that the formation of these cells is a result of the UVBR-induced changes in antigen-presenting cells (APC) in human skin caused either by the direct effects of UV radiations or by the formation of photoproducts, such as *cis*-urocanic acid, in epithelial cells of the skin [69]. To test this effect of solar radiation on the human immune system, twelve human volunteers were exposed for thirty minutes to radiations from solarium lamps [69]. This treatment resulted in a depression of natural killer (NK) cell activity against a melanoma cell line which could not be prevented by the application of a broad spectrum sunscreen lotion containing 2-ethylhexyl (4-dimethylamino)benzoate, 2-hydroxy-4-methoxybenzophenone, and 4-*tert*-butyl-4′-methoxydibenzoylmethane (BMDM, Avobenzone) with an SPF of 15 [69].

Further experiments involving irradiations of peripheral blood lymphocytes (PBL) with UV light of various wavelengths led to the conclusions that the UV light suppresses the NK activity of PBL, and that, for equivalent suppression of NK activity, a 140 times greater dose of UVA radiation than that of UVB radiation is required [69, 70]. However, when the greater proportion of UVA radiation in solar radiation and its deeper penetration into skin is taken into account, then the UVA radiation may have an equivalent or even greater direct immunosuppressive effect than the UVB radiation, although the mechanisms of their immunosuppressive effects may differ [70].

f. Cytokines

UV radiations can cause systemic suppressions of immune responses by inducing other agents, such as the cytokines, including interleukins IL-1, IL-3, IL-6, IL10, and IL12, the tumor necrosis factor (TNF), the intercellar adhesion molecule-1 (ICAM-1), and the granulocytic/macrophage colony stimulating factor (CSF) [71–75]. UV radiations stimulate the release of IL-1 [76, 77] and IL-3 [78]. The UVB radiation stimulates the formation of IL-6 either directly or via IL-1 [73, 79], with the release of IL-6 in both normal and malignant keratinocytes [80]. The UVA radiation causes the release of IL-6 in cultured fibroblasts [81], while the UVB radiation stimulates the release of TNF in cultured keratinocytes in the human skin [82, 83].

The effect of UVB irradiation on the promotion of cutaneous immunosuppression by the release of cytokines and the depletion of Langerhans cells [84–86] was investigated using sunscreen agents, such as OMC with an SPF of 12 and zinc oxide with an SPF of 6, which were applied to the forearms of human volunteers and then irradiated with a fourfold minimal erythema dose (MED) of UVB light [87]. It was found that the UVBR-induced epidermal interleukin IL-10 mRNA expression was noticeably reduced by the presence of both sunscreens, i.e., to 95% and 78%, respectively, and that the Langerhans cell depletion was partially reduced, i.e., to 47% and 50%, respectively [87]. The level of immunosuppression caused by the UVB radiation in the presence of these sunscreens was markedly lower than the level of erythema prevention [87].

iii. Efficacy of Sunscreens in the Prevention of Immunosuppression

The effect of sunscreens in reducing the suppression of CHR by UV irradiation has been reported [68, 88–99].

The elicitation of the DTH reaction by UVR was investigated in humans [100, 101]. In a study using a UVB energy absorbing sunscreen agent, no protection was found against UVR-induced suppression of DTH to recall antigens [102], whereas in other studies an immunoprotection was observed in humans with broad-spectrum UVAR and UVBR sunscreen agents [88, 103].

Human volunteers with no sunscreen protection had greatly reduced responses to DTH tests, regardless of UV exposure conditions, such as full spectrum, UVA, UVA1, and solar-simulated radiation [100, 102–105]. The use of a sunscreen agent with a UVB filter had no protective effect, whereas, with sunscreen agents containing a combination of both UVA and UVB filters, the UV-induced immune suppression was prevented [10, 102–113]. Two groups of humans received applications of sunscreen agents with the same sun protection factor, i.e., SPF = 25, but different UVA-protection factors 14 and 9. In this case, the use of the sunscreen with a high protection factor in the UVA range resulted in a noticeably reduced UV-induced immunosuppression [102]. In a comparison of two sunscreen agents with the same SPF but different UVA protection factors, the use of a sunscreen agent with the higher UVA protection factor afforded better protection against suppression of an induction of CHR [100, 101]. Thus, SPF may not be sufficient to predict the ability of sunscreens to protect from UV-induced immune suppression. In a number of studies, inconsistent results were obtained with sunscreen applications, ranging from no protection [89, 90], to partial protection [15, 91, 114, 115], and full protection [93–96,116–118]. The discrepancies are attributable to the use of different light sources and other experimental variables [1]. Determining the level of UVA protection is important, as UVA appears to have a relatively low contribution to erythema but a large contribution to immunosuppression [102, 104–107]. In general, better protection was obtained with broad-spectrum UVAR and UVBR energy absorbing sunscreen agents than with single-range compounds [88, 91, 108, 102–106, 111–113].

iv. UV-Induced Immunosuppression and Skin Cancer

a. Mutation of Cell Signaling Pathways

UV radiations induce immunosuppression, resulting in a growth of cancer cells [1, 102, 110–113, 119–123]. It is widely accepted that mutations of cell signaling pathways needed for proliferation can lead to cancer [124–126]. The Hedgehog (Hh) signaling pathway in human cells contains the Ptc protein from the Patched (PTCH) gene and is important for embryonic development [124]. Retroviral transduction of Sonic homolog of Hedgehog (SHH) into normal human keratinocytes resulted in the expression of intracellular SHH and of the known Gli-target BMP-2B and expression of Bcl-2 protein [127–130]. The Bcl-2 protein is commonly expressed in basal cell carcinoma (BCC) and is a well-known suppressor of apoptosis. SHH causes epithelial proliferation and prevents $p21^{CIP1/WAF1}$ -induced growth arrest [131].

Some melanomas (CM) can arise because of a loss of the gene INK4α on the chromosome 9p21, which disrupts two cell control pathways and causes a loss of $p16^{INK4\alpha}$ expression [124, 132]. Point mutations on the N-Ras oncogene are also associated with CM. The Ras gene induces cell senescence and cell cycle arrest in the G-1 phase and are accompanied by an accumulation of p16 and p53 [133–135]. The Ras proteins function in mitogenic pathways by activation of a receptor tyrosine kinase (RTK) at the cell membrane [124]. Squamous cell carcinoma (SCC) can arise because of a mutated p53 gene and an activated receptor tyrosine kinase-Ras oncogene (RTK)/Ras) pathway [124–126].

b. Mutation of the p53 Tumor Suppressive Gene

The p53 tumor suppressive gene is a latent, short-lived, sequence-specific DNA binding transcription factor. When UV radiation interacts with human skin and damages the DNA by forming various photoproducts such as cyclobutane pyrimidine dimers (CPDs), (6-4) photoproducts and Dewar isomers, the p53 protein is phosphorylated at one or more serine residues at the N- or C-terminus, translocates into the nucleus, binds to the enhancer/promoter elements of downstream target genes and regulates their transcription. Genes that are activated by p53 induce cell cycle arrest, DNA repair, apoptosis, inhibition of angiogenesis and metastasis [136–144]. The cell cycle arrest allows time for DNA repair before the next cycle of mitosis. This arrest occurs at the G1/S transition and the chief p53 target gene is $p21^{WAFI/CIPI}$ which inhibits the cyclin-dependent kinases 4/6 [145–147]. DNA repair occurs during the G1/S cell cycle arrest, because it allows more time for Nucleotide Excision Repair (NER) as well as the induction of transcriptional activation of several genes (GADD45 and PCNA) known to directly participate in DNA repair. When cell cycle arrest and DNA repair is impossible, then the last ditch effort to escape malignant transformation involves cell death (apoptosis) [148–150]. P53 can activate the pro-apoptotic protein Bax that is in equilibrium with anti-apoptotic Bcl-2 which inhibits apoptosis by forming a dimer with Bax [136, 137, 151–153]. The apoptotic keratinocytes produced after an exposure to UVR have been called "sunburn cells" or apoptotic cells [1, 154]. Sunburn cells are considered to be transient biomarkers of exposure to UVR, but are not in the direct pathway of photocarcinogenesis [1].

UVR-induced skin cancers in both humans and mice contain unique p53 mutations, i.e., C→T and CC→TT transitions, at high frequencies of 50–100% [1]. Studies of the p53 gene in non-melanocytic cancer-derived tissues [155–159] revealed that nearly 50% of basal cell carcinomas (BCC) and squamous cell carcinomas (SCC) contain mutations in the p53 gene, and nearly 90% of these mutations occur at pyrimidine dimer sites, consistent with UV light as the causative agent [157]. The sites of high mutation occurrences in the DNA happen almost exclusively in the nucleotides where repair is abnormally slow [160]. A low expression of the p53 gene was found in melanocytic naevi that are believed to be the pre-neoplastic lesions [161], and, thus, it can be concluded that the p53 mutation is not the initiating step in the development of melanomas. The p53 is induced by UVB radiations possibly as a response to the excision of pyrimidine dimers [162], and the UV-induced mutations of keratinocytes could give rise to an actinic keratosis [163]. In the case a second p53 allele is also mutated, an SCC may arise, while in the case that these mutations occur in the so-called hedgehog protein signaling pathway, a BCC may result [127–130]. The UVR-induced p53 mutations are considered to be important biomarkers in the development of SCC. The appearance of mutant p53-positive cells occurs well before the appearance of skin cancers [164, 165].

Cellular p53 is normally in a state of senescence because it is bound to the antagonist protein MDM2. Recent research has led to the development of small molecules that can block the p53-MDM2 interaction, producing a reactivation of p53 in cancer cells and leading to cell cycle arrest, apoptosis, and growth inhibitions [125, 166–169]. A different approach is the expression of wild type p53 by means of an adenovirus [170]. In addition, adenoviruses have been engineered to selectively kill only cancer cells with p53 mutations [171].

v. Reductions of UVR-Induced p53 Mutations by the Use of Sunscreen Agents

Because of the fact that the p53 mutations occur well before the appearance of skin cancers, they have been used as early biological markers for the evaluation of protection efficacy by sunscreen agents. In several studies, this marker was further investigated [164, 165, 172–175]. Thus, the application to mice, before irradiation with simulated solar UV light, of either the UVB sunscreens with SPF 15 (8% 2-ethylhexyl 4-methoxycinnamate (OMC), 2% 2-phenyl-5-benzimidazole sulfonic acid) or a UVB and UVA sunscreen with SPF 22 (10% octocrylene, 0.2% 2-phenyl-5-benzimidazole sulfonic acid, 3.25 % Mexoryl SX™, 1.5% 4-*tert*-butyl-4'-methoxydibenzoylmethane) resulted in an 80–100% reduction of CC → TT p53 mutations [165, 174]. The application of UVB sunscreens appeared to be as effective as the mixture of UVB and UVA sunscreen agents in inhibiting p53 mutations [165, 174]. It is unlikely that UVA-type mutations, i.e., G → T transversions can play a role in the UVR-induced skin carcinogenesis, because they are seldom present in either human or mouse UVA-induced skin cancers [1]. Mouse skin cancers induced by large doses of UVA contained no G → T transversions in the p53 gene [176]. Commercial sunscreens were shown to be effective in preventing UVB-induced mutations in basal-cell carcinomas [177].

The UVA radiation induces p53 expression mainly in the basal layer of human skin, while the UVB radiation induces p53 expression diffusely throughout the epidermis [138]. Since UVR results in an over-expression of the TP53 and $TP21^{WAF1/CIP1}$ proteins in human and mouse cells in vitro and in vivo, these two proteins have been used in studies of the protection afforded by sunscreen agents against UVR-induced DNA damage of human [172, 173, 178–180] and mouse [22, 181] skin. Thus, the use of sunscreen agents containing organic [173, 179] and inorganic [178] materials reduced the number of TP53 and TP21 proteins. The application of sunscreen agents with different SPF values [20, 155, 172] to humans can protect against nuclear TP53 protein accumulations [180]. In addition, the applications of sunscreens to mice [182–184] and male Yorkshire pigs [185] were shown to inhibit the UVB-induced formation of sunburn or apoptotic cells [182–185]. Protection against the solar-simulated UVR induced formation of sunburn cells was obtained by either a 25% or a 50% SPF 12 sunscreen agent containing a mixture of OMC, BP-3, and zinc oxide [172]. However, in but only one of these studies, was solar-simulated UVR used and was information provided about the dose-response relationship [181].

vi. Efficacy of Sunscreens in the Prevention of Skin Cancer

The use of sunscreen agents can protect mice against the UVR-induced suppression of skin cancer rejection [65–67, 88–90, 93, 96–98, 102, 104–106 109–113]. However, in studies on the effect of sunscreen agents on the growth of transplanted melanoma cells in the UV-irradiated mouse skin, it was found that the application of sunscreens containing either 7.5% of 2-ethylhexyl 4-methoxycinnamate (OMC), 8% of 2-ethylhexyl (4-dimethylamino)benzoate, (ODM-PABA), or 6% of 2-hydroxy-4-methoxybenzophenone (BP-3), failed to prevent the UVR-induced enhancement of melanoma growth [184]. The reason for this failure could be attributed to the use of unfiltered lamps as the source of UVR that caused the transmission of UVC and short-wavelength UVB radiations [1]. A possible explanation for the UVR enhancement of the melanoma growth could be attributed to the photoisomerization of *trans*-urocanic acid to the cis form [26, 27, 186], since the UVA radiations efficiently converts *trans*-urocanic acid into the cis form [29], and in the presence of a sunscreen agent with a high absorbancy of UVA radiation, the UVR-enhanced melanoma growth could be retarded in vitro and in the mouse skin [29].

The application of plant polysaccharides (*Aloe barbadensis)* to human skin was found to ameliorate the immune damage triggered by UV radiations [53]. The efficacy and mechanism of action of these agents in preserving T cell mediated immunity to antigens in humans was discussed [53, 187–190]. These plant saccharides are of interest because they can be used to target pathways activated by UV radiation [53, 187, 188]. The activity of these compounds may proceed by novel mechanisms whereby there is a blockage of signal transduction pathways and the formation of immunosuppressive cytokines [187, 188, 190]. Plant polysaccharides can preserve the T cell mediated immunity by interfering with the activation of suppressor mechanisms caused by UV radiations, and not by a general immune stimulation [53]. Xyloglucans, another class of aloe oligosaccharides, were found to regulate the mitogen-activated protein kinase (MAPK) pathways, and, thus, they could be the naturally occurring signaling molecules that are involved in the regulation of the highly conserved serine/threonine protein kinases [190]. The treatment of mice skin with aloe before UVR, resulted in a partial preservation of the numbers and morphology of $ATPase^+$ and Ia^+ Langerhans cells [191], as well as the preservation of the APC functions and blocking of events involving the activation of suppressor T cells [192].

vii. Estrogenic Activities of Sunscreens

There has been concern about the potential endocrine disrupting properties of sunscreen agents and excipients, including fragrances, such as musks. Many of these materials have been tested in vitro using recombinant yeast screens carrying the human estrogen receptors alpha (hER α) and beta (hER β), in rat hepatocytes, in MCF-7 human breast cancer cell line, and in vivo in ovariectomized rats, fish, aquatic invertebrates, and humans.

3-(4-Methylbenzylidene)camphor (4-MBC) caused a delay in male puberty, decreased adult prostate weight, and slightly increased testes weight of the rat [193]. The androgen receptor (AR), the insulin-like growth factor-1 (IGF-1), and estrogen receptor (ER alpha and ER beta) expression in the prostate were reduced at the mRNA and protein levels. Acute repression of AR and IGF-1 mRNAs by estradiol (E2), studied in the ventral prostate, was reduced by 4-MBC exposure [193]. The effect of estrogen on the expression levels of ER-alpha and ER-beta mRNAs probably involves a direct action on the developing testis, and cannot be attributed to estrogen-induced suppression of gonadotropin secretion during the neonatal period [194].

An equipotent mixture of UV filters containing 2,4-dihydroxybenzophenone (BP-1), 2-hydroxy-4-methoxybenzophenone (BP-3), 2-ethylhexyl 4-methoxycinnamate (OMC), and 4-MBC was shown to additively activate the ER-estrogen regulated pS2 gene transcription in the human breast cancer cell line MCF-7 [195]. Exposure to 4-MBC during development of prostate and accessory sex glands of the fetal rat resulted in classical growth effects associated with estrogenic endocrine disruptors [196]. The two developmental processes of ductal outgrowth in the caudal dorsal prostate and branching morphogenesis were affected by exposure to 4-MBC and OMC [196].

The UV sunscreen compounds 4-MBC, OMC, BP-3, homosalate (HMS, menthyl salicylate), 2-ethylhexyl 4-(dimethylamino)benzoate (Padimate O) were found to stimulate the MCF-7 breast cancer cells through induction of pS2 protein [197]. The proliferative effect of 4-MBC was blocked by the estrogen antagonist ICI 182,780. The uterine weight of rats was dose-dependently increased by 4-MBC and OMC, but only weakly increased by BP-3. This increase occurred by the dermal application route but not by the oral route [197, 198].

The estrogenicity of several UV filters was measured by estrogen-regulated pS2 gene transcription in MCF-7 human breast cancer cells [195]. An equipotent mixture of BP-3 and its metabolite BP-1, as well as a mixture of BP-3, BP-1, OMC, and 4-MBC, acted additively to activate the estrogen receptor; thus, the daily exposure to sunscreens may have estrogenic effects in humans [195, 199].

The sunscreens BP-3, OMC, and 4-MBC were studied in 32 healthy volunteers after daily whole-body applications of 2 mg/cm^2 of basic cream formulations, alternating week 1 without and week 2 with, the three sunscreens at 10% wt/wt of each [200]. Reproductive hormones FSH and LH were unchanged, and there were only minor differences in testosterone levels between the two weeks. Minor differences in serum estradiol and inhibin B levels were observed only in men. The conclusion was that the differences in hormone levels were not related to sunscreen exposure [200].

4-MBC was shown to induce ER-α and ER-β activity in primary rat and human hepatocytes but only in very high doses [201]. No estrogenic metabolites of 4-MBC were formed in the primary rat and human hepatocytes [201]. The two camphor sunscreens, 4-MBC and 3-benzylidene-camphor (3-BC), administered orally by gavage, were found to stimulate MCF-7 cell proliferation and to displace 16α I^{125}-estradiol from porcine uterine cytosolic receptors and from recombinant hER-β but not from hER-α [202]. This estrogen receptor subtype selectivity might be due to the formation of active metabolites with different receptor binding characteristics in vivo [202]. The camphor UV filters, 4-MBC and 3-BC, in the yeast estrogen screen test, activated hER-α [203]. Exposure of two aquatic invertebrates, *P. antipodarum* and *L. variegatus*, to these UV filters caused an increase of embryo production and mortality at high concentrations. The reproduction of both organisms was decreased by both compounds [203].

In studies of the developmental toxicities of sunscreens, a number of UV filters were found to have estrogenic and antiandrogenic activities [199]. The UV filters BP-1, 2,2',4,4'-tetrahydroxybenzophenone (BP-2), BP-3, 3-BC, 4-MBC, and OMC, administered with food, caused an increase of the uterine weight in rats [199, 204]. 3-BC and 4-MBC displaced 16-α I^{125}-estradiol from human ER-β, but not from human ER-α. The weight gain of pregnant rats was reduced by 3-BC. 4-MBC and 3-BC reduced the early postnatal survival rate and thymus weight, delayed male puberty, and dose-dependently affected reproductive organ weights of adult male and female F1 offsprings [199, 204]. Tissue-specific changes in mRNA levels of estrogen-regulated genes in prostate, uterus, and brain regions were observed in vitro [199, 204].

The interaction of several polycyclic musks and UV filters with estrogen receptor (ER), androgen receptor (AR), and progesterone receptor (PR) in reporter gene bioassays showed estrogenic effects, i.e., the musks

AHTN, HHCB, AETT, and AHMI were antagonists to ER-β, AR, and PR [205]. The filters BP-3, 3-BC, HMS, and 4-MBC were antagonists toward AR and PR. The ER-α agonist OD-PABA had no activity toward AR and PR. OMC was found to be a weak ER-α agonist but a potent PR antagonist [205]. The compound, 4-*tert*-butyl-4'-methoxydibenzoylmethane, was a weak ER-α agonist and a weak AR antagonist. Most of the effects were observed at relatively high concentrations, i.e., above 1 μM, and the anti-progestagenic effects of the musks were detected at concentrations as low as 0.01 M [205].

A number of UV filters tested positive in vitro when using reporter gene assays [206], i.e., all compounds induced estrogenic activity toward ER-α and some induced transcriptional activity of ER-β. An in vivo test, using transgenic zebra fish containing an estrogen responsive luciferase reporter gene, revealed no estrogenic activity of the UV filters. One must be mindful of predicting in vivo effects based on weak in vitro data [206].

OMC and 4-MBC were compared with 17β-estradiol (E2) for estrogenic activities [207, 208]. Both compounds had weak estrogenic effects in the uterus and in the vagina but not in the bone, where 4-MBC had antiosteoporotic effects by a different mechanism than E2 [207]. OMC and 4-MBC had different effects from E2 on several metabolic parameters, including decreased serum triglycerides, cholesterol, LDL, and HDL, increased serum LH levels, and decreased serum TH levels, leading to increased TSH levels [208]. These effects might be attributable to other than estrogen-receptive mechanisms [208].

The estrogenic effects of OMC on multiple organs of ovariectomized rats were found to exceed the threshold values recommended for use of OMC in formulations for skin protection [209]. Since nonestrogenic effects of OMC were found, it appears that there is a need for multiple-organ risk assessment of potential endocrine-active chemicals [209].

Ovariectomized rats were treated with OMC for five days, with 17-β-estradiol (E2) as a control [210]. While E2 had no effect on thyroid hormone TSH-, T4-, and T3- levels, OMC caused a dose-dependent decrease of serum concentrations of these hormones, while the TRH expression remained unaffected. In the thyroid, the TSH receptor expression, but not the sodium-iodide-symporter (NIS), was stimulated by OMC [210]. The activity of T3-responsive 5'-deiodinase (Dio 1) in the liver, but not the thyroid peroxidase (TPO) activity, was reduced by administration of OMC [210]. It was concluded that OMC causes a nonestrogenic interference within the rodent axis hypothalamo-pituitary-thyroid (HPT) with inadequate response to impaired thyroid hormone status, as indicated by decreased serum thyroid hormone and hepatic Dio l levels [210].

OMC was found to decrease the release of the luteinizing hormone-releasing hormone (LH-RH) significantly in male and female rats of both ages, to increase the release of γ-aminobutyric acid (GABA) in male rats and in female rats, and to diminish the excitatory amino acids aspartate (ASP) and glutamate (GLU) without a change in the hypothalamic GABA release [211]. Thus, during sexual maturation, the inhibitory effect of OMC on LH-RH release is related to its action on the inhibitory and excitatory amino acid neurotransmitters in male and female rats [211].

The effect of BP-2 and OMC on the immune system of mice splenocytes was studied in vitro [212]. These UV filters, at a high concentration of 10^{-5} M, shifted the Th1/Th2 balance toward a Th2 response, i.e., lower IFN-γ and higher IL-10, comparable to those of E2. Therefore, these UV filters at high doses may possess immunomodulatory effects, some of which resemble those of E2 [212].

Recombinant yeast systems, carrying either human estrogen receptor (hER-α) or human androgen receptor (hAR), were used to test for estrogenicity of 18 UV filters and one metabolite [213–215]. All compounds had hormonal activities and ten filters had agonistic effects towards hER-α. Six UV filters had androgenic activities, and many of them had pronounced antiestrogenic and antiandrogenic activities [213]. Seventeen compounds inhibited 4,5-dihydrotestosterone activity in the hAR assay, while 14 compounds inhibited estradiol activity in the hER-α assay [213]. The anti-androgenic activities of phenyl and benzyl salicylate, BP-1, BP-2, and 4-OH-BP were higher than that of flutamide, a known hAR antagonist [213].

Recombinant yeast systems containing the rainbow trout (rtER-α) and human (hER-α) estrogen receptors were used to show the estrogenicity of ethyl 4-aminobenzoate (Et-PABA) [21] as well as BP-1, BP-2, 4,4'-dihydroxybenzophenone (4,4'-$(OH)_2$–BP), 4-hydroxybenzophenone (4-OH-BP), 2,4,4'-trihydroxy-benzophenone (2,4,4'-$(OH)_3$-BP), and phenyl salicylate [216]. The activity of 17β-estradiol was lower in the rtER-α than in the hER assay, whereas the activities of the UV filters were either similar or higher in the rtER assay, indicating different binding activities of both estrogen receptors [216]. In vitro receptor-based assays of UV filters are important also for in vivo assays [216].

The UV filters 4-MBC, OMC, and the excipient *n*-propylparaben have estrogenic activity in fish as determined by increased production of vitellogenin and choriogenin, known estrogen response gene products [217]. In vivo estrogenicity activity was tested by the induction of vitellogenin in juvenile fathead minnows after 14 days of exposure [213, 224, 218]. The compounds Et-PABA [213], 3-BC, BP-1, and BP-2 [216, 218] were estrogenic by this test. BP-1 increased rat uterine weight relative to the standard ethynyl estradiol (EE) [219].

The compounds 4-MBC, ethyl 2-cyano-3,3-diphenylacrylate (etocrylene), 2-ethylhexyl-2-cyano-3,3-diphenyl acrylate (octocrylene), benzyhydrol, ethyl cinnamate, 2,2'-dihydroxy-4-methoxybenzophenone (2,2'-$(OH)_2$-4-OMe-BP) were weakly active in the MCF-7 cell proliferation assay [220]. The UV filters Tinosorb® M (Bisoctrizole) and Tinosorb® S (Bemotrizinole) were reported to have no binding to estrogen or androgen receptors and to have no activity in the immature rat uterotrophic assay [221].

Many estrogenic studies have been devoted to benzophenone (BP) and its analogs. Thus, irradiation of an aqueous solution of BP with UV or sunlight produced two estrogenic products: 3-hydroxybenzophenone (3-OH-BP) and 4-hydroxybenzophenone (4-OH-BP) [222]. The photochemically generated hydrogen peroxide and hydroxyl radical are involved in the hydroxylation of BP. The addition of hydrogen peroxide to the BP solution increased the production of 3-OH-BP and 4-OH-BP under UV irradiation [222]. BP hydroxylation with the Fenton reagent generates the hydroxyl radical without UV irradiation. Compound 4-OH-BP had more potency than 3-OH-BP in promoting ER-modulated transcription and uterotropic activity, although both had some ER-binding activity [222].

BP is enzymatically converted into benzyhydrol, 4-OH-BP, and its sulfate conjugate in rat hepatocytes [223]. Even if there is less free 4-OH-BP than benzhydrol and the sulfate conjugate in hepatocyte suspensions, 4-OH-BP acts as a weak xenoestrogen on MCF-7 human breast cancer cells [223]. BP and many of its hydroxylated derivatives were compared for their estrogenic and antiandrogenic activities [220, 224], resulting in the following order of decreasing estrogenic activity in MCF-7 human breast cancer cell lines: 2,4,4'-$(OH)_3$-BP > 2,3',4,4'-$(OH)_4$-BP > 4,4'-$(OH)_2$-BP > BP-2 > BP-1 [32], while BP had little activity. BP and some of its derivatives have significant antiandrogenic activity against the dihydrotestosterone in the rat fibroblast cell line NIH 3T3: 2,4,4'-$(OH)_3$-BP > 2,3',4,4'-$(OH)_4$-BP > BP-2 > 3-OH-BP > BP-1, while 2,3,4,4'-$(OH)_4$-BP and 2,3,4-$(OH)_3$-BP had little activity [224]. In the uterotropic assay using ovariectomized rats, positive responses were obtained with the compounds 2,4,4'-$(OH)_3$-BP and BP [224]. In the Hershberger assay using castrated rats, a positive response was obtained with the compound 2,4,4'-$(OH)_3$-BP. The conclusion from this research was that the 4-OH group on the phenyl ring of BP derivatives is essential for high hormonal activities, and the presence of other OH groups markedly alters these activities [224].

The gene expression of marker genes after oral applications of BP-2 in adult ovariectomized rats over five days revealed a dose-dependent estradiol (E2) activity, resulting in an increased weight of the uterus, an increased IGF 1 expression in the vagina, a reduced LH synthesis in the pituitary, an increased IGF 1 expression in the liver, and a reduced level of cholesterol, HDL, and LDL in the lipoproteins [225]. A non-E2-like action of BP-2 was observed for the thyroid hormone T4 and T3 levels that were significantly reduced. Nevertheless, BP-2 clearly exerts E2 agonistic actions [225]. The effect on the thyroid hormone levels could be attributed to an inhibition of the thyroid peroxidase enzyme (TPO) [225]. The effects of BP-2 on the serum, pituitary, and uterus of ovariectomized rats were comparable to changes in the E2 controls [226].

Although BP-2 is rapidly metabolized in rats to its glucuronide and sulfate conjugates, the amount of unconjugated BP-2 is sufficiently high to induce a dose-dependent estrogenic effect in the uterotropic assay [227]. BP-2 was shown to inhibit the human recombinant thyroid peroxidase (hrTPO) [228]. Thus, the total serum T4 was significantly decreased and serum thyrotropin was significantly increased. The TPO enzyme activation in the thyroids of treated animals was unchanged, and the effects were more pronounced in the absence of iodide [228].

In rat hepatocytes, 2-hydroxy-4-methoxybenzophenone (BP-3) is converted into 2,4-dihydroxybenzophenone (BP-1) and a hydroxylated intermediate 2,2'-dihydroxy-4-methoxybenzophenone (2,2'-$(OH)_2$-4-OMe-BP) [229]. These compounds are rapidly conjugated as their glucuronides. The compounds BP-1 and 2,3,4-$(OH)_3$-BP displaced 17β-estradiol bound to the recombinant hER-α, and BP-1 caused a concentration-dependent proliferation of MCF-7 human breast cancer cells [229]. 2,2'-$(OH)_2$-4-OMe-BP and 2,3,4-$(OH)_3$-BP caused a slight increase in cancer cell numbers, whereas BP-3 was inactive [229]. Based on the relative inhibitory constant (IC_{50}) for the competitive binding and the proliferative effect on MCF-7 cells, the order of estrogenic potency is: BP-1 > 2,3,4-$(OH)_3$-BP > 2,2'-$(OH)_2$-4-OMe-BP; hence, it was concluded that the hydroxylated intermediates rather than the parent compound, BP-3, function as xenoestrogens via biotransformation [229].

The possibilities of estrogenic activity of the excipients parabens and fragrances, e.g., musks, used in sunscreen preparations were investigated. The binding capacity to the ER of 37 components of sunscreen lotions was determined by the use of two in vitro assays, i.e., an ELISA-based ER competitive binding assay and a modified yeast two-hybrid estrogen assay, with and without addition of a rat liver preparation S9 mix [230]. Eleven of the compounds, mostly BP derivatives and parabens, were found to bind to the ER without addition of the S9 preparation. The compounds 4-octylphenyl salicylate and BP2 appeared to acquire estrogenic activity by metabolic activation [230]. Eight parabens were active without the addition of the liver SP mix. It was found that benzophenones with para-hydroxyl groups and parabens with branched and/or linear chains were generally more potent in both bioassays [230]. Weak antagonistic activity with S9 treatment was observed for 4-*tert*-butylphenyl salicylate, 2-ethylhexyl dimethyl PABA, and α-tocopherol acetate [230].

As mentioned previously, the interaction of several polycyclic musks and UV filters with estrogen receptor (ER), androgen receptor (AR), and progesterone receptor (PR) in reporter gene bioassays have estrogenic effects [206]. The antiprogestagenic effects of the musks were detected at low concentrations of 0.01 μM [206]. Fragrances had no activation of ER-β. Methylparaben, ethylparaben, the musks moskene, celestolide and cashmeran, and musk ketone and BP-3 were not considered estrogenic at 10^{-5} M [231]. The order of potency on ER-α against three reporter cell lines was as follows: butylparaben > *n*-propylparaben > homosalate = dimethyl-PABA = 4-MBC = OMC = ethylparaben = galaxolide [231].

The polycyclic musks have very weak estrogenic activity in vitro and no activity in vivo, when tested in rats and zebra fish [232]. However, these musks possess antiestrogenic (ER-β selective), antiandrogenic, and antiprogestagenic activities. Using human cell-based reporter gene assays, the musks had agonistic rather than antagonistic effects [232].

In conclusion, the various UV filters have shown some estrogenic activity in the in vitro screens, including activation of the human estrogen receptors alpha and beta. The in vivo screens relied mainly on rats and fish, and only in one reported case [201] were human volunteers used. In the latter case, only minor differences in reproductive hormone levels were observed, and these were not related to sunscreen exposure [201].

viii. Environmental Effects of Estrogenic Sunscreens and Metabolites

There is increasing concern about the presence of estrogenic sunscreens in the environment. (See **Section 2F.vii**.) These UV filters are added to many cosmetics, body lotions, and other personal care products resulting in increased exposure of humans to these materials. The sunscreen 2-hydroxy-4-methoxybenzophenone (BP-3) was detected in about 97% of the analyzed 2,517 human urine samples from United States residents [233].

After topical application of 3-benzylidene camphor (3-BC) to rats, this sunscreen was found in adipose tissue, brain, liver, muscle, plasma, and testis, and it was concluded that such absorption through the skin could occur in humans [234].

A study involving the topical application of BP-3 to 25 human volunteers, both with and without UV irradiation, revealed that a large amount of BP-3 was absorbed in the body since it was excreted in the urine three to five days after the last application [235]. Furthermore, there was no significant difference in absorption between the irradiated and unirradiated groups [235].

The estrogenic sunscreens 4-methylbenzylidene camphor (4-MBC) and 3-benzylidene camphor (3-BC) were tested for transdermal passage from mother to offspring through breast milk [236]. The results obtained during the years 2004 and 2005 showed that 79% of women reported use of these cosmetic UV filters and 76% of milk samples contained these filters. This result represents a significant correlation, and it was stated that it might be possible to reduce human exposure to these UV filters between pregnancy and lactation by abstaining from their use [236].

These sunscreens undergo metabolic transformations that add a further level of complexity to the picture [237, 238]. For example, the metabolism of BP-3 in rats led to three metabolites: 2,4-dihydroxybenzophenone (DHB), formed by O-demethylation of BP-3, 2,2'-dihydroxy-4-methoxybenzophenone (DHMB), formed by hydroxylation of BP-3, and 2,3,4-trihydroxybenzophenone (THB), formed by hydroxylation of DHB [237, 238]. Benzophenone in rats was metabolized to benzhydrol and 4-hydroxybenzophenone [238]. The concentration of the metabolites in the blood of rats over time was greater than that of the parent compounds, leading to the conclusion that the transformed products could have more adverse environmental effects over longer time periods [238].

Polycyclic musks are fragrances that are widely used in perfumes, cosmetics, and laundry detergents. The ubiquitous presence of these materials in the aquatic environment was demonstrated [239, 240]. The C-14 ring labeled musks, 7-acetyl-1,1,3,4,4,6-hexamethyl-1,2,3,4-tetrahydronaphthalene (AHTN) and 1,3,4,6,7,8-hexahydro-4,6,6,7,8,8-hexamethylcyclopenta-gamma-2-benzopyran (HHCB), were tested for their absorption through the skin in humans [241]. Over a five-day period, the levels of the two musks in blood and plasma were below levels of detection. The total absorbed amount of these musks was approximately 1 and 0.1%, respectively, based on excretion in urine. However, during that period, 14.5% of AHTN and 19.5% of HHCB were recovered from the skin over the sites of application, indicating that a reservoir of musks had formed in the skin but these materials were subsequently lost by various processes and not available for absorption. The amounts that evaporated from the skin were 24% and 22%, respectively [241].

In order to determine the trace amounts of sunscreens found in the environment, sensitive analytical methods and assays had to be developed [242–246]. Lipophilic sunscreens were analyzed by gas chromatography–electroionization mass spectrometry, and polar and mid-polar compounds by liquid chromatography–electrospray ionization mass spectrometry [243]. A chromatographic method was devised for estimating the amount of percutaneous absorption of the water-soluble UV filters, phenylbenzimidazole sulfonic acid, disodium phenyl dibenzimidazole tetrasulfonate, BP-4, and terephthalylidene dicamphor sulfonic acid (Mexoryl® SX) [244].

Enantioselective gas chromatography–mass spectrometry was used to determine the stereoisomer composition of 4-MBC in untreated and treated wastewater, lakes, rivers, and in fish from the lakes [245]. Three sunscreens, benzylidene camphor sulfonic acid (Mexoryl® SL), camphor benzalkonium methosulfate (Mexoryl® SO), and Mexoryl® SX, were exposed to UVA and/or UVB radiations, and were not photomutagenic by either a bacterial reverse mutation or a mammalian chromosome aberration assay [246].

The concentrations of the lipophilic sunscreens 2-ethylhexyl 4-methoxycinnamate (OMC), octocrylene, 4-MBC, 4-*tert*-butyl-4'-methoxydibenzoylmethane (BMDM), and BP-3 at bathing areas around Lake Zurich, a typical midland lake in Switzerland, and Lake Huttersee, a small bathing lake, were determined by gas chromatography–mass spectrometry [247]. The concentrations of the UV filters in the lakes were lower than predicted from input estimates based on the number of swimmers and the usage of sunscreens. This result could be explained by (1) overestimation of the inputs, e.g., wash-off of the UV filters assumed to occur during swimming, and (2) removal of compounds by degradation and/or sorption/sedimentation [247]. The UV filters in the lakes were also detected by semipermeable membrane devices (SPMDs), confirming that sunscreens were present in surface waters and could bioaccumulate. However, no filters were found in a remote mountain lake [247, 248].

A number of studies have been conducted on the amount of UV filters found in wastewater. In untreated wastewater, the loads of UV filter levels were in the order OMC > 4-MBC = BP-3 > octocrylene (OC) [248]. In treated wastewater, the order of prevalence was 4-MBC > BP-3, OMC, and OC [248]. Fish from these Swiss lakes contained only low concentrations of these UV filters. The fact that the concentrations of 4-MBC, relative to methyl triclosan, a chemical marker for lipophilic contamination from wastewater treatment plants (WWTPs), were lower in fish than in SPMDs exposed in the same lakes, could be explained if it is assumed that 4-MBC is either less bioaccumulated or is metabolized in fish [248].

A higher concentration of several UV filters in Swiss rivers than in lakes was traced to the discharge from WWTPs into the rivers [249]. The fact that the compound OC was mostly absent from lake fish, and found in higher concentration in river fish than 4-MBC, was interpreted to suggest that there is a difference in the bioaccumulation of these two UV filters [249].

The removal of UV filters by separate units of a WWTP differed according to the method used [250]. Thus, the ozonation treatment removed the most filters (16–28%), followed by coagulation–flocculation (8–21%), and continuous microfiltration (4–8%). The total removal efficiencies in the plants varied from 28% to 43%, indicating that there is considerable carryover of these materials into the environment [250].

The amounts of the UV filters 4-MBC, OMC, OC, and octyltriazone (OT) in sewage sludge were determined [251]. These materials originated mainly from private households, but other environmental sources, such as industries and surface runoffs, must be considered [251]. The removal efficiency of the sunscreen preservatives butylparaben and benzylparaben by WWTPs and their acute/chronic toxicities in fish and algae were investigated in further studies [252].

In a short-term study, the sunscreen filter 4-MBC, at environmental concentrations, caused lower stress protein (Hsp70) levels in adult amphipod crustaceans; however, long-term exposures and the presence of juvenile crustaceans could result in toxic effects [253].

The photochemistry of the UV filters 2-ethylhexyl salicylate (ES), 2-ethylhexyl 4-(dimethylamino)benzoate (EH-PABA), and BP-3 in different aquatic conditions was described [254, 255]. The photochemical reaction rates were pseudo-first-order for the following concentrations of filters: distilled water as reference > swimming pool water > seawater, based mainly on the amount of dissolved organic matter. The isolated products were determined by gas chromatography–mass spectrometry, and were derived mainly through dealkylation and hydroxylation reactions of the filters [254]. In addition, the swimming pool water contained chlorinated products [254, 255]. Thus, in the case of BP-3, mono- and di-halogenated aromatic derivatives, as well as halogenated forms of 3-methoxyphenol, were isolated [255].

The photoreaction of methylparaben with sunlight produced two products, *para*-hydroxybenzoic acid (PHBA) and 3-hydroxymethylparaben (MP-3OH) [256]. A simulated MP metabolism using dermal tissue produced these two photoproducts and a metabolite, proto-catechuic acid, that was formed by the action of the skin esterase on MP-3OH. This metabolite caused damage to the DNA as determined by an in vitro damage assay [256]. The metabolite, in the presence of cellular divalent copper ion and the reductant NADH, could generate active oxygen species that, in turn, could damage cellular DNA and lead to carcinogenesis [256].

Sunscreens and ingredients of commercial sunscreen products have been implicated in the process of coral bleaching [257]. These materials, especially those containing parabens, cinnamates, benzophenones, and camphor derivates, can cause the bleaching of corals. The treatment of hard corals with sunscreen solutions causes the release of viruses from the corals to the surrounding sea water. The subsequent coral bleaching is caused by the sunscreen's induction of the lytic viral cycle in symbiotic zooxanthelliae with latent infections [257]. This process has great significance for the tropical areas of the world, as it is estimated that up to 10% of the world reefs are potentially threatened by sunscreen-induced coral bleaching [257].

A number of very lipophilic benzotriazole UV filters were found distributed throughout the marine food chain in the Arike Sea in western Japan [258]. These compounds accumulate in oysters, tidal flat species, marine mammals, and seabirds. In addition, high concentrations of these sunscreens were found in mussels collected from Korea, Hong Kong, and Japan [258]. The synthetic musks HHCB and AHTN have been found in many marine organisms collected from Japanese coastal waters as well as in seals and dolphins in US waters [259].

A review of the physicochemical properties, mechanisms of photodegradation, metabolites, quantitative analysis, and environmental levels of UV filters has been published [260].

References

1. Vainio H. and Bianchini F. (eds.) (2001) Sunscreens. In: *IARC Handbooks of Cancer Prevention*, Vol. 5, International Agency for Research on Cancer, WHO, Lyon.
2. Halliday G. M. and Rana S. (2007) The effects of solar radiation on the immune response. In: *Biophysical and Physiological Effects of Solar Radiation on Human Skin*, pp 127–163, Giacomoni P. U. (ed.), RSC Publishing, Cambridge.
3. Halliday G. M. and Honigsmann H. (2009) Sunscreens, photoimmunosuppression, and photoaging. In: *Clinical guide to sunscreens*

and photoprotection, pp 101–116, Lim H. W. and Draelos Z. D. (eds.), Informa Healthcare, New York.
4. Norval M. (2001) Effects of solar radiation on the human immune system. In: *Sun Protection in Man*, pp 91–115, Giacomoni P. U. (ed.), Elsevier, Amsterdam.
5. De Gruijl F. R. and Van Kranen H. J. (2001) UV radiation, mutations and oncogenic pathways in skin cancer. In: *Sun Protection in Man*, pp 287–302, Giacomoni P. U. (ed.), Elsevier, Amsterdam.
6. Hanneman K. K., Cooper K. D. and Baron E. D. (2006) Ultraviolet immunosuppression: mechanisms and conseqences. *Dermatol. Clin.* **24**: 19–25.
7. Tornaletti S. and Pfeifer G. P. (1994) Slow repair of pyrimidine dimers at p53 mutation hotspots in skin cancer. *Science* **263**: 1436–1438.
8. Peak M. J., Peak J. G. and Carnes B. A. (1987) Induction of direct and indirect single-strand mechanisms. *Photochem. Photobiol.* **45**: 381–3871.
9. Applegate L. A., Ley R. D., Alcalay J. and Kripke M. L. (1989) Identification of the molecular target for the suppression of contact hypersensitivity by UVR. *J. Exp. Med.* **170**: 1117–1131.
10. Kripke M. L., Cox P. A., Alas L. G. and Yarosh D. B. (1992) Pyrimidine dimers in DNA initiate systemic immunosuppression in UV-irradiated mice. *Proc. Natl. Acad. Sci. U. S. A.* **89**: 7516–7520.
11. Vink A. A., Yarosh D. B. and Kripke M. L. (1996) Chromophore for UV-induced immunosuppression: DNA. *Photochem. Photobiol.* **63**: 383–386.
12. Vinck A. A., Moodycliffe A. M., Shreedhar V., Ullrich S. E., Roza L., Yarosh D. B. and Kripke M. L. (1997) The inhibition of antigen-presenting activity of dendritic cells resulting from UV irradiation of murine skin is restored by in vitro photorepair of cyclobutane pyrimidine dimers. *Proc. Natl. Acad. Sci. U. S. A.* **94**: 5255–5260.
13. Stege H., Roza L., Vink A. A., Grewe M., Ruzicka T., Grether-Beck S. and Krutmann J. (2000) Enzyme plus light therapy to repair DNA damage in ultraviolet-B-irradiated human skin. *Proc. Natl. Acad. Sci. U. S. A.* **97**: 1790–1795.
14. Mees A., Klar T., Gnau P., Hennecke U., Eker A. P., Carell T. and Essen L. O. (2004) Crystal structure of a photolyase bound to a CPD-like DNA lesion after in situ repair. *Science* **306**: 1789–1793.
15. Wolf P., Yarosh D. B. and Kripke M. L. (1993) Effects of sunscreens and a DNA excision repair enzyme on ultraviolet radiation-induced

inflammation, immune suppression, and cyclobutane pyrimidine dimer formation in mice. *J. Invest. Dermatol.* **101**: 523–527.
16. Freeman S. E., Ley R. D. and Ley K. D. (1988) Sunscreen protection against UV-induced pyrimidine dimers in DNA of human skin in situ. *Photodermatol.* **5**: 243–247.
17. Van Praag M. C. G., Roza L., Boom B. W., Out-Luijting C., Bergen Henegouwen J. B. A., Vermeer B. J. and Mommaas A. M. (1993) Determination of the photoprotective efficacy of a topical sunscreen against UVB-induced DNA damage in human epidermis. *J. Photochem. Photobiol.* **19**: 129–134.
18. Bykov V. J., Marcusson J. A. and Hemminki K. (1998) Ultraviolet B-induced DNA damage in human skin and its modulation by a sunscreen. *Cancer Res.* **58**: 2961–2964.
19. Young A. R., Sheehan J. M., Chadwick C. A. and Potten C. S. (2000) Protection by UVA and UVB sunscreens against in situ dipyrimidine photolesions in human epidermis is comparable to protection against sunburn. *J. Invest. Dermatol.* **115**: 37–41.
20. Walter J. F. (1981) Evaluation of seven sunscreens on hairless mouse skin. *Arch. Dermatol.* **117**: 547–550.
21. Walker J. F. and DeQuoy P. R. (1980) The hairless mouse as a model for evaluating sunscreens. Prevention of ultraviolet B inhibition of epidermal DNA synthesis. *Arch. Dermatol.* **116**: 419–421.
22. Ley R. D. and Fourtanier A. (1997) Sunscreen protection against ultraviolet radiation-induced pyrimidine dimers in mouse epidermal DNA. *Photochem. Photobiol.* **65**: 1007–1011.
23. Suzuki M. (1987) Protective effect of fine particle titanium dioxide on UVB-induced DNA damage in hairless mouse skin. *Photodermatol.* **4**: 209–211.
24. McVean M. and Liebler D. C. (1997) Inhibition of UVB induced DNA photodamage in mouse epidermis by topically applied α-tocopherol. *Carcinogenesis* **18**: 1617–1622.
25. McVean M. and Liebler D. C. (1999) Prevention of DNA photodamage by vitamin E compounds and sunscreens: roles of ultraviolet absorbance and cellular uptake. *Mol. Carcinog.* **24**: 169–176.
26. De Fabo E. C. and Noonan F. P. (1983) Mechanism of immune suppression by ultraviolet irradiation in vivo. 1. Evidence for the existence of a unique photoreceptor in skin and its role in photoimmunology. *J. Exp. Med.* **157**: 84–98.
27. Noonan F. P. and De Fabo E. C. (1992) Immunosuppression by ultraviolet B radiation: initiation by urocanic acid. *Immunol. Today* **13**: 250–254.

28. Reeve V. E., Boehm-Wilcox C., Bosnic M. and Reilly W. G. (1994) Differential photoimmunoprotection by sunscreen ingredients is unrelated to epidermal *cis*-urocanic acid formation in hairless mice. *J. Invest. Dermatol.* **103**: 801–806.
29. Gibbs N. K., Norval M., Traynor N. J., Wolf M., Johnson B. E. and Crosby J. (1993) Action spectra for the trans to cis photoisomerisation of urocanic acid in vitro and in mouse skin. *Photochem. Photobiol.* **57**: 584–590.
30. Duthie M. S., Kimber I. and Norval M. (1999) The effects of ultraviolet radiation on the human immune system. *Br. J. Dermatol.* **140**: 995–1009.
31. Reeve V. E. (1997) The relationship between sunscreen protection from erythema, photoimmunosuppression and photocarcinogenesis in the hairless mouse. In: *Sunscreen photobiology: molecular, cellular and physiological aspects*, pp 157–176, Gasparro F. P. (ed.), Springer-Verlag/Landes Bioscience, Berlin.
32. Norval M. and El-Ghorr A. A. (2002) Studies to determine the immuno-modulating effects of cis-urocanic acid. *Methods* **28**: 63–70.
33. Rigas B. and Sun Y. (2008) Induction of oxidative stress as a mechanism of action of chemopreventive agents against cancer. *Br. J. Cancer* **98**: 1157–1160.
34. Hemelarr P. J. and Beijersbergen van Henegouwen G. M. (1996) The protective effect of *N*-acetylcysteine on UVB-induced immunosuppression by inhibition of the action of *cis*-urocanic acid. *J. Photochem. Photobiol.* **63**: 322–327.
35 Van den Broeke L. T. and Beijersbergen van Henegouwen G. M. (1995) Topically applied *N*-acetylcysteine as a protector against UVB-induced systemic immunosuppression. *J. Photochem. Photobiol. B.* **27**: 61–65.
36. Trautinger F. (2001) Mechanisms of photodamage of the skin and its functional consequences for skin ageing. *Clin. Exp. Dermatol.* **26**: 573–577.
37. Hanson K. M. and Simon J. D. (1998) Epidermal *trans*-urocanic acid and the UV-A-induced photoaging of the skin. *Proc. Natl. Acad. Sci. U. S. A.* **95**: 10576–10578.
38. Kuchel M., Barnetson R. S. and Halliday G. M. (2003) Nitric oxide appears to be a mediator of solar-stimulated ultraviolet radiation-induced immunosuppression in humans. *J. Invest. Dermatol.* **121**: 587–593.
39. Yuen K. S., Nearn M. R. and Halliday G. M. (2002) Nitric oxide-mediated depletion of Langerhans cells from the epidermis may be

involved in UV radiation-induced immunosuppression. *Nitric Oxide* **6**: 313–318.

40. Halliday G. M., Russo P. A., Yuen K. S. and Robertson B. O. (1999) Effect of inhibitors of oxygen radical and nitric oxide formation on UV radiation-induced erythema, immunosuppression and carcinogenesis. *Redox Rep.* **4**: 316–318.
41. Halliday G. M., Byrne S. N., Kuchel J. M., Poon T. S. and Barnetson R. S. (2004) The suppression of immunity by ultraviolet radiation: UVA, nitric oxide and DNA damage. *Photochem. Photobiol. Sci.* **3**: 736–740.
42. Moison R. M., Steenvoorden D. P. and Beijersbergen van Henegouwen G. M. (2001) Topically applied eicosapentaenoic acid protects against local immunosuppression induced by UVB irradiation, *cis*-urocanic acid and thymidine dinucleotides. *Photochem. Photobiol.* **73**: 64–70.
43. Steenvoorden D. P. and Beijersbergen van Henegouwen G. (1999) Protection against UV-induced systemic immunosuppression in mice by a single topical application of the antioxidant vitamins C and E. *Int. J. Radiat. Biol.* **75**: 747–755.
44. Russo P. A. and Halliday G. M. (2006) Inhibition of nitric oxide and reactive oxygen species production improves the ability of a sunscreen to protect from sunburn, immunosuppression and photocarcinogenesis. *Br. J. Dermatol.* **155**: 408–415.
45. Walterscheid I. P., Ullrich S. E. and Nghiem D. X. (2002) Platelet-activating factor: a molecular sensor for cellular damage, activates systemic immune suppression. *J. Exp Med.* **195**: 171–179.
46. Shreedhar V., Giese T., Sung V. W. and Ullrich S. E. (1998) A cytokine cascade including prostaglandin E-2, IL-4 and IL-10 is responsible for UV-induced systemic immune suppression. *J. Immunol.* **160**: 3783–3789.
47. Ullrich S. E. (2002) Photoimmune suppression and photocarcinogenesis. *Front. Biosci.* **7**: D684–D703.
48. Niizeki H., Allard P. and Streilein J. W. (1997) Calcitonin gene-related peptide is necessary for ultraviolet B-impaired induction of contact hypersensitivity. *J. Immunol.* **159**: 5183–5186.
49. Misery L. (2000) The neuro-immuno-cutaneous system and ultraviolet radiation. *Photodermatol. Photoimmunol. Photomed.* **16**: 78–81.
50. Bergstresser P. R., Toews G. B. and Streilein J. W. (1980) Natural and perturbed distribution of Langerhans cells: responses to ultraviolet light, heterotopic skin grafting and dinitrofluorobenzene sensitization. *J. Invet. Dermatol.* **75**: 73–77.

51. Moodycliffe A. M., Kimber I. and Norval M. (1992) The effects of ultraviolet B irradiation and urocanic acid isomers on dendritic cell migration. *Immunology* **77**: 394–399.
52. Vink A. A., Moodycliffe A. M., Shreedhar V., Ullrich S. E., Roza L., Yarosh D. B. and Kripke M. L. (1997) The inhibition of antigen-presenting activity of dendritic cells resulting from irradiation of murine skin is restored by in vitro photorepair of cyclobutane pyrimidine dimers. *Proc. Natl. Acad. Sci. U. S. A.* **94**: 5255–5260.
53. Strickland F. M. (2001) Immune regulation by polysaccharides: implications for skin cancer. *J. Photochem. Photobiol., B* **63**: 132–140.
54. Toews G. B., Bergstresser P. R. and Streilein J. W. (1980) Epidermal Langerhans cell density determines whether contact hypersensitivity or unresponsiveness follows skin painting with DNFB. *J. Immunol.* **124**: 445–453.
55. Simon J. C., Tigelaar R. E., Bergstresser P. R., Edelbaum P. and Cruz P. D. (1991) Ultraviolet B radiation converts Langerhans cells from immunogenic to tolererogenic antigen-presenting cells. *J. Immunol.* **146**: 485–491.
56. Elmets C. A., Bergstresser P. R., Tigelaar R. E., Wood P. J. and Streilein J. W. (1983) Analysis of the mechanism of unresponsiveness produced by haptens painted on skin exposed to low dose ultraviolet radiation. *J. Exp. Med.* **158**: 781–794.
57. Schwarz T. (2005) Regulatory T cells induced by ultraviolet radiation. *Int. Arch. Allergy Immunol.* **137**: 187–193.
58. Byrne S. N. and Halliday G. M. (2005) B cells activated in lymph nodes in response to ultraviolet irradiation or by interleukin-10 inhibit dendritic cell induction of immunity. *J. Invest. Dermatol.* **124**: 570–578.
59. Moodcliffe A. M., Nghiem D., Clydesdale G. and Ullrich S. E. (2000) Immune suppression and skin cancer development: regulation by NKT cells. *Nature Immunol.* **1**: 521–525.
60. Yoshikawa T., Rae V., Bruins-Slot W., Van den Berg J. W., Taylor J. R. and Streilein J. W. (1990) Susceptibility to effects of UVB radiation on induction of contact hypersensitivity as a risk factor for skin cancer in humans. *J. Invest. Dermatol.* **95**: 530–536.
61. Kripke M. L. (1974) Antigenicity of murine skin tumors induced by ultraviolet light. *J. Natl. Cancer Inst.* **53**: 1333–1336.
62. Fisher M. S. and Kripke M. L. (1982) Suppressor T lymphocytes control the development of primary skin cancers in ultraviolet-irradiated mice. *Science* **216**: 1133–1134.

63. Noonan F. P., De Fabo E. C. and Kripke M. L. (1981) Suppression of contact hypersensitivity by ultraviolet radiation: an experimental model. *Springer Semin. Immunopathol.* **4**: 293–304.
64. Fisher M. S. and Kripke M. L. (1978) Further studies on the tumor specific suppressor cells induced by ultraviolet radiation. *J. Immunol.* **121**: 1139–1144.
65. Kripke M. L. (1981) Immunologic mechanisms in UV radiation carcinogenesis. *Adv. Cancer Res.* **34**: 69–106.
66. Noonan F. P., De Fabo E. C. and Kripke M. L. (1981) Suppression of contact hypersensitivity by ultraviolet radiation and its relationship to UV-induced suppression of tumor immunity. *Photochem. Photobiol.* **34**: 683–689.
67. Ullrich S. E. (1986) Suppression of the immune response to allogeneic histocompatibility antigens by a single exposure to ultraviolet radiation. *Transplantation* **42**: 287–291.
68. Hayag M. V., Chartier T., Devoursney J., Tie C., Machler B. and Taylor J. R. (1997) A high SPF sunscreen's effects on UVB-induced immunosuppression of DNCB contact hypersensitivity. *J. Dermatol. Sci.* **16**: 31–37.
69. Hersey P., MacDonald M., Burns C., Schibeci S., Matthews H. and Wilkinson F. J. (1987) Analysis of the effect of a sunscreen agent on the suppression of natural killer cell activity induced in human subjects by radiation from solarium lamp. *J. Invest. Dermatol.* **88**: 271–276.
70. Hersey P., Magrath H. and Wilkinson F. (1993) Development of an in vitro system for the analysis of ultraviolet radiation-induced suppression of natural killer cell activity. *Photochem. Photobiol.* **57**: 279–284.
71. Schwarz T. and Luger T. A. (1992) Pharmacology of cytokines in the skin. In: *Pharmacology of the skin*, pp 283–313, Mukhtar H. (ed.), CRC Press, Boca Raton.
72. Stratton S. P., Dorr R. T. and Alberts D. S. (2000) The state-of-the-art in chemoprevention of skin cancer. *Eur. J. Cancer* **36**: 1292–1297.
73. Schwarz T. and Luger T. A. (1989) New trends in photobiology (invited review). Effect of UV irradiation on epidermal cell cytokine production. *J. Photochem. Photobiol., B* **4**:1–13.
74. Clingen P. H., Berneburg M., Petit-Frere C., Woolons A., Lowe J. E., Arlett C. F. and Greene M. H. (2001) Contrasting effects of an ultraviolet B and an ultraviolet A tanning lamp on interleukin-6, tu-

mour necrosis factor-alpha and intercellular adhesion molecule-1 expression. *Br. J. Dermatol.* **145**: 54–62.
75. Ahrens C., Grewe M., Berneburg M., Grether-Beck S., Quillet X., Mezzina M., Sarazin A., Lehmann A. R., Arlett C. F. and Krutman J. (1997) Photocarcinogenesis and inhibition of intercellular adhesion molecule 1 expression in cells of DNA-repair-defective individuals. *Proc. Natl. Acad. Sci. U. S. A.* **94**: 6837–6841.
76. Kupper T. S., Chua A. O., Flood P., McGuire J. and Gubler U. (1987) Interleukin 1 gene expression in cultured human keratinocytes is augmented by ultraviolet radiation. *J. Clin. Invest.* **80**: 430–437.
77. Nozaki S., Abrams J. S., Pearce M. K. and Sauder D. N. (1991) Augmentation of granulocyte/macrophage colony-stimulating factor expression by ultraviolet irradiation is mediated by interleukin 1 in Pam 212 keratinocytes. *J. Invest. Dermatol.* **97**: 10–14.
78. Gallo R. L., Brounstein E. and Granstein R. D. (1989) Secretion of interleukin 3 activity from a transformed murine keratinocyte cell line after exposure to ultraviolet radiation: role of membrane signal transduction mechanisms. *J. Invest. Dermatol.* **92**: 432.
79. Kirnbauer R., Kock A., Krutmann J., Schwarz T., Urbanski A. and Luger T. A. (1989) Different effects of UVA and UVB irradiation on epidermal cell IL6 expression and release. *J. Invest. Dermatol.* **92**: 459.
80. Kirnbauer R., Kock A., Neuner P., Forster E., Krutmann J. and Urbanski A. (1991) Regulation of epidermal cell interleukin-6 production by UV light and corticosteroids. *J. Invest. Dermatol.* **96**: 484–489.
81. Wlaschek M., Bolsen K., Herrman G., Schwarz A., Wilmroth F., Henrich P. C., Goerz G. and Scharffetter-Kochanek K. (1993) UVA-induced autocrine stimulation of fibroblast-derived collagenase by IL-6: a possible mechanism in dermal photodamage. *J. Invest. Dermatol.* **101**: 164–168.
82. Oschholm A., Oschholm P., Staberg B. and Bendtzen K. (1988) Immunohistological detection of interleukin-1 like molecules and tumor necrosis factor in human epidermis before and after UVB irradiation in vivo. *Br. J. Dermatol.* **118**: 369–377.
83. Koch A., Urbanski A. and Luger T. A. (1989) mRNA expression and release of tumor necrosis factor by human epidermal cells. *J. Invest. Dermatol.* **92**: 462.
84. Ho, K. K., Halliday G. M. and Barnetson R. S. (1992) Sunscreens protect epidermal Langerhans cells and Thy-1$^+$ cells but not local

contact sensitization from the effects of ultraviolet light. *J. Invest. Dermatol.* **98**: 720–724.

85. Walker S. L., Morris J., Chu A. C. and Young A. R. (1994) Relationship between the ability of sunscreens containing 2-ethylhexyl-4'-methoxycinnamate to protect against UVR-induced inflammation, depletion of epidermal Langerhans (Ia^+) cells and suppression of alloactivating capacity of murine skin in vivo. *J. Photochem. Photobiol., B* **22**: 29–36.
86. Beasley D. G., Montgomery M. A., Moloney S. J., Edmonds S. and Roberts L. K. (1998) Commercial sunscreen lotions prevent ultraviolet radiation-induced depletion of epidermal Langerhans cells in Skh-1 and C3H mice. *Photodermatol. Photoimmunol. Photomed.* **14**: 90–99.
87. Hochberg M. and Enk C. D. (1999) Partial protection against epidermal IL-10 transcription and Langerhans cell depletion by sunscreens after exposure of human skin to UVB. *Photochem. Photobiol.* **70**: 766–772.
88. Damian D. L., Halliday G. M. and Barnetson R. S. (1997) Broad-spectrum sunscreens provide greater protection against ultraviolet-radiation-induced suppression of contact hypersensitivity to a recall antigen in humans. *J. Invest. Dermatol.* **109**: 146–151.
89. Fisher M. S., Menter J. M. and Willis I. (1989) Ultraviolet radiation-induced suppression of contact hypersensitivity in relation to Padimate O and oxybenzone. *J. Invest. Dermatol.* **92**: 337–341.
90. Ho K. K., Halliday G. M. and Barnetson R. S. (1992) Sunscreen protect epidermal Langerhans cells and Thy-1^+ cells but not local contact sensitization from the effects of ultraviolet light. *J. Invest. Dermatol.* **98**: 720–724.
91. Bestak R., Barnetson R. S., Nearn M. R. and Halliday G. M. (1995) Sunscreen protection of contact hypersensitivity responses from chronic solar-simulated ultraviolet irradiation correlates with the absorption spectrum of the sunscreen. *J. Invest. Dermatol.* **105**: 345–351.
92. Reeve V. E., Bosnic M., Boehm-Wilcox C. and Ley R. D. (1991) Differential protection by two sunscreens from UV radiation-induced immunosuppression. *J. Invest. Dermatol.* **97**: 624–628.
93. Wolf P., Donawho C. K. and Kripke M. L. (1993) Analysis of the protective effects of different sunscreens on ultraviolet radiation-induced local and systemic suppression of contact hypersensitivity and inflammatory responses in mice. *J. Invest. Dermatol.* **100**: 254–259.

94. Wolf P., Hoffmann C., Quehenberger F., Grinschgl S. and Kerl H. (2003) Immune protection factors of chemical sunscreens measured in the local contact hypersensitivity model in humans. *J. Invest. Dermatol.* **121**: 1080–1087.
95. Cooper K. D., Baron E. D., LeVee G. and Stevens S. R. (2002) Protection against UV-induced suppression of contact hypersensitivity responses by sunscreens in humans. *Exp. Dermatol.* **11**: 20–27.
96. Morison W. L. and Kelley S. P. (1985) Sunlight suppressing rejection of 280 to 320-nm UV-radiation induced skin tumors in mice. *JNCI, J. Natl. Cancer Inst.* **74**: 525–527.
97. Roberts L. K. and Beasley D. G. (1995) Commercial sunscreen lotions prevent ultraviolet-radiation induced immune suppression of contact hypersensitivity. *J. Invest. Dermatol.* **105**: 339–344.
98. Roberts L. K. and Beasley D. G. (1997) Sunscreen lotions prevent ultraviolet radiation-induced suppression of antitumor immune responses. *Int. J. Cancer* **71**: 94–102.
99. Walker S. L. and Young A. R. (1997) Sunscreens offer the same UVB protection factors for inflammation and immunosuppression in the mouse. *J. Invest. Dermatol.* **108**: 133–138.
100. Moyal C., Coubiere C., Le Corre Y., de Lacharriere O. and Hourseau C. (1997) Immunosuppression induced by chronic solar-simulated irradiation in humans and its prevention by sunscreens. *Eur. J. Dermatol.* **7**: 223–225.
101. Moyal C. (1998) Immunosuppression induced by chronic ultraviolet irradiation in humans and its prevention by sunscreens. *Eur. J. Dermatol.* **8**: 209–211.
102. Moyal D. D. and Fourtanier A. M. (2001) Broad-spectrum sunscreens provide better protection from the suppression of the elicitation phase of delayed-type hypersensitivity response in humans. *J. Invest. Dermatol.* **117**: 1186–1192.
103. Serre I., Cano J. P., Picot M. C., Meynadier J. and Meunier L. (1997) Immunosuppression induced by acute solar-simulated ultraviolet exposure in humans: prevention by a sunscreen with a sun protection factor of 145 and high UVA protection. *J. Am. Acad. Dermatol.* **37**: 187–194.
104. Moyal D. D. and Fourtanier A. M. (2002) Effects of UVA radiation on an established immune response in humans and sunscreen efficacy. *Exp. Dermatol.* **11** (Suppl. 1): 28–32.
105. Moyal D. D. and Fourtanier A. M. (2003) Efficacy of broad-spectrum sunscreens against the suppression of elicitation of de-

layed-type hypersensitivity responses in humans depends on the level of ultraviolet A protection. *Exp. Dermatol.* **12**: 153–159.
106. Baron E. D., Fourtanier A., Compan D., Medaisko C., Cooper K. D. and Stevens S. R. (2003) High ultraviolet A protection affords greater immune protection confirming that ultraviolet A contributes to photoimmunosuppression in humans. *J. Invest. Dermatol.* **121**: 869–875.
107. Fourtanier A., Gueniche A., Compan D., Walker S. L. and Young A. R. (2000) Improved protection against solar-simulated radiation-induced immunosuppression by a sunscreen with enhanced ultraviolet A protection. *J. Invest. Dermatol.* **114**: 620–627.
108. Seite S., Moyal D., Richard S., de Rigal J., Leveque J. L., Hourseau C. and Fourtanier A. (1998) Mexoryl SX: a broad absorption UVA filter protects human skin from the effects of repeated suberythemal doses of UVA. *J. Photochem. Photobiol., B* **44**: 69–76.
109. Gueniche A. and Fourtanier A. (1997) Mexoryl SX protects against photoimmuno-suppression. In: *Skin cancer and UV radiation*, pp 249–262, Altmeyer P., Hoffmann K. and Stucker M. (eds.), Springer-Verlag, Heidelberg.
110. Fourtanier A., Moyal D. and Seite S. (2008) Sunscreens containing the broad-spectrum UVA absorber, Mexoryl SX, prevent the cutaneous detrimental effects of UV exposure: a review of clinical study results. *Photodermatol. Photoimmunol. Photomed.* **24**: 164–174.
111. Moyal D. D. and Fourtanier A. M. (2008) Broad-spectrum sunscreens provide better protection from solar ultraviolet-stimulated radiation and natural sunlight-induced immunosuppression in human beings. *J. Am. Acad. Dermatol.* **58** (5 Suppl. 2): S149–154.
112. Nghiem D. X., Kazimi N., Clydesdale G., Ananthaswamy H. N., Kripke M. L. and Ullrich S. E. (2001) Ultraviolet A radiation suppresses an established immune response: implications for sunscreen design. *J. Invest. Dermatol.* **117**: 1193–1199.
113. Poon T. S., Barnetson R. S. and Halliday G. M. (2003) Prevention of immunosuppression in humans is unrelated to protection from erythema and dependent on protection from ultraviolet A in the face of constant ultraviolet B protection. *J. Invest. Dermatol.* **12**: 184–190.
114. Whitmore S. E. and Morison W. L. (1995) Prevention of UVB-induced immunosuppression in humans by a high sun protection factor sunscreen. *Arch. Dermatol.* **131**: 1128–1133.
115. Beasley D. G., Beard J., Stanfield J. W. and Roberts L. K. (1996) Evaluation of an economical sunlamp that emits a near solar UV

power spectrum for conducting photoimmunological and sunscreen immune protection studies. *Photochem. Photobiol.* **64**: 303–309.
116. Roberts L. K., Beasley D. G., Learn D. B., Giddens L. D., Beard J. and Stanfield J. W. (1996) Ultraviolet spectral energy differences affect the ability of sunscreen lotions to prevent ultraviolet-radiation-induced immunosuppression. *Photochem. Photobiol.* **63**: 874–884.
117. Roberts L. K. and Beasley D. G. (1997) Sunscreens prevent local and systemic immunosuppression of contact hypersensitivity in mice exposed to solar-simulated ultraviolet radiation. *J. Photochem. Photobiol., B* **39**: 121–129.
118. Ullrich S. E., Kim T. H., Ananthaswamy H. N. and Kripke M. L. (1999) Sunscreen effects on UV-induced immune suppression. *J. Invest. Dermatol. Symp. Proc.* **4**: 65–69.
119. Ullrich S. E., Kripke M. L. and Ananthaswamy H. N. (2002) Mechanisms underlying UV-induced immune suppression: implications for sunscreen design. *Exp. Dermatol.* **11**: 13–16.
120. Strickland F. M. and Kripke M. L. (1997) Immune response associated with nonmelanoma skin cancer. *Clin. Plastic Surg.* **24**: 637–647.
121. Garland C. F., Garland F. C. and Gorham E. D. (1994) Effect of sunscreens on the UV radiation-induced enhancement of melanoma growth in mice. *JNCI, J. Natl. Cancer Inst.* **86**: 798–800.
122. Wolf P. and Kripke M. L. (1996) Sunscreens and immunosuppression. *J. Invest. Dermatol.* **106**: 1152–1154.
123. Gill E. M. and Kim T. H. (2000) UV-induced immune suppression and sunscreen. *Photodermatol., Photoimmunol. Photomed.* **16**: 101–110.
124. De Gruijl F. R. and Van Kranen H. J. (2001) UV radiation, mutations and oncogenic pathways in skin cancer. In: *Sun Protection in Man*, pp 287–302, Giacomoni P. U. (ed.), Elsevier, Amsterdam.
125. Xie J. (2008) Molecular biology of basal and squamous cell carcinoma. In: *Sunlight, Vitamin D and Skin Cancer*, pp 241–251, Reichrath J. (ed.), Springer Science + Business Media, LLC, New York, and Landes Bioscience, Austin, TX.
126. Dominago D. S. and Baron E. D. (2008) Melanoma and nonmelanoma skin cancers and the immune system. In: *Sunlight, Vitamin D and Skin Cancer*, pp 187–202, Reichrath J. (ed.), Springer Science + Business Media, LLC, New York, and Landes Bioscience, Austin, TX.
127. Bale A. E. and Yu K. P. (2001) The hedgehog pathway and basal cell carcinomas. *Hum. Mol. Genet.* **10**: 757–762.

128. Aszterbaum M., Beech J. and Epstein E. J. Jr. (1999) Ultraviolet radiation mutagenesis of hedgehog pathway genes in basal cell carcinomas. *J. Invest. Dermatol. Symp. Proc.* **4**: 41–45.
129. Fan H., Oro A. E., Scott M. P. and Khavari P. A. (1997) Induction of basal cell carcinoma features in transgenic human keratinocytes expressing Sonic Hedgehog. *Nat Med.* **3**: 788–792.
130. Dahmane N., Lee J., Robins P., Heller P., Ruiz A. and Altaba I. (1997) Activation of the transcription factor Gli1 and the Sonic Hedgehog signaling pathway in skin tumours. *Nature* **389**: 876–881.
131. Fan H. and Khavari P. A. (1999) Sonic hedgehog opposes epithelial cell cycle arrest. *J. Cell Biol.* **147**: 71–76.
132. Funk J. O., Schiller P. T., Barrett M. T., Wong D. J., Kind P. and Sander C. A. (1998) P16INK4α expression is frequently decreased and associated with 9p21 loss of heterozygosity in sporadic melanoma. *J. Cutaneous Pathol.* **25**: 291–296.
133. Van Elsas A., Zerp S. F., van der Flier S., Kruse K. M., Aarnoudse C., Hayward N. K., Ruiter D. J. and Schrier P. I. (1996) Relevance of ultraviolet-induced N-ras oncogene point mutations in development of primary human cutaneous melanoma. *Am. J. Pathol.* **143**: 883–893.
134. Van't Veer L. J., Burgering B. M. T., Versteeg R., Boot A. J. M., Ruiter D. J., Osanto S., Schrier P. I. and Bos J. L. (1989) N-ras mutations in human cutaneous melanoma from sun-exposed body sites. *Mol. Cell. Biol.* **9**: 3114–3116.
135. Serrano M., Lin W. A., McCurrach M. E., Beach D. and Lowe S. W. (1997) Oncogenic ras provides premature cell senescence associated with accumulation of p53 and $p16^{INK4\alpha}$. *Cell* **88**: 593–602.
136. Decraeme D., Agostinis P., Pupe A., De Haes P. and Garmyn M. (2001) p53 protein and the response of human skin to UV. In: *Sun protection in Man*, pp 407–418, Giacomoni P. U. (ed.), Elsevier, Amsterdam.
137. Benjamin C. L., Melnikova V. O. and Ananthaswamy H. N. (2008) p53 protein and pathogenesis of melanoma and nonmelanoma skin cancer. In: *Sunlight, vitamin D and skin cancer*, pp 265–282, Reichrath J. (ed.), Springer Science+Business Media, LLC, New York, and Landes Bioscience, Austin, TX.
138. Maltzman W. and Czyzk L. (1984) UV irradiation stimulates levels of p53 cellular tumor antigen in nontransformed mouse cells. *Mol. Cell. Biol.* **4**: 1689–1694.

139. Campbell C., Quinn A. G., Angus B., Farr P. M. and Rees J. L. (1993) Wavelength specific patterns of p53 induction in human skin following exposure to UV radiation. *Cancer Res.* **53**: 2697–2699.
140. Hall P. A., McKee P. H., Menage H. D. P., Dover R. and Lane D. P. (1993) High levels of p53 protein in UV-irradiated normal human skin. *Oncogene* **8**: 203–207.
141. Lu X. and Lane D. P. (1993) Differential induction of transcriptionally active p53 following UV or ionizing radiation: defects in chromosome instability syndromes? *Cell* **75**: 765–778.
142. Zhan Q., Carrier F. and Fornace A. J. Jr. (1993) Induction of cellular p53 activity by DNA-damaging agents and growth arrest. *Mol. Cell. Biol.* **13**: 4242–4250.
143. Kastan M. B., Onyekewere O., Sidransky D., Vogelstein B. and Craig R. W. (1991) Participation of p53 protein in the cellular response to DNA damage. *Cancer Res.* **51**: 6304–6311.
144. Kastan M. B., Canman C. E. and Leonard C. J. (1995) P53, cell cycle control and apoptosis: implications for cancer. *Cancer Metastasis Rev.* **14**: 3–15.
145. El-Deiry W. S., Tokino T., Velculescu V. E., Levy D. B., Parsons R., Trent J. M., Lin D., Mercer W. E., Kinzler K. W. and Vogelstein B. (1993) WAF1, a potential mediator of p53 tumor suppression. *Cell* **75**: 817–825.
146. Harper J. W., Adami G. R., Wei N., Keyomarsi K. and Elledge S. J. (1993) The p21 Cdk-interacting protein Cip1 is a potent inhibitor of G1 cyclin-dependent kinases. *Cell* **75**: 805–816.
147. Xiong Y., Hannon G. J., Zhang H., Casso D., Kobayashi R. and Beach D. (1993) p21 is a universal inhibitor of cyclin kinases. *Nature* **366**: 701–704.
148. Reed J. C. (1994) Bcl-2 and the regulation of programmed cell death. *J. Cell. Biol.* **124**: 1–6.
149. Ziegler A., Jonason A. S., Lafell D. H., Simon J. A., Sharma H. W., Kimmelmann J., Remington L., Jacks T. and Brash D. E. (1994) Sunburn and p53 in the onset of skin cancer. *Nature* **372**: 773–776.
150. Erb P., Jingmin J., Kump E., Mielgo A. and Wernli M. (2008) Apoptosis and pathogenesis of melanoma and nonmelanoma skin cancer. In: *Sunlight, vitamin D and skin cancer*, pp 283–295, Reichrath J. (ed.), Springer Science+Business Media, LLC, New York, and Landes Bioscience, Austin, TX.
151. Gillaradon F., Eschenfelder C., Uhlmann E., Hartschuh W. and Zimmermann M. (1994) Differential regulation of c-fos, fosB, c-jun, junB, bcl-2 and bax expression in rat skin following single or chronic

ultraviolet irradiation and in vivo modulation by antisense oligodeoxynucleotide superfusion. *Oncogene* **9**: 3219–3225.
152. Miyashita T., Krajewski S., Krajewska M., Wang H. G., Lin H. K., Liebermann D. A., Hoffman B. and Reed J. C. (1994) Tumor suppressor p53 is a regulator of bcl-2 and bax gene expression in vitro and in vivo. *Oncogene* **9**: 1799–1805.
153. Miyashita T. and Reed J. C. (1995) Tumor suppressor p53 is a direct transcriptional activator of the human bax gene. *Cell* **80**: 293–299.
154. Hoffmann-Wellenhof R., Smolle J., Roschger A., Strunk D., Hubmer M., Hoffmann C., Quehenberger F., Horn M., Kerl H. and Wolf P. (2004) Sunburn cell formation, dendritic cell migration, and immunomodulatory factor production after solar-simulated irradiation of sunscreen-treated human skin explants in vitro. *J. Invest. Dermatol.* **123**: 781–787.
155. Brash D. E., Rudolph J. A., Simon J. A., Linn A., McKenna G. J., Baden H. P., Halperin A. P. and Pontén J. (1991) A role for sunlight in skin cancer: UV induced p53 mutations in squamous cell carcinoma. *Proc. Natl. Acad. Sci. U. S. A.* **88**: 10124–10128.
156. Pierceall W. E., Mukhopadhyay T., Goldberg C. H. and Ananthaswamy H. A. (1991) Mutation in the p53 suppressor gene in human cutaneous squamous cell carcinomas. *Mol. Carcinog.* **4**: 445–449.
157. Rady P., Scinicariello F., Wagner R. F. and Tyring S. K. (1992) p53 mutations in basal cell carcinomas. *Cancer Res.* **52**: 3804–3806.
158. Moles J. P., Moyret C., Guillot B., Jeanteur P., Guilhou J. J., Theillet C. and Basset-Seguin N. (1993) p53 mutations in human epithelial skin cancers. *Oncogene* **8**: 583–588.
159. Ziegler A. M., Leffell D. J., Kunala S., Sharma H. W., Gailani M., Simon J. A., Halperin A. J., Baden H. P., Shapiro P. E. and Bale A. E. (1993) Mutation hotspots due to sunlight in the p53 gene of nonmelanoma skin cancers. *Proc. Natl. Acad. Sci. U. S. A.* **90**: 4216–4220.
160. Tornaletti S. and Pfeifer G. P (1994) Slow repair of pyrimidine dimers at p53 mutation hotspots in skin cancer. *Science* **263**: 1436–1438.
161. Yu C. C., MacGregor J. M., Dublin E. A., Barnes D. M., Macdonald D. M. and Levison D. A. (1992) Patterns of immunostaining for p53 in benign and malignant melanocytic lesions (meeting abstract). *J. Pathol.* **167** (Suppl.): 130A.
162. Goukassian D. A., Eller M. S., Yaar M. and Gilchrest B. A. (1999) Thymidine dinucleotide mimics the effect of solar simulated irradia-

tion on p53 and p53-regulated proteins. *J. Invest. Dermatol.* **112**: 25–31.
163. Ziegler A., Jonason A. S., Leffell D. J., Simon J. A., Sharma H. W., Kimmelman J., Remington L., Jacks T. and Brash D. E. (1994) Sunburn and p53 in the onset of skin cancer. *Nature* **372**: 773–776.
164. Berg R. J. W., van Kranen H. J., Rebel H. G., de Vries A., van Vloten W. A., van Kreijl C. F., Van der Leun J. C. and De Gruijl F. R. (1996) Early p53 alterations in mouse skin carcinogenesis by UVB radiation: immunohistochemical detection of mutant p53 protein in clusters of preneoplastic epidermal cells. *Proc. Natl. Acad. Sci. U. S. A.* **93**: 274–278.
165. Ananthaswamy H. N., Loughlin S. M., Cox P., Evans R. L., Ullrich S. E. and Kripke M. L. (1997) Sunlight and skin cancer: Inhibition of p53 mutations in UV-irradiated mouse skin by sunscreens. *Nature Med.* **3**: 510–514.
166. Shangary S. and Wang S. (2009) Small-molecule inhibitors of the MDM2-p53 protein-protein interaction to reactivate p53 function: a novel approach for cancer therapy. *Annu. Rev. Pharmacol. Toxicol.* **49**: 223–241.
167. Vassilev L. T., Vu B. T., Graves B., Carvajal D., Podlaski F., Filipovic Z., Kong N., Kammlott U., Lukacs C., Klein C., Fotouhi N. and Liu E. A. (2004) In vivo activation of the p53 by small-molecule antagonists of MDM2. *Science* **303**: 844–848.
168. Baoying H., Dayanard D., Mingxuan X. and Vansilev L. T. (2009) Pharmacologic p53 activation blocks cell cycle progression but fails to induce senescence in epithelial cancer cells. *Mol. Cancer Res.* (MCR) **7**: 1497–1509.
169. Lane D. P. (2004) p53 from pathway to therapy. *Carcinogenesis* **25**: 1077–1081.
170. Roth J. A. (2006) Adenovirus p53 gene therapy. *Expert Opin. Biol. Ther.* **6**: 55–61.
171. McCormick F. (2003) Cancer-specific viruses and the development of ONYX-015. *Cancer Biol. Ther.* **2**: S157–S160.
172. Ponten F., Berne B., Ren Z. P., Mister M. and Ponten J. (1995) Ultraviolet light induces expression of p53 and p21 in human skin: effect of sunscreen and constitutive p21 expression in skin appendages. *J. Invest. Dermatol.* **105**: 402–406.
173. El Deiry W. S., Tokino T., Waldman T., Oliner J. D., Velculescu V. E., Burrell M., Hill D. E., Healy E., Rees J. L., Hamilton S. R., Kinzler K. W. and Vogelstein B. (1995) Topological control of

p21k$^{WAF1/CIP1}$ expression in normal and neoplastic tissues. *Cancer Res.* **55**: 2901–2919.

174. Ananthaswamy H. N., Ullrich S. E., Mascotto R. E., Fourtanier A., Loughlin S. M., Khaskina P., Bucana C. D and Kripke M. L. (1999) Inhibition of solar simulator-induced p53 mutations and protection against skin cancer development in mice by sunscreens. *J. Invest. Dermatol.* **112**: 764–768.
175. Ananthaswamy H. N., Loughlin S. M., Ullrich S. E. and Kripke M. L. (1998) Inhibition of UV-induced p53 mutations by sunscreens implications for skin cancer prevention. *J. Invest. Dermatol. Symp. Proc.* **3**: 52–56.
176. Van Kranen H. J., de Laat A., van de Ven J., Wester P. W., de Vries A., Berg R. J., Van Kreijl C. F. and De Gruijl F. R. (1997) Low incidence of p53 mutations in UVA (365-nm)-induced skin tumors in hairless mice. *Cancer Res.* **57**: 1238–1240.
177. Rosenstein B. S., Phelps R. G., Weinstock M. A., Bernstein J. L., Gordon M. L., Rudikoff D., Kantor I., Shelton R. and Lebwohl M. G. (1999) p53 mutations in basal cell carcinomas arising in routine users of sunscreens. *Photochem. Photobiol.* **70**: 798–806.
178. Berne B., Ponten J. and Ponten F. (1998) Decreased p53 expression in chronically sun-exposed human skin after topical photoprotection. *Photodermatol., Photoimmunol. Photomed.* **14**: 148–153.
179. Seite S., Moyal D., Verdier M.-P., Hourseau C. and Fourtanier A. (2000) Accumulated p53 protein and UVA protection levels of sunscreens. *Photodermatol., Photoimmunol. Photomed.* **16**: 3–9.
180. Krekels G., Voorter C., Kuik F., Verhaegh M., Ramaekers F. and Neumann M. (1997) DNA-protection by sunscreens: using p53-immunostaining. *Eur. J. Dermatol.* **7**: 259–262.
181. Sambuco C. P., Forbes P. D., Davies R. E. and Urbach F. (1984) An animal model to determine sunscreen protectiveness against both vascular injury and epidermal cell damage. *J. Am. Acad. Dermatol.* **10**: 737–743.
182. Wolf P., Donawho C. K. and Kripke M. L. (1994) Effect of sunscreens on UV radiation-induced enhancement of melanoma growth in mice. *JNCI, J. Natl. Cancer Inst.* **86**: 99–105.
183. Wolf P., Cox P., Yarosh D. B. and Kripke M. L. (1995) Sunscreens and T4N5 liposomes differ in their ability to protect against ultraviolet-induced sunburn cell formation, alterations of dendritic epidermal cells, and local suppression of contact hypersensitivity. *J. Invest. Dermatol.* **104**: 287–292.

184. Darr D., Dunston S., Faust H. and Pinnell S. (1996) Effectiveness of antioxidants (vitamin C and E) with and without sunscreens as topical photoprotectants. *Acta Derm.-Venereol.* **76**: 264–268.
185. Okamoto H., Mizuno K., Itoh T., Tanaka K. and Horio T. (1999) Evaluation of apoptotic cells induced by ultraviolet light B radiation in epidermal sheets stained by the TUNEL technique. *J. Invest. Dermatol.* **113**: 802–807.
186. Donawho C. K., Norval M. and Yarosh D. B. (1998) Molecular target of UV-B radiation in the melanoma enhancing effect of UV irradiation in a murine model. *Photochem. Photobiol.* **6**: 64S.
187. Strickland F. M., Darvill A., Albersheim P., Eberhard S., Pauly M. and Pelley R. P. (1999) Inhibition of UV-induced immune suppression and Interleukin-10 production by plant polysaccharides. *Photochem. Photobiol.* **69**: 141–147.
188. Afaq F., Adhami V. M. and Mukhtar H. (2005) Photochemoprevention of ultraviolet B signaling and photocarcinogenesis. *Mutat. Res.* **571**: 153–173.
189. Strickland F. M., Kuchel J. M. and Halliday G. M. (2004) Natural products as aids for protecting the skin's immune system against UV damage. *Cutis* **74** (5 Suppl): 24–28.
190. Hirt H. (1997) Multiple roles of MAP kinases in plant signal transduction. *Trends Plant Sci.* **2**: 11–15.
191. Strickland F. M., Pelley R. P. and Kripke M. L. (1994) Prevention of ultraviolet radiation-induced suppression of contact and delayed hypersensitivity by Aloe barbadensis gel extract. *J. Invest. Dermatol.* **102**: 197–204.
192. Shreedhar V. K., Pride M. W., Sun Y., Kripke M. L. and Strickland F. M. (1998) Origin and characteristics of UV-B radiation-induced suppressor T lymphocytes. *J. Immunol.* **161**: 1327–1335.
193. Durrer S., Ehnes C., Fuetsch M., Maerkel K., Schlumpf M. and Lichtensteiger W. (2007) Estrogenic sensitivity of target genes and expression of nuclear receptor co-regulators in rat prostate after pre- and postnatal exposure to the ultraviolet filter 4-methylbenzylidene camphor. *Environ. Health Perspect.* **115** (Suppl 1): 42–50.
194. Tena-Sempere M., Navarro J., Pinilla L., Gonzalez L. C., Huhtaniemi I. and Aguilar E. (2000) Neonatal exposure to estrogen differentially alters estrogen receptor alpha and beta mRNA expression in rat testis during postnatal development. *J. Endocrinol.* **165**: 345–357.
195. Heneweer M., Muusse M., van den Berg M. and Sanderson J. T. (2005) Additive estrogenic effects of mixtures of frequently used UV

filters on pS2-gene transcription in MCF-7 cells. *Toxicol. Appl. Pharmacol.* **208**: 170–177.
196. Hofkamp L., Bradley S., Tresguerres J., Lichtensteiger W., Schlumpf M. and Timms B. (2008) Region-specific growth effects in the developing rat prostate following fetal exposure to estrogenic ultraviolet filters. *Environ. Health Perspect.* **116**: 867–872.
197. Schlumpf M., Cotton B., Conscience M., Heller V., Steinmann B. and Lichtensteiger W. (2001) In vitro and in vivo estrogenicity of UV screens. *Environ. Health Perspect.* **109**: 239–244.
198. Tinwell H., Lefevre P. A., Moffat G. J., Burns A., Odum J., Spurway T. D., Orphanides G. and Ashby J. (2002) Confirmation of uterotrophic activity of 3-(4-methoxybenzylidene)camphor in the immature rat. *Environ. Health Perspect.* **110**: 533–536.
199. Schlumpf M., Schmid P., Durrer S., Conscience M., Maerkel K., Henseler M., Gruetter M., Herzog I., Reolon S., Ceccatelli R., Faass O., Stutz E., Jarry H., Wuttke W. and Lichtensteiger W. (2004) Endocrine activity and developmental toxicity of cosmetic UV filters – an update. *Toxicology* **205**: 113–122.
200. Janjua N. R., Mogensen R., Andersson A. M., Petersen J. H., Henriksen M., Skakkebaek N. E. and Wulf H. C. (2004) Systemic absorption of the sunscreens benzophenones-3, octylmethoxycinnamate, and 3-(4-methylbenzylidene)camphor after whole-body topical application and reproductive hormone levels in humans. *Invest. Dermatol.* **123**: 57–61.
201. Mueller S. O., Kling M., Arifin Firzani P., Mecky A., Duranti E., Shields-Botella J., Delansorne R., Broschard T. and Kramer P. J. (2003) Activation of estrogen receptor alpha and ERbeta by 4-methylbenzylidenecamphor in human and rat cells: comparison with phylo- and xenoestrogens. *Toxicol. Lett.* **142**: 89–101.
202. Schlumpf M., Jarry H., Wuttke W., Ma R. and Lichtensteiger W. (2004) Estrogenic activity and estrogenic receptor beta binding of the UV filter 3-benzylidenecamphor. Comparison with 4-methylbenzylidenecamphor. *Toxicology* **199**: 109–120.
203. Schmitt C., Oetken M., Dittberner O., Wagner M. and Oehlmann J. (2008) Endocrine modulation and toxic effects of two commonly used UV screens on the aquatic invertebrates *Potamopyrgus antipodarum* and *Lumbriculus variegatus*. *Environ. Pollut.* **152**: 322–329.
204. Schlumpf M., Durrer S., Faass O., Ehnes C., Fuetsch M., Gaille C., Henseler M., Hofkamp L., Maerkel K., Reolon S., Timms B., Tresguerres J. A. and Lichtensteiger W. (2008) Development and toxicity

of UV filters and environmental exposure: a review. *Int. J. Androl.* **31**: 144–151.
205. Schreurs R. H., Sonneveld E., Jansen J. H., Seinen W. and van der Burg B. (2005) Interaction of polycyclic musks and UV filters with the estrogen receptor (ER), androgen receptor (AR), and progesterone receptor (PR) in reporter gene bioassays. *Toxicol. Sci.* **83**: 264–272.
206. Schreurs R., Lanser P., Seinen W. and van der Burg B. (2002) Estrogen activity of UV filters determined by an in vitro reporter gene assay and an in vivo transgenic zebra fish assay. *Arch. Toxicol.* **76**: 257–261.
207. Seidlova-Wuttke D., Jarry H., Christoffel J., Rimoldi G. and Wuttke W. (2006) Comparison of effects of estradiol (E2) with those of octylmethoxycinnamate (OMC) and 4-methylbenzylidene camphor (4MBC) - 2 filters of UV light on several uterine, vaginal and bone parameters. *Toxicol. Appl. Pharmacol.* **210**: 246–254.
208. Seidlova-Wuttke D., Christoffel J., Rimoldi G., Jarry H. and Wuttke W. (2006) Comparison of effects of estradiol with those of octylmethoxycinnamate and 4-methylbenzylidene camphor on fat tissue, lipids and pituitary hormones. *Toxicol. Appl. Pharmacol.* **214**: 1–7.
209. Klammer H., Schlecht C., Wuttke W. and Jarry H. (2005) Multi-organic risk assessment of estrogenic properties of octylmethoxycinnamate in vivo. A 5-day sub-acute pharmacodynamic study with ovariectomized rats. *Toxicology* **215**: 90–96.
210. Klammer H., Schlecht C., Wuttke W., Schmutzler C., Gotthardt J., Kohrle J. and Jarry H. (2007) Effects of a 5-day treatment with the UV-filter octyl-methoxycinnamate (OMC) on the function of the hypothalamo-pituitary-thyroid function in rats. *Toxicology* **238**: 192–199.
211. Szwarcfarb B., Carbone S., Reynoso R., Boltero G., Ponzo O., Moguilevsky J. and Scacchi P. (2008) Octyl-methoxycinnamate (OMC), an ultraviolet (UV) filter, alters LHRH and amino acid neurotransmitters release from hypothalamus of immature rats. *Exp. Clin. Endocrinol. Diabetes* **116**: 94–98.
212. Rachon D., Rimoldi G. and Wuttke W. (2006) In vitro effects of benzophenone-2 and octyl-methoxycinnamate on the production of interferon-gamma and interleukin-10 by murine splenocytes. *Immunopharmacol. Immunotoxicol.* **28**: 501–510.
213. Kunz P. Y. and Fent K. (2006) Multiple hormonal activities of UV filters and comparison of in vivo and in vitro estrogenic activity of ethyl 4-aminobenzoate in fish. *Aquat. Toxicol.* **79**: 305–324.

214. Kunz P. Y. and Fent K. (2009) Estrogenic activity of ternary UV filter mixtures in fish (Pimephales promelas) – an analysis with non-linear isobolograms. *Toxicol. Appl. Pharmacol.* **234**: 77–88.
215. Kunz P. Y. and Fent K. (2006) Estrogenic activity of UV filter mixtures. *Toxicol. Appl. Pharmacol.* **217**: 86–99.
216. Kunz P. Y., Galicia H. F. and Fent K. (2006) Comparison of in vitro and in vivo estrogenic activity of UV filters in fish. *Toxicol. Sci.* **90**: 349–361.
217. Inui M., Adachi T., Takenaka S., Inui H., Nakazawa M., Ueda M., Watanabe H., Mori C., Iguchi T. and Miyatake K. (2003) Effect of UV screens and preservatives on vitellogenin and choriogenin production in male madeka (Oryzias latipes). *Toxicology* **194**: 43–50.
218. Weisbrod C. J., Kunz P. Y., Zenker A. K. and Fent K. (2007) Effects of the UV filter benzophenone-2 on reproduction in fish. *Toxicol. Appl. Pharmacol.* **225**: 255–266.
219. Koda T., Umezu T., Kamata R., Morohoshi K., Ohta T. and Morita M. (2005) Uterotrophic effects of benzophenone derivatives and *p*-hydroxybenzoate used in ultraviolet screens. *Environ. Res.* **98**: 40–45.
220. Matsumoto H., Adachi S. and Suzuki Y. (2005) Estrogenic activity of ultraviolet absorbers and the related compounds. *Yakugaku Zasshi* **125**: 643–652.
221. Ashby J., Tinwell H., Plautz J., Twomey K. and Lefevre P. A. (2001) Lack of binding to isolated estrogen or androgen receptors, and inactivity in the immature rat uterotrophic assay, of the ultraviolet sunscreen filters Tinosorb M-active and Tinosorb S. *Regul. Toxicol. Pharmacol.* **34**: 287–291.
222. Hayashi T., Okamoto Y., Ueda K. and Kojima N. (2006) Formation of estrogenic products from benzophenone after exposure to sunlight. *Toxicol. Lett.* **167**: 1–7.
223. Nakagawa Y., Suzuki T. and Tayama S. (2000) Metabolism and toxicity of benzophenone in isolated rat hepatocytes and estrogenic activity of its metabolites in MCF-7 cells. *Toxicology* **156**: 27–36.
224. Suzuki T., Kitamura S., Khota R., Sugihara K., Fujimoto N. and Ohta S. (2005) Estrogenic and antiandrogenic activities of 17 benzophenone derivatives used as UV stabilizers and sunscreens. *Toxicol. Appl. Pharmacol.* **203**: 9–17.
225. Jarry H., Christoffel J., Rimoldi G., Koch L. and Wuttke W. (2004) Multi-organic endocrine disrupting activity of the UV screen benzophenone-2 (BP2) in ovariectomized adult rats after 5 days treatment. *Toxicology* **205**: 87–93.

226. Schlecht C., Klammer H., Wuttke W. and Jarry H. (2006) A dose-response study of the estrogenic activity of benzophenone-2 on various endpoints in the serum, pituitary and uterus of female rats. *Arch. Toxicol.* **80**: 656–661.
227. Schlecht C., Klammer H., Frauendorf H., Wuttke W. and Jarry H. (2008) Pharmacokinetics and metabolism of benzophenone-2 in the rat. *Toxicology* **245**: 11–17.
228. Schmutzler C., Bacinski A., Gotthardt I., Huhne K., Ambrugger P., Klammer H., Schlecht C., Hoang-Vu C., Grüters A., Wuttke W., Jarry H. and Köhrle J. (2007) The ultraviolet filter benzophenone-2 interferes with the thyroid hormone axis in rats and is a potent in vitro inhibitor of human recombinant thyroid peroxidase. *Endocrinology* **148**: 2835–2844.
229. Nakagawa Y. and Suzuki T. (2002) Metabolism of 2-hydroxy-4-methoxybenzophenone in isolated rat hepatocytes and xenoestrogenic effects of its metabolites on MCF-7 human breast cancer cells. *Chem.-Biol. Interact.* **139**: 115–128.
230. Morohoshi K., Yamamoto H., Kamata R., Shiraishi F., Koda T. and Morita M. (2005) Estrogenic activity of 37 compounds of commercial sunscreen lotions evaluated by in vitro assays. *Toxicol. In Vitro* **19**: 457–469.
231. Gomez E., Pillon A., Fenet H., Rosain D., Duchesne M. J., Nicolas J. C., Balaguer P. and Casellas C. (2005) Estrogenic activity of cosmetic components in reporter cell lines: parabens, UV screens, and musks. *J. Toxicol. Environ. Health, Part A.* **68**: 239–251.
232. Van der Burg B., Schreurs R., van der Linden S., Seinen W., Brouwer A. and Sonneveld E. (2008) Endocrine effects of polycyclic musks: do we smell a rat? *Int. J. Androl.* **31**: 188–193.
233. Calafat A. M., Wong L.-Y., Ye X., Reidy J. A. and Needham L. L. (2008) Concentrations of the sunscreen agent benzophenone-3 in residents of the United States: national health and nutrition examination survey 2003–2004. *Environ. Health Perspect.* **116**: 893–897.
234. Søeborg T., Ganderup N. C., Kristensen J. M., Bjerregaard P., Pedersen K. L., Bollen P., Hansen S. H. and Halling-Sørensen B. (2006) Distribution of the UV filter 3-benzylidene camphor in rat following topical application. *J. Chromatogr. B: Anal. Technol. Biomed. Life Sci.* **834**: 117–121.
235. Gonzalez H., Farbrot A., Larko O. and Wennberg A. M. (2006) Percutaneous absorption of the sunscreen benzophenone-3 after repeated whole body applications, with and without ultraviolet irradiation. *Br. J. Dermatol.* **154**: 337–340.

236. Schlumpf M., Kypke K., Vökt C. C., Birchler M., Durrer S., Faass O., et al. (2008) Endocrine active UV filters: developmental toxicity and exposure through breast milk. *CHIMIA–Int. J. Chem.* **62**: 345–351.
237. Okereke C. S., Kadry A. M., Abdel-Rahman M. S., Davis R. A. and Friedman M. A. (1993) Metabolism of benzophenone-3 in rats. *Drug Metab. Dispos.* **21**: 788–791.
238. Jeon H. K., Sarma S. N., Kim Y. J. and Ryu J. C. (2008) Toxicokinetics and metabolisms of benzophenone-type UV filters in rats. *Toxicology* **248**: 89–95.
239. Rimkus G. G. (1999) Polycyclic musk fragrances in the aquatic environment. *Toxicol. Lett.* **111**: 37–56.
240. Balk F. and Ford R. A. (1999) Environmental risk assessment for the polycyclic musks, AHTN and HHCB. II. Effect assessments and risk characterization. *Toxicol. Lett.* **111**: 81–94.
241. Ford R. A., Hawkins D. R., Schwarzenbach R. and Api A. M. (1999) The systemic exposure of the polycyclic musks, AHTN and HHCB, under conditions of use as fragrance ingredients: evidence of lack of complete absorption from a skin reservoir. *Toxicol. Lett.* **111**: 133–142.
242. Giokas D. L., Salvador A. and Chisvert A. (2007) UV filters: from sunscreens to human body and the environment. *TrAC, Trends Anal. Chem.* **26**: 360–374.
243. Zenker A., Schmutz H. and Fent K. (2008) Simultaneous trace determination of nine organic UV-absorbing compounds (UV filters) in environmental samples. *J. Chromatogr. A* **1202**: 64–74.
244. Leon Z., Balaguer A., Chisvert A., Salvador A., Herraez M. and Diez O. (2008) A reversed-phase ion-interaction chromatographic method for in-vitro estimation of the percutaneous absorption of water-soluble UV filters. *Anal. Bioanal. Chem.* **391**: 859–866.
245. Buser H. R., Muller M. D., Balmer M. E., Polger T. and Buerge I. J. (2005) Stereoisomer composition of the chiral UV filter 4-methylbenzylidene camphor in environmental samples. *Environ. Sci. Technol.* **39**: 3013–3019.
246. Dean S. W., Dunmore R. H., Ruddock S. P., Dean J. C., Martin C. N. and Kirkland D. J. (1992) Development of assays for the detection of photomutagenicity of chemicals during exposure to UV light. II. Results of testing three sunscreen ingredients. *Mutagenesis* **7**: 79–82.
247. Poiger T., Buser H. R., Balmer M. E., Bergqvist P. A. and Muller M. D. (2004) Occurrence of UV filter compounds from sunscreen in sur-

face waters: regional mass balance in two Swiss lakes. *Chemosphere* **55**: 951–963.
248. Balmer M. E., Buser H. R., Muller M. D. and Polger T. (2005) Occurrence of some organic UV filters in wastewater, in surface waters, and in fish from Swiss Lakes. *Environ. Sci. Technol.* **39**: 953–962.
249. Buser H. R., Balmer M. E., Schmid P. and Kohler M. (2006) Occurrence of UV filters 4-methylbenzylidene camphor and octocrylene in fish from various Swiss rivers with inputs from wastewater treatment plants. *Environ. Sci. Technol.* **40**: 1427–1431. Comment in *Environ. Sci. Technol.* **40**: 1377–1378.
250. Li W., Ma Y., Guo C., Hu W., Liu K., Wang Y. and Zhu T. (2007) Occurrence and behavior of four of the most used sunscreen UV filters in a wastewater reclamation plant. *Water Res.* **41**: 3506–3512.
251. Plaggellat C., Kupper T., Furrer R., de Alencastro L. F., Grandjean D. and Tarradellas J. (2006) Concentrations and specific loads of UV filters in sewage sludge originating from a monitoring network in Switzerland. *Chemosphere* **62**: 915–925.
252. Yamamoto H., Watanabe M., Hirata Y., Nakamura Y., Nakamura Y., Kitani C., Sekizawa J., Uchida M., Nakamura H., Kagami Y., Koshio M., Hirai N. and Tatarazako N. (2007) Preliminary ecological risk assessment of butylparaben and benzylparaben. Removal efficiency in wastewater treatment, acute/chronic toxicity for aquatic organisms, and effects on medaka gene expression. *Environ. Sci.* **14** (Suppl.): 73–87.
253. Scheil V., Triebskorn R. and Kohler H. R. (2008) Cellular and stress protein responses to the UV filter 3-benzylidene camphor in the amphipod crustacean Gammarus fossarum (Koch 183). *Arch. Environ. Contam. Toxicol.* **54**: 684–689.
254. Sakkas V. A., Giokas D. L., Lambropoulou D. A. and Albanis T. A. (2003) Aqueous photolysis of the sunscreen agent octyl-dimethyl-*p*-aminobenzoic acid. Formation of disinfection byproducts in chlorinated swimming pool water. *J. Chromatogr. A.* **1016**: 211–222.
255. Negreira N., Canosa P., Rodriguez L., Ramil M., Rubi E. and Cela R. (2008) Study of some UV filters stability in chlorinated water and identification of halogenated by-products by gas chromatography-mass spectrometry. *J. Chromatogr. A.* **1178**: 206–214.
256. Okamoto Y., Hayashi T., Matsunami S., Ueda K. and Kojima N. (2008) Combined activation of methyl paraben by light irradiation and esterase metabolism toward oxidative DNA damage. *Chem Res. Toxicol.* **21**: 1594–1599.

257. Danovaro R., Bongiorni L., Corinaldesi C., Giovannelli D., Damiani E., Astolfi P., Greci L. and Pusceddu A. (2008) Sunscreens cause coral bleaching by promoting viral infections. *Environ. Health Perspect.* **116**: 441–447.
258. Nakata H., Murata S., Shinohara R., Filatreau J., Isobe T., Takahashi S. and Tanabe S. (2009) Occurrence and concentrations of persistent personal care products, organic UV filters, in the marine environment. *Interdisciplinary Studies on Environmental Chemistry – Environmental Research in Asia*, pp 239–246, Obayashi Y., Isobe A., Subramanian A., Suzuki S. and Tanabe S. (eds.), TERRAPUB.
259. Kannan K., Reiner J., Yun S. H., Perrotta E. E., Tao L., Johnson-Restrepo B. and Rodan B. D. (2005) Polycyclic musk compounds in higher trophic level aquatic organisms and humans from the United States. *Chemosphere* **61**: 693–700.
260. Diaz-Cruz M. S., Llorca M. and Barcelo D. (2008) Organic UV filters and their photodegradates, metabolites and disinfection by-products in the aquatic environment. *TrAC Trends Anal. Chem.* **27**: 873–88.

G. Cancerous Dermatologic Changes. Human Skin Cancers Induced by UV Radiation, Effects of Sunscreen Agents, Topical Applications of DNA Repair Enzymes, and Mechanisms of Anticancer Drugs

i. Types of Cancers

Although solar radiation has the all-encompassing benign effects that are essential for the sustenance of life on this planet, it has also malign streaks, i.e., it is a prooxidant, a mutagen, and a carcinogen. The most important consequence of the properties of solar radiation is the induction of cutaneous cancerous growth in humans, other mammals, and other species [1–9].

The human body has a large skin surface area of about 1.5–2.0 square meters. This area is the target of sunrays and of all sorts of xenobiotics that damage the skin. The average U.S. citizen receives about 25000–33000 J/m^2 of ultraviolet dose per year. In recent years, more than one million of new skin cancer cases per year have been diagnosed in the USA, as compared to about 1.3 million cases of all other cancers combined. Hence, the incidence of skin cancers is about one-half of all other cancers that have been diagnosed per year. The most prevalent skin cancers are the basal cell carcinoma (BCC), the squamous cell carcinoma (SCC) and melanomas. The nonmelanoma skin cancers are mainly found on the head, neck, hands, and forearms; however, they can also appear on any other part of the skin [1–5]. The more aggressive types of skin cancer are the malignant cutaneous T lymphoma that can spread through the entire skin and can metastasize to other organs, and Kaposi sarcoma, a vascular malignancy that appears first on the skin, and has become a marker of the acquired immune deficiency syndrome, i.e., the AIDS disease, and the melanomas. Actually, there are four known histologic types of cutaneous melanoma, i.e., lentigo maligna melanoma, superficial spreading melanoma, nodular melanoma, and acral-lentiginous melanoma [3, 4]. The first three melanomas are the more common cancers of the skin. The lentigo maligna melanoma is definitely caused by cumulative life-long exposures to solar radiations. In the other melanomas, the inductions of the diseases are not certain. The melanomas are composed of more than 90% as cutaneous lesions. However, they can also occur as noncutaneous growth in the retina, mucous membranes, and other parts of the body. In the United States, 68180 cases of melanoma were diagnosed in 2009, resulting in 8700 deaths, i.e., 12.8% [5].

Although, over the years, the incidence of melanoma was on the average about 5% of that of nonmelanoma cancers, the melanoma cancers caused about three times as many death as the nonmelanoma cancers, e.g., 7600 for melanoma against 2200 for nonmelanoma in 2003 to 2008.

Melanoma was barely known at the beginning of the twentieth century. Thus, in 1935, the chance of suffering from the incidence of melanoma was about 1 in 1500, while 35 years later the ratio was about 1 in 70. Anecdotally, the increase in incidences of melanoma coincides with the increase of sales and consumption of sunscreen products. These figures are frequently quoted in various articles stressing the apparently unabated growth of incidences of melanoma, and a possible role of sunscreen agents in the proliferation of skin cancers, seemingly without consulting some pertinent statistical data [3–6]. Thus, the incidence of melanoma over the past thirty years in the USA among the so-called "whites", i.e., people with light-colored skin, rose during the period 1975 to 2003 from about 8 to 24 per 100,000; while the rates for persons of African origin remained unchanged at approximately 1 to 2 per 100,000; and for people with other colored skin like Hispanic, Asia/Pacific Islanders, American Indians, and Alaska natives, the incidence remained unchanged during the period 1993 to 2003, from 2 to 5 per 100,000. It is also of interest that the incidences of melanoma among the "white" male and female populations of age groups 50–54 to 85 declined during the years 2001 to 2003 in comparison with the period 1992 to 1994. Further, it is also significant that, in spite of the steep increase of incidences of melanoma in light-colored populations, the mortality rate in the USA remained practically unchanged during the period 1975 to 2003, between 2–2.5 per 100,000 for the light-colored population, and even lower for people with other colored skin, between 1 to 2 per 100,000 [5–9].

Sometimes alarmistic statements can be found in the press, such as "one person with melanoma dies every 68 minutes." However, it amounts actually to a death of 7624 per one million incidences of all skin cancers per year in the USA, which is one of the lowest of all cancers. Thus, such statements convey a possible epidemic that is not real [10]. It is further instructive to assess and make comparisons of the percentages of patients who will succumb to the respective cancers based on the diagnosed cases in the USA in 2008 [4]. In the following evaluation, the first entries in the brackets are the incidences per year, the second entries are the associated deaths, and the third entries are the percentages of those who died of a particular cancer [5]: pancreatic (37170, 33370, 90%), esophageal (16470, 14280, 87%), lung (220020, 162610, 74%,), multiple myeloma (19920, 10690, 54%), acute leukemias (44270, 21710, 49%), ovarian (21650, 15520, 72%), gastric (21000, 10880, 52%), non-Hodgkin (56120, 19160, 29%), colorectal/anal (148810, 49960, 34%), kidney (54390, 13010, 24%), cervical (11070, 3670, 33%), urethelial (68810, 14100, 21%), breast (182460, 40480, 22%), endometrial (39080, 7400, 19%), prostate (186320, 28600, 15%), all skin cancers about one million were diagnosed, resulting in 8700 deaths, i.e., ~ 1% [4]. Based on 68180 incidences of melanoma cases in 2009 and associated deaths of 8700, the mortality would be about 12% [5].

Thus, the skin cancers, in spite of the highest incidences of all cancers, are among the lowest in mortality. Furthermore, in contrast to most other cancers, the skin cancers and their precursors can be early visually detected and readily clinically diagnosed. Most melanomas and nearly all nonmelanoma skin cancers that are diagnosed at an early stage can be readily cured by surgery, radiations, and chemotherapy. The five-year survivals, i.e., a period that is considered as a cure, are 87% for melanoma when it is localized and 99% for nonmelanoma cancers. In the case of regional spread, the survival figures for melanoma are 35% and 50% for nonmelanomas, while for a delayed treatment, resulting in a distant spread to other organs, i.e., metastasis, the survival figures for melanoma are only 2% and for the nonmelanomas <10%. However, metastasis occurs only in about 2% of SCC patients and in about 0.1% of BCC patients [3–6].

ii. Induction of Cancerous Dermatological Changes by Ultraviolet Radiation

The UVA and UVB radiations are both potent immunosuppressors. The immunosuppression is probably relevant to the induction of skin cancers. In addition, other factors are believed to be involved in the progress of carcinogenesis, such as p53 gene mutations, contact hypersensitivity (CHR), delayed-type hypersensitivity (DTH), depression of NK killer cell activity, Langerhans cell depletion, induced epidermal interleukin-10, urocanic acid trans–cis isomerization, and many other factors. The various effects of solar radiation on the human body will depend on the intensity of solar radiation at the skin, that, in turn, will be determined by prevailing conditions, such as the time of the day, the season, the altitude, the parts of the body which are exposed to direct irradiation, the duration of exposure, i.e., whether it was chronic or intermittent, and whether the skin was topically covered with cosmetics, sunscreen agents, medications, antioxidants or orally administered medications that will, inadvertently, surface at the skin either unchanged or, most likely, as metabolites [7–9, 11–25].

For some time, it was considered that the UVB part of the solar radiation is the sole cause of damages to the DNA, mutations, and immunosuppressive effects that, eventually, culminate in carcinogenesis and skin cancers. However, in extensive studies over the past decades, evidence has been accumulating that the UVA radiation also exerts injurious effects on the DNA in humans and contributes substantially to the pathogenesis of skin cancers [11–18]. This conclusion is based on the following evidence. The UVA radiation causes DNA damages via the photosensitized reactions that produce reactive oxygen species (ROS). The UVA radiation can induce in vitro mutations in cells and in vivo mutations, e.g., in the hybrid fish *Xiphophorus* and the opossum *Mondelphis domestica* [14]. Melanoma precursors and melanoma can be induced with UVA radiation and the UVA radiation produces immunosuppression in humans and other mammals. Further, it was established by epidemiologic studies that there is an increase of melanoma cases in users of cosmetic indoor tanning [14,16], which may involve up to 100% of UVA radiation with about ten times higher doses than those found in solar radiation. The same increase is true of the adjunct use of psoralenes, which are known to be carcinogenic, and the psoralenes are also used clinically in combination with UVA radiation for the treatment of psoriasis, i.e., PUFA therapy [11, 13, 14]. The exceedingly complex details of the initiation and progression of skin cancers have been critically discussed in excellent reviews [11–18].

Many conclusions on the propagation of skin cancers are based on experiments with small, short-lived mammals, usually with specially bred mice, because one can obtain results in a much shorter time than with human volunteers. Thus, one can observe the evolution of a cancer in a small mammal over a period of two years while it would require with human volunteers a period of up to 60 to 80 years. Clearly, it is risky to form definite conclusions on the basis of experiments with small mammals.

It is not unreasonable to assume that all skin cancers would be preceded by some lesions, i.e., pathologically altered tissues of the skin that might be viewed as precursors or precancers. While in cases of SCC and melanoma such recognizable precursors are observed, in the case of BCC no such precursors can be found. The BCC and SCC are very common slow-growing cancers that rarely metastasize. The precursors of SCC are dysplasias in the form of actinic (solar) keratosis, which appears at the sun-exposed areas of the skin and is well identifiable in clinical oncology. Patients with solar keratosis can have a 30–50% deficit in DNA repair of photoproducts. These solar keratoses often regress. The SCC appearance may occur twenty or forty years after the initial appearances of dysplasias, and they seldom, if ever, regress. The mechanism of regression is not fully understood. However, it is believed that the cause of regression could be the recovery of the immune system, coupled with a possible induction of apoptosis, since the solar keratosis and the SCC are frequently found in patients on immunosuppressive drugs. The p53 gene that regulates the cell cycle and cell death, i.e., apoptosis, and the PTCH gene, which is part of the signaling pathways, are mutated in BCC and SCC. The p53 gene is also mutated in dysplasias and in at least one-half of all human cancers. Dysplasias can be clinically treated with 5-fluorouracil, which, apparently, is somehow involved as an apoptosis-inducing agent [17–25].

Ultraviolet solar radiation enhances the growth of melanoma. The mechanism of this enhancement is not fully understood; however, it is known that solar radiation can function not only as an initiator but also as a promoter of cancer development.

The effects of intermittent exposure to solar radiation are more prevalent in melanoma cases than those from chronic exposures. Induction usually occurs during childhood, and sunlight can also function as a promoter in the following years. Persons with chronic solar exposure are at lower risks of developing melanoma than persons with intermittent exposures. Thus, melanoma incidences are more common in indoor working persons than in outdoor workers, occurring on parts of the body that are only occasionally exposed to sunlight. Almost all BCC and SCC of human nonmelanoma cancers occur on chronic exposures to sunlight, mainly on the head, neck, and hands. There is a clear association between the cumulative sun exposures and incidences of the nonmelanoma cancers.

The precursors of melanoma may appear at an early age of one to five years, either as melanocytic naevi (Greek *naevi*, i.e., moles, birthmarks) which increase in numbers and disappear by the age of 15 to 25, or as dysplastic naevi, i.e., atypical moles that can have malignant characteristics. The typical benign moles, i.e., melanocytic naevi are regularly shaped with tan or brown color. Persons with this type of mole are at some risk of eventually developing melanoma. Atypical moles, i.e., dysplastic naevi are large and irregularly shaped with tan and brown color. Persons with this type of moles are at about 80% risk of developing melanoma. These pigmented lesions may appear in childhood at ages 5 to 6 years. The number of naevi is directly proportional to the exposure to sunlight during the early ages of life. Moles usually regress by the age of 15 to 25, and, at advanced ages, the moles are usually absent. Thus, it was found that each year out of 7000 cases with common naevi and 80 with dysplastic naevi, only one melanoma case is diagnosed. About 5 percent of melanomas also regress. Since it is believed that melanomas are caused in part by a convoluted mechanism involving immunosuppression, the regression is probably associated with the restoration of the immune system and apoptosis. The progression of naevi to melanomas is a slow process and may commence at the age of 30 or later. Many mammalian melanomas contain mutations and inactivations in the p53 gene and in the tumor suppressor gene CDKN2A involving methylation processes of the cytosine sites and resulting in the formation of 5-methylcytosines that are converted into thymines by a deamination process [17–25].

Although the cancer precursors; such as the solar keratoses, moles, papillomas, naevi, and other lesions of the skin; and, finally, the manifestation of the cancerous growth can be clinically well diagnosed and treated, the ultimate question arises whether all of these visual signs and possible markers, such as the mutated genes, are propagated during the whole process over many decades until the appearance of the cancerous lesions, or is one, at present, following the wrong trails.

How can one be sure that skin cancer formation is prevented by elimination of the precursors, such as keratinocytes and naevi? It is possible that, besides these and other markers that may or may not develop into the cancerous state after decades of incubation following induction by solar radiation, there exist precancerous cell types, such as cancerous pluripotent stem cells, which cannot be detected and clinically treated at the present time [17, 18, 26–45].

Unlike normal healthy cells, which are continuously dividing, producing progeny copies, and eventually dying out, the cancerous stem cells can undergo differentiation, divide only occasionally, can remain in a resting phase for prolonged periods of time, and are not affected by regular treatments with anticancer drugs. It is possible that these stem cells, which comprise only a small fraction of all cells, are determining the outcome of skin cancers, and the bulk of other cells are inconsequential. The challenge, then, is to be able clinically to recognize these cancerous stem cells and to devise methods for clinical treatments at the early stages of cutaneous cancer development, i.e., at the precursor and precancerous stages.

iii. Topical Applications of Sunscreens for the Prevention of Human Skin Cancers. A Critical Evaluation of the Present Status

At present, there is uncertainty concerning the cancer-preventing effectiveness of sunscreen applications to the human skin [13, 16, 47–63]. Frequently, the experimental results and conclusions of various investigations are at variance because of the differing experimental conditions, such as the sources of UV radiations, modes of application of sunscreen agents, and the selection of sunscreens and their sunscreen protection factor (SPF). These, in turn, are affected by variables, such as the type of human skin, sweating, amount of sunscreen, frequency of application, and duration of the experiments, which ideally should be conducted over a period of years [13, 16, 47]. However, it was shown in several randomized trials that sunscreen use can moderately reduce the occurrence of squamous cell carcinoma, while no such effect was observed with basal cell carcinoma and cutaneous malignant melanoma [62, 63]. There is also some evidence that the use of sunscreens can reduce the risk of developing actinic keratosis that might be viewed as a precancerous state for the SCC lesions [62, 63]. However, the transformation rate of actinic keratosis to SCC appears to be low [17]. Nevertheless, these lesions could be considered as possible markers for SCC [59–76]. In cases of malignant melanomas, statistical analyses of case-control studies render no clear support for a causal relationship between the use of sunscreens and the development of malignant melanomas [59–75]. The mutagenicity and carcinogenicity of sunscreen agents have been reported [17, 77, 78].

With the advent of heavy use of sunscreen products, there has been promulgated a fallacious belief that sunscreens with high SPF values, diligently applied to the human body according to rules by the FDA, will enable not only the prediction of the onset of erythema but also the onsets of immunosuppression, UV degradation of DNA, skin cancers, and other maladies. However, it has been slowly recognized that the onsets of immunosuppression and other maladies occur at suberythemal doses of solar-simulating radiations and, hence, knowing the SPF value of the sunscreen formulation, one cannot use it to predict the onset of, for example, the UV-induced skin cancers [56, 79].

iv. Repair of the UV Radiation Damaged Components of Human Skin by Topical Applications of Photolyase Enzymes, the Endonuclease T4N5, and T-Oligonucleotides

The topical applications to the skin of ultraviolet light energy absorbing substances, such as sunscreens, have a purely prophylactic effect; i.e., after damage to the skin has occurred, no sunscreen application can revert the damage. Recently, it was shown that topical applications to the human skin of a DNA repair enzyme, i.e., a photolyase, can mediate the removal of cyclobutane pyrimidine dimers, and even prevent the UVB radiation-induced immunosuppressive effects [80–93]. The photolyase enzyme is not found in the human skin. In active form, this enzyme is found in many prokaryotes and in certain eukaryotes, such as fish and poach animals.

Similar results were obtained with liposomal preparations containing the DNA repair enzymes T4 endonuclease V (T4N5) and T-oligonucleotides. These enzymes, applied topically to the skin of patients were studied for their penetration into the skin and their effects on repairs of UV light induced DNA damages [25, 93].

v. The Chemotherapy of Skin Cancers

The medicinal treatments of human skin cancers in clinical oncology are surgery, radiation, and chemotherapy, often in combination with radiation, such as photodynamic therapy [1–4, 15, 95, 96]. The anticancer drugs against skin cancers can be categorized into several diverse chemical classes [3, 4] such as chloroethylnitroso alkylating agents CCNU (lomustine, **1**), MeCNU (semustine, **2**), BCNU (carmustine, **3**), and fotemustine; various antibiotics and alkaloids, such as vincristine, actinomycin and rubomycin (**10**); antimetabolites such as 5-fluorouracil (5-FU); and the alkylating drugs, triazene, 5-(3,3-dimethyl-1-triazenyl)-*H*-imidazole-4-carboxamide (dacarbazine, DTIC, **9**) [97–102], and temozolomide (Temodar®), an analog of DTIC [94]. The combinations of the drugs DTIC, BCNU, and vincristine; or MeCNU and fotemustine; or CCNU and DTIC; seem to be the most effective treatments of melanomas in clinical oncology [101]. Unfortunately, the alkylating drugs are very toxic, causing bone marrow toxicities and other side effects. In addition, the drugs fluorouracil, vinblastine, an analog of vincristine, dacarbazine (**9a**), and methotrexate can undergo photosensitization reactions similar to the photodynamic therapy drugs, i.e., absorption of solar energy radiations, resulting in structural changes and formation of reactive oxygen species [103, 104]. Further drugs for melanoma chemotherapy are the cyclophosphamide (Endoxan, **11**), bleomycin, the platinum compound cisplatin, vinblastine, interferon-alpha 2b, tamoxifen, and interleukin-2. Various combinations of these drugs, including carmustine and DTIC have been clinically evaluated and compared with DTIC against the metastatic melanoma [3, 4, 94, 105, 106]. The humanized monoclonal antibody drugs Cetuximab® (Erbitux®) and Bevacizumab were introduced into clinical oncology to target and block the epidermal growth factor receptor (EGFR) for the treatment of various cancers, including the squamous cell carcinoma (SCC) of the neck and head [94, 105, 106], and malignant melanoma [94]. The antibody treatment is more effective in combination with cisplatin, 5-FU, and methotrexate, and other combinations [105, 106].

No efforts have been spared during the past decades to find biological entities for the cure of skin cancers, in particular the malignant melanoma. Since the malignant melanoma can be considered an immunogenic cancer, the applications of immunotherapeutic entities have been intensively explored with some success, i.e., interleukin-2, interferon-alpha-2b, and the humanized antibodies Erbitux®, Cetuximab® and Bevacizumab. In addition, a series of small molecules for various biological targets have been introduced into clinical trials [20, 22, 94, 105, 106].

Investigations have also been aimed at restoring the inactivated cancer suppressor gene p53. Thus, adenovirus entities were developed either to restore the deactivated p53 or to kill the cells that contain the p53 mutations. Numerous attempts have been made to develop melanoma vaccines using melanoma antigens, albeit with mixed results.

The humanized papilloma virus (HPV) was found to be active against SCC cancer cells. In another approach, substances with antiangiogenic and immune-modulating properties, such as thalidomide alone or in combination with temozolomide, have been tested in phase II trials against melanoma and brain tumor. Unfortunately, most of these and other trials have not culminated to date in persuasive results, except for brain tumors. Nevertheless, in spite of the limited advances in immunotherapy of melanoma, there is well-founded hope that melanoma cancerous stem cells will be sensitive to immunotherapy [26–46].

vi. The Influences of Nitroxyl Radical Moieties on the Lipophilicities, Activities, and Detoxifying Effects of Anticancer Drugs

During the past forty years, extensive efforts have been made in search of parameters that would enable one to make predictive designs of anticancer drugs [101, 107]. To achieve this goal, some studies were aimed at the correlations of structure–activity relationship (SAR and QSAR) parameters, involving the correlations of lipophilicity, i.e., hydrophilic and hydrophobic properties of drugs obtained in vitro, with the anticancer activities of drugs obtained in vivo [98, 100]. Thus, the correlations of logarithmic plots of the partition coefficient parameters of drugs in vitro against the percent increase in life span (% ILS) parameter in vivo using mice infected with either the lymphocytic P388 or the lymphoid L1210 leukemia ranged in cases of the most active drugs on average between log *P* values of –1.5 and +2.5 [98]. The following experimental data may serve to clarify the aim of such correlations: activities (% ILS) for anticancer drugs: SLCNU-1 (**4**) 542 > SLCNU-2 (**5**) 514 > CCNU (**1**) 192 > MeCCNU (**2**) 145, and the corresponding lipophilicities, log *P* (**4**) 1.58, (**5**) 1.67, (**1**) 2.55, (**2**) 3.25 [**Fig. 2G.vi-1**]. These types of study have been primarily conducted with the clinically used alkylating drugs, such as thio-TEPA, nitrosoureas, and chloroethylnitrosoureas and their nitroxyl (aminoxyl) congeners [98, 99, 108–110]. The modifications of clinical drugs by introduction of the nitroxyl moiety have been shown on many occasions to enhance the activities and lower the toxicities of the spin-labeled congener drugs [98–100, 107]. Further analogs of these spin-labeled drugs include amino acids and peptides [101–107], carbohydrates [108–110], triazenoimidazole derivatives [111–116], and the antibiotic rubomycin [117–119].

The nitroxyl (aminoxyl) radicals have been used in organic chemistry, medicinal chemistry [97, 101, 126–137], and biological and industrial [129–132] applications, and a huge literature has been generated over the years. The nitroxyl species are sterically hindered paramagnetic organic free radicals that are stable at room temperatures and can be stored for prolonged periods of time. However, they can be readily reduced to the corresponding hydroxylamine derivatives [133]. In extra- and intracellular biological environments, the reduction can be caused by the ubiquitous ascorbic acid, which is present in many organs of the human body in concentrations of 1–40 μg/mL [12]. The nitroxyl radicals, with structures that have been used in the syntheses of most spin-labeled anticancer drugs, were found to be nontoxic and nonmutagenic [127, 128]. Because of their paramagnetic properties, nitroxyl-labeled compounds have been extensively studied in biomedical environments by electron paramagnetic resonance (EPR) spectroscopy, and there exists an extensive literature on applications of EPR spectroscopy in biological systems [101, 134–139]. (See **Section 1C** on melanins.)

In connection with the present topic, EPR spectroscopy can be applied to measurements of the partition coefficients of spin-labeled drugs [100, 107, 135], their reducibility and permeability of cell membranes, and of the extra- and intracellular content of molecular oxygen [136, 137]. The permeability of spin-labeled drugs through cell membranes will depend, in part, not only on the reducibility of the nitroxyl function [137–139], but also on the nature of other substituents in the molecule [138]. Thus, it was found that ionizable weak acid and amine substituents would not hinder a rapid equilibration across erythrocyte membranes, whereas strong acid and quaternary substituents would prevent the migration [138]. The activity of spin-labeled drugs and their reduced congeners will also be affected by their p*Ka* values. Thus, it was shown that the neutral nitroxyl labeled drugs will have higher activities and lower partition coefficients than the reduced congeners, i.e., the hydroxylamines with p*Ka* values of 4.0–6.3 and the secondary amines with p*Ka* values of 7.7–11.7 [140].

On the basis of results obtained with spin-labeled drugs and leukemias, it was anticipated that the spin-labeled anticancer drugs would be as effective against the malignant melanomas. Indeed, this prediction was realized [106, 144–147]. Thus, the spin-labeled 2-chloroethyl-1-nitrosoureas SLCNU-1 (**4**), SLCNU-2 (**5**), the amino acid derivatives **6a–f**, the tyrosine derivatives TNU (**7a**) and MTNU (**7b**), the 1-alkyl-1-nitroso spin-labeled ureas **8a–d**, the spin-labeled analog SL-DTIC (**9b**) of DTIC (**9a**), and the spin-labeled rubomycin (**10b**), which had a lower cardiotoxicity than **10a**, were all more active and less toxic than the precursor parent drugs against the B16 melanoma [101, 121–125, 141–147]. All spin-labeled drugs were characterized by low carbamoylating properties, in contrast to the unlabeled precursor drugs, which, in general, have higher carbamoylating and lower alkylating properties.

Sometimes, a simple addition of a nitroxyl radical to a drug can have a potentiating effect on the drug. Thus, the addition of 4-hydroxy-2,2,6,6-tetramethylpiperidin-1-oxyl (TEMPO) to 6-mercaptopurine, an antineoplastic and immunosuppressive drug used primarily for the treatment of acute leukemia, augmented the activity and reduced the toxicity of the drug to some extent [148]. This effect of the nitroxyl radical was attributed to its general antioxidant property.

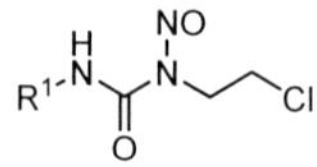

No.	R^1	Abbrev.
1	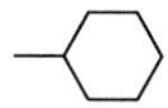	CCNU
2	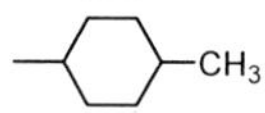	MeCCNU
3	$-CH_2CH_2Cl$	BCNU
4	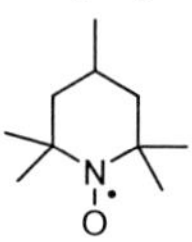	SLCNU-1
5	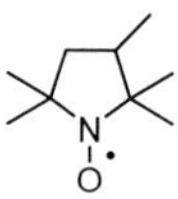	SLCNU-2

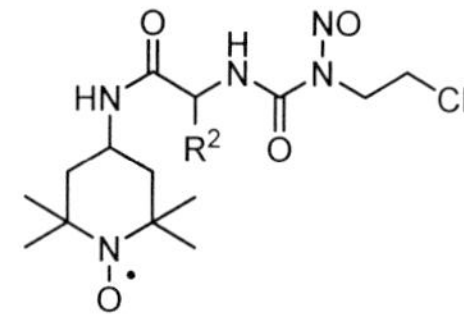

No.	R^2	Abbrev.
6a	H	SLCNU-gly
6b	CH_3	SLCNU-ala
6c	$(CH_3)_2CHCH_2$	SLCNU-leu
6d	$CH_3SCH_2CH_2$	SLCNU-met
6e	$PhCH_2$	SLCNU-phe
6f	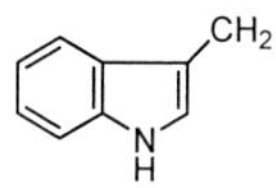	SLCNU-trp

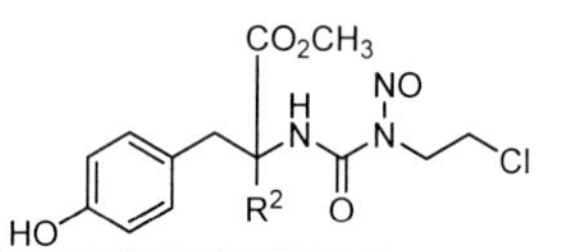

No.	R^2	Abbrev.
7a	H	TNU
7b	CH_3	MTNU

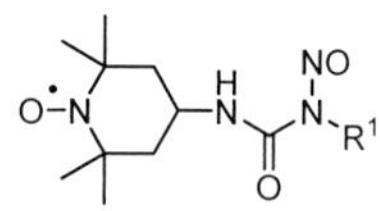

No.	R^1	Abbrev.
8a	CH_3	SLMNU
8b	CH_3CH_2	SLENU
8c	$(CH_3)_2CH$	SLPNU
8d	$CH_3(CH_2)_3$	SLBNU

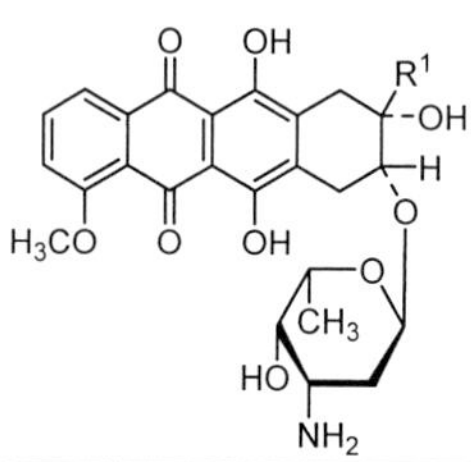

No.	R^1
10a	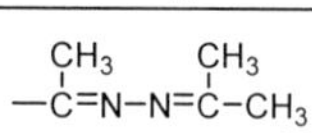
10b	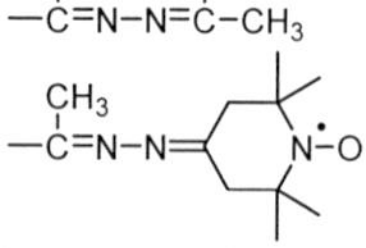

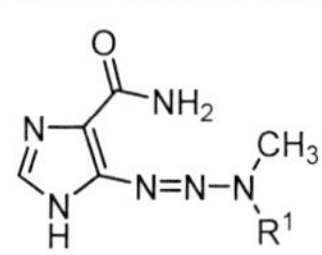

No.	R^1	Abbrev.
9a	CH_3	DTIC
9b	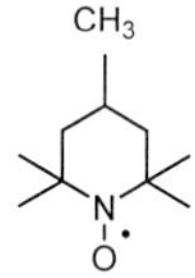	SLDTIC

Fig. 2G.vi-1. Structures of anticancer drugs.

In another case, a pretreatment of rabbits with TEMPO prior to administering CCNU (**1**) caused a lowering of the general toxicity as compared to the effect of CCNU alone. This result was explained by the reactions of nitroxyls with the toxic, metabolically produced free radical species [148]. Similarly, the nitroxyl radical species of the spin-labeled rubomycin (**10b**) undergo reactions with unstable radicals that are formed during the metabolism of the drug [101].

Nitroxyl radicals and nitric oxide have some similarities in their chemical and biochemical properties, and the presence of nitroxyl radicals can have a modulatory effect on the toxicity of nitric oxide. Nitric oxide, a radical species, resembles nitroxyls. It is formed in human endothelial cells, in neurons of the brain, and in macrophages during inflammation processes [150]. Nitric oxide is a neurotransmitter, a blood pressure regulator, a vasodilator, an inhibitor of adhesion, and is involved in the activation and aggregation of platelets, programmed cell death, and many other functions in human health and diseases, in particular, in cancers [147,150–152]. Nitric oxide is also produced during the metabolism of anticancer drugs containing the nitrosourea moiety, such as the clinically used CCNU (**1**). The reaction of nitric oxide with the superoxide anion radical ($O_2\cdot^-$) results in the formation of the very toxic peroxynitrite species O–N–O–O^- H^+. (See **Sections 3** and **4** and references therein.) However, since the nitroxyl species is a mimic of the superoxide dismutase enzyme (SOD), the competitive reaction of nitroxyl radicals with the superoxide anion radical ($O_2\cdot^-$) can prevent, to some extent, the formation of the peroxynitrite species. (See **Sections 3** and **4**.) It was hypothesized that such competitive reactions occur in the case of spin-labeled drugs, such as SLCNU-1 (**4**), resulting in higher activity and lower toxicity values than those obtained with the clinically used CCNU drug [147]. The role of nitric oxide in sunscreens as either a mitigating or promoting agent in skin cancers, such as melanoma, is somewhat controversial [153, 154]. However, it is believed that nitric oxide is involved in the inhibitory process of malignant cells, and extensive studies have been conducted on the therapeutic effects of nitric oxide on cancers, in particular, the malignant melanoma [155–163]. It was found that addition of nitric oxide in the form of a donor compound, such as 3,3-bis(nitroxylmethyl)oxetane (**12**) [**Fig. 2G(vi)-2**], can also have a modulatory enhancing effect on the anticancer activities of various anticancer drugs [165].

Thus, a combination of clinically used drugs, such as cyclophosphamide (**11**), cisplatin and adriamycin, with certain nitric oxide (NO) donors, e.g., compound **12**, results in a synergistic effect on the effectiveness of the chemotherapy, as measured by the percent increase in life span parameter (% ILS) in vitro using the lymphocytic leukemia P388, lymphoid leukemia L1210, and the transplantable intracerebral leukemia P388 in vivo [165]. In addition, the drug combination was found to have an inhibitory effect on the development of drug resistance [165]. The combination therapy also had an antimetastatic effect in the inhibition of melanoma B16 in vivo. Thus, the metastatic inhibition index, using a 30mg/kg dose of cyclophosphamide (**11**), was 50%, while the combination of the drug with a nitric oxide donor resulted in an improvement of the index to about 80% [155].

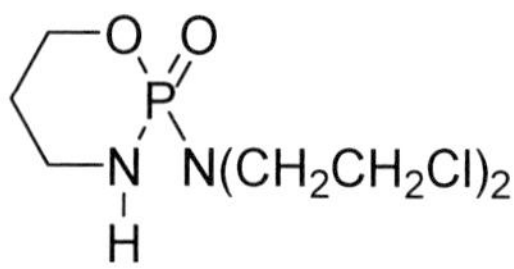

11

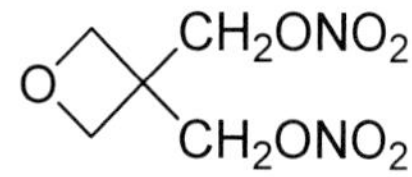

12

Fig. 2G(vi)-2. Clinically used drug cyclophosphamide (**11**) and donor compound 3,3-bis(nitroxylmethyl)oxetane (**12**).

vii. The Effects of Nitroxyl Radical Species on the Tyrosinase-Mediated Oxidations of L-Tyrosine and L-Dopa to L-Dopaquinone and on the Alkylating and Carbamoylating Properties of Anticancer Drugs

The facile interactions of nitroxyl labeled drugs with melanins and melanomas, their increased alkylating and decreased carbamoylating properties, their decreased toxicity and increased anticancer activities as compared to the unlabeled congeners, and the influence of the nitroxyl species on the tyrosinase enzyme mediated oxidation have been investigated in a series of studies [165–169].

The tyrosinase enzyme, composed of three isozymes and copper cations, mediates, in the presence of oxygen, the oxidations of the initial intermediates, i.e., L-tyrosine and L-DOPA, in the multistage process of formation of eumelanin polymers. This radicaloid-type oxidation is a copper cation catalyzed reaction, i.e., the catalytic amounts of copper cations are the actual oxidant, and molecular oxygen is destined to serve to restore the reduced cuprous cation to the cupric cation. (See section on melanins.) Based on such a mechanism, it would be intuitively expected that the nitroxyl species, either alone or as part of a spin-labeled drug, could exert an enhancing effect on this oxidative process. Thus, taking into account **Schemes 1C-8** to **1C-10** and **1C-14** of the melanin section (Section 1C), one could envisage the following oxidative redox processes [**Sch 2G(vii)-1**].

Thus, in an intracellular environment, in the case of nitroxyl-labeled drugs, the toxic superoxide anion radicals ($O_2{\cdot}^-$) would be continuously eliminated, while in the presence of unlabeled drug analogs an accumulation of the toxic species ($O_2{\cdot}^-$) would inevitably occur. Indeed, it has been found that most nitroxyl-labeled compounds, including anticancer drugs, have this enhancing property [101, 143, 145, 166–169]. In contrast, the clinically used unlabeled drugs, such as CCNU (**1**) and DTIC (**9a**), are lacking the superoxide anion radical ($O_2{\cdot}^-$) scavenging activity, and are more toxic than the spin-labeled congeners, perhaps, in part, because of this deficiency.

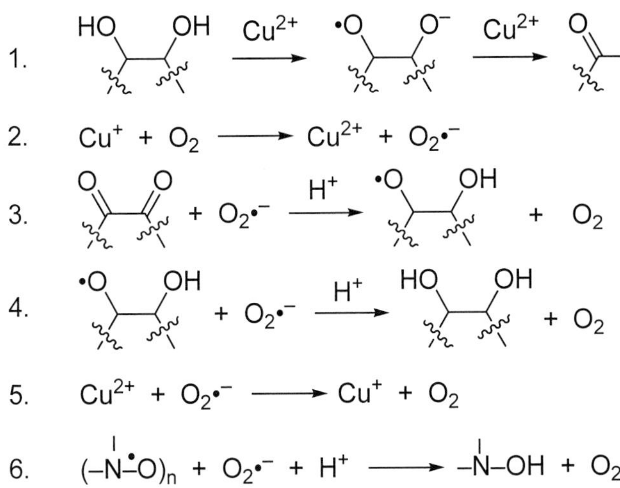

Sch 2G(vii)-1. Mechanisms of tyrosine enzyme mediated oxidations and the enhancing effect of nitroxyl species. Step 1: oxidations of hydroquinones to quinones via semiquinones; Step 2: restoration of the cupric cation; Steps 3–5: retroactive, inhibitory reactions; Step 6: nitroxyl radicals as superoxide dismutase mimic, an enhancing reaction (n = excess of nitroxyl species).

Furthermore, the enhancement of the conversion of L-tyrosine and L-DOPA to L-dopaquinone could also involve an additional, nonenzymatic pseudo superoxide dismutase reaction of nitroxyl moieties with the hydroxyl groups of L-tyrosine and L-DOPA, whereby the nitroxyl radical could function as an acceptor of hydrogen atoms, according to **Sch. 1C-11** (melanin Section 1C), thereby enhancing the formation of L-dopaquinone without the formation of superoxide anion radicals.

The clinical drugs CCNU (**1**), and the antimelanoma active experimental tyrosine derivatives TNU (**7a**) and MTNU (**7b**), all devoid of the nitroxyl moiety, had highly inhibitory activities in the tyrosinase-mediated oxidations, while the spin-labeled compounds SLMNU (**8a**), SLPNU (**8c**), SLENU (**8b**), SLBNU (**8d**), and SLCNU-tyr (**6f**) were found to have strongly activating effects up to 90 minutes of an incubation period [101]. SLCNU-1 (**4**) and most spin-labeled amino acid derivatives (**6a–e**) had a two-stage effect, i.e., up to 60 minutes of incubation, an activating and, after 90 minutes, a deactivating effect. This dualism of effects was attributed to the formation, during the sixty minutes, of alkylating species causing the activating effect, while the deactivating effect was attributed to a carbamoylating reaction resulting from the slowly emerging isocyanate species, after sixty minutes of the incubation period [101]. Compounds that are devoid of 2-chloroethyl groups usually have longer half-lives and no inhibitory phase, since their degradations produce either little or no isocyanate species. The spin-labeled 2-chloroethylnitrosoureas have, in general, shorter half-lives and lower carbamoylation and higher alkylation potentials than the unlabeled congeners, such as the clinically used CCNU (**1**).

In a biological environment, the metabolic fragmentation of the 2-chloroethylnitrosourea drugs, such as CCNU (**1**), proceeds by various and exceedingly complex mechanisms, resulting in the formation of a number of entities [98].

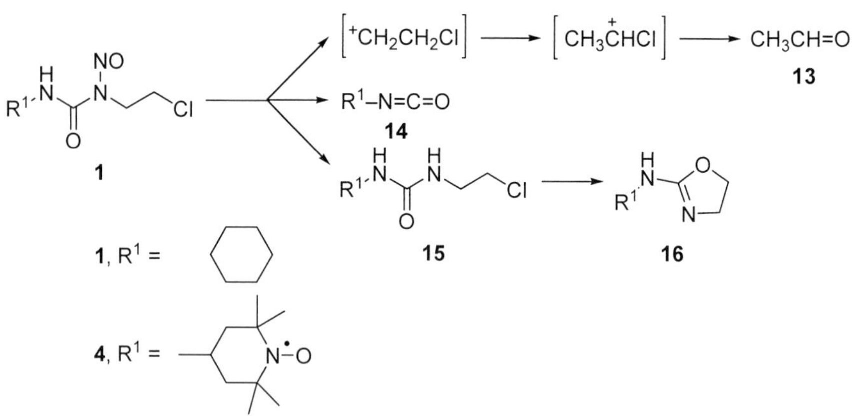

Sch 2G(vii)-2. Simplified metabolic fragmentation of 1-(2-chloroethyl)-3-cyclohexyl-1-nitrosourea.

In one such metabolic fragmentation of CCNU (**1**) under physiological conditions at 37 °C and pH 7.4, the following metabolites, among other products, were analytically elucidated: acetaldehyde (**13**), cyclohexyl isocyanate (**14**), 1-(2-chloroethyl)-3-cyclohexylurea (**15**), and 2-(cyclohexylamino)-3-oxazoline (**16**) [**Sch 2G(vii)-2**] [98].

The drug CCNU (**1**) and the congener drugs are classified as alkylating drugs, i.e., they are, in part, metabolized to electrophilic species [**Sch 2G(vii)-2**], which are then supposed to selectively interact with the DNA in cancer cells. In addition, the metabolic fragmentation yields the isocyanate species that undergo carbamoylation reactions with hydroxyl, amino, and mercapto groups of biological entities. The general toxicity of the alkylating drugs is mainly attributed to these carbamoylation reactions. Metabolite **16** could be considered a trap for the isocyanate species, thereby either delaying, diminishing, or precluding the formation of the isocyanate metabolite in quantity. One could hypothesize that analogous metabolic fragmentation of the nitroxyl-labeled congeners, such as SLCNU-1 (**4**) would result in analogous nitroxyl-labeled metabolites **14** and **16**.

Unlike the metabolites derived from CCNU (**1**), these spin-labeled metabolites would have additional powerful properties. Thus, they could undergo oxidative reactions by hydrogen atom abstraction, reactions as superoxide dismutase mimics thus inhibiting the production of superoxide anion radical ($O_2{\cdot}^-$) in a biological environment. This hypothesis may serve to explain a number of reactions of spin-labeled drugs as compared to those of unlabeled congeners.

References

1. Carter S. K., Bakowski M. T. and Hellmann K. (1987) *Chemotherapy of Cancer*, 3rd ed. Churchill Livingstone, New York.
2. Taleisnik A. (1994) Malignancies of the skin. In: *Practical Oncology - a Lange Clinical Manual*, 1st ed., pp 133–143, Cameron R. B. (ed.), Appleton & Lange, Norwalk.
3. Pazdur R., Coia L. R., Hoskins W. J. and Wagman L. D. (eds.) (2003) *Cancer Management: A Multidisciplinary Approach*, 7th ed., The Oncology Group, a Division of SCP Communications, Inc., New York.
4. Pazdur R., Wagman L. D., Camphausen K. A. and Hoskins W. J. (eds.) (2008) *Cancer Management: A Multidisciplinary Approach,* 11th ed., Medical, Surgical & Radiation Oncology, CMPMedica LLC, a United Business Media Company.

5. Ries L. A. G., Harkins D., Krapcho M., Mariotto A., Miller B. A., Feuer E. J., Clegg L., Eisner M. P., Horner M. J., Howlader N., Hayat M., Hankey B. F. and Edwards B. K. (eds.) (2009) Surveillance Epidemiology and End Results. *SEER Cancer Statistics Review, 1975–2003*, National Cancer Institute, Bethesda.
6. Jemal A., Siegel R., Ward E., Murray T., Xu J. and Thun M. J. (2007) Cancer statistics, 2007. *Ca-Cancer J. Clin.* **57**: 43–46.
7. Grant W. B. (2008) Solar ultraviolet irradiance and mortality. In: *Sunlight, Vitamin D and Skin Cancer*, pp 16–30, Reichrath J. (ed.), Springer Science + Business Media, LLC, New York, and Landes Bioscience, Austin, TX.
8. Leiter U. and Garbe C. (2008) Epidemiology of melanoma and non-melanoma skin cancer – the role of sunlight. In: *Sunlight, Vitamin D and Skin Cancer*, pp 89–103, Reichrath J. (ed.), Springer Science + Business Media, LLC, New York, and Landes Bioscience, Austin, TX.
9. Berwick M., Lachiewicz A., Pestak C. and Thomas N. (2008) Solar UV exposure and mortality from skin tumors. In: *Sunlight, Vitamin D and Skin Cancer*, pp 117–124, Reichrath J. (ed.), Springer Science + Business Media, LLC, New York, and Landes Bioscience, Austin, TX.
10. Beddingfield F. C., 3rd (2003) The melanoma epidemic: res ipsa loquitur. *Oncologist* **8**: 448–450 and **8**: 459–465.
11. Tyrrell R. M. (1994) The molecular and cellular pathology of solar ultraviolet radiations. *Mol. Aspects Med.* **15**: 1–77.
12. Fuchs J. (1992) *Oxidative injury in dermatopathology*, Springer Verlag, Berlin.
13. Vainio H. and Bianchini F. (eds.) (2001) Sunscreens. In: *IARC Handbooks of Cancer Prevention*, Vol. 5, International Agency for Research on Cancer, WHO, Lyon.
14. Wang S. Q., Setlow R., Berwick M., Polsky D., Marghoob A. A., Kopf A. W. and Bart R. S. (2001) Ultraviolet A and melanoma: a review. *J. Am. Acad. Dermatol.* **44**: 837–846.
15. Francis S. O., Mahlberg M. J., Johnson K. R., Ming M. E. and Dellavalle R. P. (2006) Melanoma chemoprevention. *J. Am. Acad. Dermatol.* **55**: 849–861.
16. IARC (1992) Solar and Ultraviolet Radiation. In: *IARC Monograph on the Evaluation of Carcinogenic Risks to Humans*, Vol. 55, pp 1–316, International Agency for Research on Cancer, Lyon.

17. Brash D. E. and Ponten J. (1998) Skin precancer. In: *Cancer Surveys*, Vol. 32, pp 69–113, Precancer: Biology, Importance and Possible Prevention, Imperial Cancer Research Fund.
18. Ponten J. (1998) Cell biology of precancer. In: *Cancer Surveys*, Vol. 32 pp 5–35, Precancer: Biology, Importance and Possible Prevention, Imperial Cancer Research Fund.
19. De Gruijl F. R. and van Kranen H. J. (2001) UV radiation, mutations and oncogenic pathways in skin cancer. In: *Sun Protection in Man*, pp 287–302, Giacomoni, P. U. (ed.), Elsevier, Amsterdam.
20. Domingo D. S. and Baron E. (2008) Melanoma and nonmelonoma skin cancers and the immune system. In: *Sunlight, Vitamin D and Skin Can*cer, pp 187–202, Reichrath J. (ed.), Springer Science + Business Media, LLC, New York, and Landes Bioscience, Austin, TX.
21. Hoban P. and Strange R. (2007) Genetic background and UVR-induced skin cancer. In: *Biophysical and Physiological Effects of Solar Radiation on Human Skin*, pp 165–189, Giacomoni P. U. (ed.), The Royal Society of Chemistry, Cambridge, U.K.
22. Xie J. (2008) Molecular biology of basal and squamous cell carcinomas. In: *Sunlight, Vitamin D and Skin Cancer*, pp 241–251, Reichrath J. (ed.), Springer Science + Business Media, LLC, New York, and Landes Bioscience, Austin, TX.
23. Erb P., Ji J., Kump E., Mielgo A. and Wernli M. (2008) Apoptosis and pathogenesis of melanoma and nonmelanoma skin cancer. In: *Sunlight, Vitamin D and Skin Cancer*, pp 283–295, Reichrath J. (ed.), Springer Science + Business Media, LLC, New York, and Landes Bioscience, Austin, TX.
24. Rass K. and Reichrath J. (2008) UV damage and DNA repair in malignant melanoma and nonmelonoma skin cancer. In: *Sunlight, Vitamin D and Skin Cancer*, pp 162–178, Reichrath J. (ed.), Springer Science + Business Media, LLC, New York, and Landes Bioscience, Austin, TX.
25. Yarosh D. B. and Smiles K. A. (2009) DNA repair and photoprotection. In: *Clinical Guide to Sunscreen and Photoprotection*, pp 168–179, Lim H. W. and Draelos Z. D. (eds.), Informa Healthcare, New York.
26. Reya T., Morrison S. J., Clarke M. F. and Weissman I. L. (2001) Stem cells, cancer, and cancer stem cells. *Nature* **414**: 105–111.
27. Weissman I. (2005) Stem cell research: paths to cancer therapies and regenerative medicine. *JAMA* **294**: 1359–1366.

28. Wang J. C. and Dick J. E. (2005) Cancer stem cells: lessons from leukemia. *Trends Cell Biol.* **15**: 494–501.
29. Hurt E. M. and Farrar W. L. (2008) Cancer stem cells: the seeds of metastasis? *Mol. Interventions* **8**: 140–142.
30. Chan W. Z. and Huntly B. J. (2008) Leukemia stem cells in acute myeloid leukemia. *Semin. Oncol.* **35**: 326–335.
31. Zabierowski S. E. and Herlyn M. (2008) Melanoma stem cells: the dark seed of melanoma. *J. Clin. Oncol.* **26**: 2890–2894.
32. Houben R., Wischhusen J., Menaa F., Synwoldt P., Schrama D., Bröcker E. B. and Becker J. C. (2008) Melanoma stem cells: targets for successful therapy? *J. Dtsch. Dermatol. Ges.* **6**: 541–546.
33. Schatton T. and Frank M. H. (2008) Cancer stem cells and human malignant melanoma. *Pigm. Cell Melanoma Res.* **21**: 39–55.
34. Lomas J., Martin-Duque P., Pons M. and Quintanilla M. (2008) The genetics of malignant melanoma. *Front Biosci.* **13**: 5071–5093.
35. Mimeault M. and Batra S. K. (2008) Targeting of cancer stem/progenitor cells plus stem cell-based therapies: the ultimate hope for treating and curing aggressive and recurrent cancers. *Panminerva Med.* **50**: 3–18.
36. Aboody K. S., Najbauer J. and Danks M. K. (2008) Stem and progenitor cell-mediated tumor selective gene therapy. *Gene Ther.* **15**: 739–52.
37. Schatton T., Murphy G. F., Frank N. Y., Yamaura K., Waaga-Gasser A. M., Gasser M., Zhan Q., Jordan S., Duncan L. M., Weishaupt C., Fuhl-brigge R. C., Kupper T. S., Sayegh M. H. and Frank M. H. (2008) Identification of cells initiating human melanomas. *Nature* **451**: 345–349.
38. Klein W. M., Wu B. P., Zhao S., Wu H., Klein-Szanto A. J. and Tahan S. R. (2007) Increased expression of stem cell markers in malignant melanoma. *Mod. Pathol.* **20**: 102–107.
39. Keshet G. I., Goldstein I., Itzhaki O., Cesarkas K., Shenhav L., Yakirevitch A., Treves A. J., Schachter J., Amariglio N. and Rechavi G. (2008) MDR1 expression identifies human melanoma stem cells. *Biochem. Biophys. Res. Commun.* **368**: 930–936.
40. Yu J. and Thomson J. A. (2008) Pluripotent stem cells lines. *Genes Dev.* **22**: 1987–1997.
41. Aboody K. S., Najbauer J., Schmidt N. O., Yang W., Przylecki W., Wu J. K., Zhuge Y., Carroll R., Black P. M. and Perides G. (2006) Targeting of melanoma brain metastases using engineered neural stem/progenitor cells. *Neuro. Oncol.* **8**: 119–126.

42. Crowe D. L., Parsa B. and Sinha U. K. (2004) Relationships between stem cells and cancer stem cells. *Histol. Histopathol.* **19**: 505–509.
43. Fang D., Nguyen T. K., Leishear K., Finko R., Kulp A. N., Hotz S., Van Belle P. A., Xu X., Elder D. E. and Herlyn M. (2005) A tumorigenic subpopulation with stem cell properties in melanomas. *Cancer Res.* **65**: 9328–9337.
44. Grichnik J. M., Burch J. A., Schulteis R. D., Shan S., Liu J., Darrow T. L., Vervaert C. E. and Seigler H. F. (2006) Melanoma, a tumor based on a mutant stem cell? *J. Invest. Dermatol.* **126**: 142–153.
45. Mimeault M., Hauke R., Mehta P. P. and Batra S. K. (2007) Recent advances in cancer stem/progenitor cell research: therapeutic implications for overcoming resistance to the most aggressive cancers. *J. Cell Mol. Med.* **11**: 981–1011.
46. Kirkwood J. M., Tarhini A. A., Panelli M. C., Moschos S. J., Zarour H. M., Butterfield L. H. and Gogas H. J. (2008) Next generation of immunotherapy for melanoma. *J. Clin. Oncol.* **26**: 3445–3455.
47. Edlich R. F., Winters K. L., Lim H. W., Cox M. J., Becker D. G., Horowitz J. H., Nichter L. S., Britt L. D. and Long W. B. (2004) Photoprotection by sunscreens with topical antioxidants and systemic antioxidants to reduce sun exposure. *J. Long-Term Eff. Med. Implants* **14**: 317–340.
48. Diffey B. L. (2005) Sunscreens and melanoma: the future looks bright. *Br. J. Dermatol.* **153**: 378–381.
49. Wolf P., Donawho C. K. and Kripke M. L. (1994) Effect of sunscreens on UV radiation-induced enhancement of melanoma growth in mice. *JNCI, J. Natl. Cancer Inst.* **86**: 99–105.
50. Al Mahroos M., Yaar M., Phillips T. J., Bhawan J. and Gilchrest B. A. (2002) Effect of sunscreen application on UV-induced thymine dimers. *Arch. Dermatol.* **138**: 1480–1485.
51. Dobak J. and Liu F. T. (1992) Sunscreens, UVA, and cutaneous malignancy: adding fuel to the fire. *Int. J. Dermatol.* **31**: 544–548.
52. Naylor M. F. and Farmer K. C. (1997) The case for sunscreens. A review of their use in preventing actinic damage and neoplasia. *Acta Dermatol.* **133**: 1146–1154.
53. Hemminki K., Xu G. and Le Curieux F. (2001) Ultraviolet radiation-induced photoproducts in human skin DNA as biomarkers of damage and its repair. In: *Biomarkers in Cancer Chemoprevention*, pp 69–73, Miller A. B., Bartsch H., Boffetta P., Dragsted L. and Vainio H. (eds.), IARC Scientific Publications No. 154, International Agency for Research on Cancer, Lyon.

54. Garland C. F., Garland F. C. and Gorham E. D. (1993) Rising trends in melanoma. An hypothesis concerning sunscreen effectiveness. *Ann. Epidemiol.* **3**: 103–110.
55. Rigel D. S. (2002) The effect of sunscreen on melanoma risk. *Dermatol. Clin.* **20**: 601–606.
56. Burren R., Scaletta C., Frenk E., Panizzon R. G. and Applegate L. A. (1998) Sunlight and carcinogenesis: expression of p53 and pyrimidine dimers in human skin following UVA I, UVA I + II and solar stimulating radiation. *Int. J. Cancer* **76**: 201–206.
57. Bastuji-Garin S. and Diepgen T. L. (2002) Cutaneous malignant melanoma, sun exposure, and sunscreen use: epidemiological evidence. *Br. J. Dermatol.* **146** (Suppl. 61): 24–30.
58. Lund L. P. and Timmins G. S. (2007) Melanoma, long wavelength ultraviolet and sunscreens: controversies and potential resolution. *Pharmacol. Ther.* **114**: 198–207.
59. Gefeller O. and Pfahlberg A. (2002) Sunscreen use and melanoma: a case of evidence-based prevention? *Photodermatol., Photoimmunol. Photomed.* **18**: 153–156.
60. Huncharek M. and Kupelnick B. (2002) Use of topical sunscreens and the risk of malignant melanoma meta-analysis of 9067 patients from 11 case-control studies. *Am. J. Public Health* **92**: 1173–1177.
61. Murphy G. M. and Hawk J. L. M. (2009) Sunscreens and photocarcinogenesis. In: *Clinical Guide to Sunscreens and Photoprotection*, pp 89–99, Lim H. W. and Draelos Z. D. (eds.), Informa Healthcare, New York.
62. Autier P. (2009) Sunscreen abuse for intentional sun exposure. *Br. J. Dermatol.* **161** (Suppl. 3): 40–45.
63. Autier P., Boniol M. and Dore J. F. (2007) Sunscreen use and increased duration of intentional sun exposure: Still a burning issue. *Int. J. Cancer.* **121**: 1–5.
64. Diffey B. L. (2001) Sunscreens: use and misuse. In: *Sun Protection in Man*, pp 521–534, Giacomoni, P. U. (ed.), Elsevier, Amsterdam.
65. Autier P. (2005) Cutaneous malignant melanoma: facts about sunbeds and sunscreen. *Expert Rev. Anticancer Ther.* **5**: 821–833.
66. Naldi L., Gallus S., Imberti G. L., Cainelli T., Negri E. and La Vecchia C. (2000) Sunscreens and cutaneous malignant melanoma: an Italian case-control study. *Int. J. Cancer* **86**: 879–882.
67. Gil E. M. and Kim T. H. (2000) UV-induced immune suppression and sunscreen. *Photodermatol., Photoimmunol. Photomed.* **16**: 101–110.

68. Westerdahl J., Ingvar C., Masback A. and Olsson H. (2000) Sunscreen use and malignant melanoma. *Int. J. Cancer* **87**: 145–150.
69. Vainio H., Miller A. B. and Bianchini F. (2000) An international evaluation of the cancer-preventive potential of sunscreens. *Int. J. Cancer* **88**: 838–842.
70. Vainio H. and Bianchini F. (2000) Cancer-preventive effects of sunscreens are uncertain. *Scand. J. Work, Environ. Health* **26**: 529–531.
71. Bens, G. (2008) Sunscreens. In: *Sunlight, Vitamin D and Skin Cancer*, pp 137–161, Reichrath J. (ed.), Springer Science and Business Media LLC, New York, and Landes Bioscience, Austin, TX.
72. Haywood R., Wardman P., Sanders R. and Linge C. (2003) Sunscreens inadequately protect against ultraviolet-A-induced free radicals in skin: implications for skin aging and melanoma? *J. Invest. Dermatol.* **121**: 862–868.
73. Dennis L. K., Beane Freeman L. E. and VanBeek M. J. (2003) Sunscreen use and the risk for melanoma: a quantitative review. *Ann. Intern. Med.* **139**: 966–978.
74. Maier T. and Korting H. C. (2005) Sunscreens – which and what for? *Skin Pharmacol. Physiol.* **18**: 253–262.
75. Diffey B. L. and Ferguson J. (2009) Assessment of photoprotective properties of sunscreens. In: *Clinical Guide to Sunscreens and Photoprotection*, pp 53–63, Lim H. W. and Draelos Z. D. (eds.), Informa Healthcare, New York.
76. Orentreich D., Leone A.-S., Arpino G. and Burack H. (2001) Sunscreens: practical applications. In: *Sun protection in Man*, pp 535–559, Giacomoni, P. U. (ed.), Elsevier Science, Amsterdam.
77. Knowland J., McKenzie E. A., McHugh P. J. and Cridland N. A. (1993) Sunlight-induced mutagenicity of common sunscreen ingredient. *FEBS Letters* **324**: 309–313.
78. McHugh P. J. and Knowland J. (1997) Characterization of DNA damage inflicted by free radicals from mutagenic sunscreen ingredients and its location using an in vitro genetic reversion assay. *Photochem. Photobiol.* **66**: 276–281.
79. Halliday G. M. and Hönigsmann (2009) Sunscreens, photoimmunosuppression, and photoaging. In: *Clinical Guide to Sunscreen and Photoprotection*, pp 101–116, Lim H. W. and Draelos Z. D. (eds.), Informa Healthcare, New York.
80. Krutmann J. (2001) New developments in photoprotection of human skin. *Skin Pharmacol. Appl. Skin Physiol.* **14**: 401–407
81. Krutmann J. (2001) Die Verwendung von topisch applizierten DNS-Reparaturenzymen zum Schutz der menschlichen Haut gegen UVB-

induzierte Schaden. *Bundesgesundheitsblatt-Gesundheitsforschung-Gesundheitsschutz* **44**: 480–483.

82. Stege H., Roza L., Vink A. A., Grewe M., Ruzicka T., Grether-Beck S. and Krutmann J. (2000) Enzyme plus light therapy to repair DNA damage in ultraviolet-B-irradiated human skin. *Proc. Natl. Acad. Sci. U. S. A.* **97**: 1790–1795.
83. Decome L., De Meo M., Geffard A., Doucet O., Dumenil G. and Botta A. Evaluation of photolyase (Photosome) repair activity in human keratinocytes after a single dose of ultraviolet B irradiation using the comet assay. *Photochem. Photobiol.* **79**: 101–108.
84. Hidema J., Taguchi T., Ono T., Teranishi M., Yamamoto K. and Kumagai T. (2007) Increase in CPD photolyase activity functions effectively to prevent growth inhibition caused by UVB radiation. *Plant J.* **50**: 70–79.
85. Butenandt J., Epple R., Wallenborn E. U., Eker A. P., Gramlich V. and Carell T. (2000) A comparative repair study of thymine- and uracil-photodimers with model compounds and a photolyase repair enzyme. *Chemistry* **6**: 62–72.
86. Schul W., Jans J., Rijksen Y. M., Klemann K. H., Eker A. P., de Wit J., Nikaido O., Nakajima S., Yasui A., Hoeijmakers J. H. and van der Horst G. T. (2002) Enhanced repair of cyclobutane pyrimidine dimers and improved UV resistance in photolyase transgenic mice. *EMBO J.* **21**: 4719–4729.
87. Sancar G. B. (1990) DNA photolyases: physical properties, action mechanism, and roles in dark repair. *Mutat. Res.* **236**: 147–160.
88. Garinis G. A., Jans J. and van der Horst G. T. (2006) Photolyases: capturing the light to battle skin cancer. *Future Oncol.* **2**: 191–199.
89. Garinis G. A., Mitchell J. R., Moorhouse M. J., Hanada K., de Waard H., Vandeputte D., Jans J., Brand K., Smid M., van der Spek P. J., Hoeijmakers J. H., Kanaar R. and van der Horst G. T. (2005) Transcriptome analysis reveals cyclobutane pyrimidine dimers as a major source of UV-induced DNA breaks. *EMBO J.* **24**: 3952–3962.
90. Essen L. O. and Klar T. (2006) Light-driven DNA repair by photolyases. *Cell Mol. Life Sci.* **63**: 1266–1277.
91. Jans J., Schul W., Sert Y. G., Rijksen V., Rebel H., Eker A. P. Nakajima S., van Steeg H., de Gruijl F. R., Yasui A., Hoeijmakers J. H. and van der Horst G. T. (2005) Powerful skin cancer protection by a CPD-photolyase transgene. *Curr. Biol.* **15**: 105–115.
92. Jans J., Garinis G. A., Schul W., van Oudenaren A., Moorhouse M., Smid M., Sert Y. G., van der Velde A., Rijksen Y., de Gruijl F. R., van der Spek P. J., Yasui A., Hoeijmakers J. H., Leenen P. J. and van

der Horst G. T. (2006) Differential role of basal keratinocytes in UV-induced immunosuppression and skin cancer. *Mol. Cell Biol.* **26**: 8515–8526.
93. Wolf P. (2007) DNA repair therapy. In: *Biophysical and Physiological Effects of Solar Radiation on Human Skin*, pp 321–332, Giacomoni P. U. (ed.), The Royal Society of Chemistry, Cambridge.
94. Rass K. and Tilgen W. (2008) Treatment of melanoma and nonmelanoma skin cancer. In: *Sunlight, Vitamin D and Skin Cancer*, pp 296–318, Reichrath J. (ed.), Springer Science+Business Media, LLC, New York, and Landes Bioscience, Austin, TX.
95. Dougherty T. J. (1981) Photosensitization of malignant tumors. *Semin. Surg. Oncol.* **2**: 24–37.
96. Kroon B. B. and Nieweg O. E. (2000) Management of malignant melanoma. *Ann. Chir. Gynaecol.* **89**: 242–250.
97. Sosnovsky G., Li S. W. and Rao N. U. M. (1987) In the search for new anticancer drugs. XXI spin labeled nitrosoureas. *Z. Naturforsch.* **42c**: 921–931.
98. Gnewuch C. T. and Sosnovsky G. (1997) A critical appraisal of the evolution of *N*-nitrosoureas as anticancer drugs. *Chem. Rev.* **97**: 829–1013.
99. Sosnovsky G. and Li S. W. (1985) 1-(2-Chloroethyl)-3-(1-oxyl-2,2,6,6-tetramethylpiperidinyl)-1-nitrosourea. *Drugs Future* **10**: 211–212.
100. Sosnovsky G. (1990) The quest for a predictive design of anticancer drugs. *Pure Appl. Chem.* **62**: 289–294.
101. Raikov Z. D., Raikova E. T., Zheleva A. M. and Gadzheva V. G. (2000) *Spin-labelled antitumor compounds*, pp 1–183, Robev S. K. (ed.).
102. Comis R. L. (1976) DTIC (NSC-54388) in malignant melanoma: a perspective. *Cancer Treat. Rep.* **60**: 165–176.
103. Moore D. E. (2002) Drug-induced cutaneous photosensitivity. Incidence, mechanism, prevention and management. *Drug Safety* **25**: 345–372.
104. Marrot L. and Meunier J.-R. (2008) Skin DNA photodamage and its biological consequences. *J. Am. Acad. Dermatol.* **58** (5 Suppl. 2): S139–S148.
105. Harding J. and Burtness B. (2005) Cetuximab: an epidermal growth factor receptor chemeric human-murine monoclonal antibody. *Drugs Today* (Barc.) **41**: 107–127.

106. Vallbohmer D. and Lenz H. J. (2005) Epidermal growth factor receptor as a target for chemotherapy. *Clin. Colorectal Cancer* **5** (Suppl 1): S19–27.
107. Gnewuch C. T. and Sosnovsky G. (2002) Critical appraisals of approaches for predictive designs in anticancer drugs. *Cell. Mol. Life Sci.* **59**: 959–1023.
108. Konovalova N. P., Diatchkovskaya R. F., Volkova L. M. and Varfolomeev V. N. (1991) Nitroxyl radicals decrease toxicity of cytostatic agents. *Anticancer Drugs* **2**: 591–595.
109. Emanuel N. and Konovalova N. (1992) Nitroxyl radicals for cancer chemotherapy. In: *Bioactive spin-labels*, pp 439–460, Zhdanov, R. I. (ed.), Springer-Verlag, Berlin.
110. Gadzheva V., Ilarionova M., Raikov Z. and Todorov D. (1991). Biological activity and toxicity of new alkyl-nitro-3-cyclohexylurea derivatives of CCNU. *Oncology* **28**: 18.
111. Ilarionova M., Todorov D. K., Zheleva A. and Raikov Z. (1993) Third generation potential antimelanomic drugs. *Oncologia* **30** (Suppl. 1): 73.
112. Zheleva A., Raikov Z., Ilarionova M., Carpenter B., Todorov D. and Armstrong N. (1996) Potential antimelanomic drugs. I. Synthesis and anti-melanomic effect of a spin label D,L-amino acid containing a 2-chloro-ethylnitrosocarbamoyl group. *Pharmazie* **51**: 602.
113. Zheleva A., Raikov Z., Ilarionova M. and Todorov D. (1995) Spin labeled amino acid nitrosourea derivatives – synthesis and antitumour activity. *Pharmazie* **50**: 25.
114. Sosnovsky G., Baysal M. and Erciyas E. (1994) In the search for new anticancer drugs 28. Synthesis and evaluation of highly active aminoxyl labeled amino acid derivatives containing the [*N*'-(2-chloroethyl)-*N*'-nitrosoamino]carbonyl group. *J. Pharm. Sci.* **83**: 999–1005.
115. Sosnovsky G., Prakash I. and Rao N. U. M. (1993) In the search for new anticancer drugs. XXIV: Synthesis and anticancer activity of amino acids and dipeptides containing the 2-chloroethyl- and [*N*'-(2-chloroethyl)-*N*'-nitrosoamino]carbonyl groups. *J. Pharm. Sci.* **82**: 1–10 and **82**: 1300.
116. Sosnovsky G. and Rao N. U. M. (1990) In the search for new anticancer drugs. XXII. Synthesis and anticancer evaluation of some dipeptides containing *N*-nitrosochloroethylamino and chloroethylamino moieties. *J. Pharm. Sci.* **79**: 369–370.
117. Sosnovsky G. and Gnewuch C. T. (1994) In the search for new anticancer drugs. 27. Synthesis and comparison of anticancer activity *in*

vivo of amino acids, carbohydrates, and carbohydrate-amino acid conjugates containing the [*N*'-(2-chloroethyl)-*N*'-nitrosoamino]-carbonyl group. *J. Pharm. Sci.* **83**: 989–998.

118. Sosnovsky G. and Rao N. U. M. (1991) In the search for new anti-cancer drugs. XXIII: Exploration of a predictive design for anti-cancer drugs of carbohydrates containing *N*-nitrosochloro-ethylamino, *N*-nitrosomethyl, and *N*-nitrosoaminoxyl components. *J. Pharm. Sci.* **80**: 693–699.
119. Sosnovsky G. and Rao N. U. M. (1986) Synthesis of 2-deoxy-2-[3-(2,2,6,6-tetramethyl-piperidine-1-oxyl-4-yl)-3-nitrosoureido]-D-glucopyranose (SLGNU). *Drugs Future* **11**: 285.
120. Hansch C., Smith N., Engle R. and Wood H. (1972) Quantitative structure-activity relationships of antineoplastic drugs: nitrosoureas and triazeno-imidazoles. *Cancer Chemother. Rep.* **56**: 443–456.
121. Emmanuel N. M., Konovalova N. P. and Diatchovskaya R. F. (1985) Potential anticancer agents-nitroxyl derivatives of Rubomycin. *Neo-plasma* **32**: 285–292.
122. Bogdanov G. N., Orlov V. S. and Duzhkov V. B. (1987) Specialties of the free radical mechanism of biological action of Rubomicine ni-troxyl derivative. *Chemico-Pharmaceutical Y.* (Russ.) 1042.
123. Konovalova N. P., Diatchkovskaya R. F. and Kukushkina G. V. (1988) Pharmacokinetics of spin-labeled rubomycin analog. *Neo-plasma* **35**: 185–189.
124. Franchi F., Konovalova N. P., Seminara P., Diatchkovskaya R. F., Volkova L. M. and Bonomo L. (1992) Ruboxyl as a potential anti-tumor agent in the therapy of colorectal cancer. *Cancer Res. Ther. Control* **2**: 199–205.
125. Leonetti C., Arrone T., Konovalova N., Diatchkovskaya R. F., Shapiro A. B. and Franchi F. (1993) Ruboxyl, a new nitroxyl deriva-tive of Daunorubicin: acute toxicity and antitumor effect in animals. *Intern. J. Oncol.* **3**: 615–618.
126. Gnewuch C. T. and Sosnovsky G. (1986) Spin-labeled carbohy-drates. *Chem. Rev.* **86**: 203–238.
127. Zhdanov R. I. (1992) The toxicity of aminoxyl radicals. In: *Bioactive spin labels*, Zhdanov R. I. (ed.), Springer Verlag, New York.
128. Sosnovsky G. (1992) A critical evaluation of the present status of toxicity of aminoxyl radicals. *J. Pharm. Sci.* **81**: 496–499.
129. Sosnovsky G., Jawdosiuk M. and Clumpner J. M. (2000) Di-*tert*-alkyl nitroxyl radicals. Synthesis, physical properties and applica-tions as inhibitors of vinyl polymerization at elevated temperatures. *Z. Naturforsch.* **55b**: 109–126.

130. Jawdosiuk M., Sosnovsky G., Clumpner J. M. and O'Lenick Jr. A. J. (2006) Hindered spiro-ketal nitroxides. *U.S. Patent* 7,132,540 B1.
131. Hideg K., Kálai T. and Sár C. P. (2005) Recent results in chemistry and biology of nitroxides. *J. Heterocycl. Chem.* **42**: 437–450.
132. Greci L., Damiani E. and Astolfi P. (2007) Synthesis of a novel nitroxide antioxidant and methods of use in cosmetic and dermatological compositions. *Int. Patent* WO2007068759 A2.
133. Sosnovsky G. and Konieczny M. (1977) Preparation of 4-phosphorylated 1,4-dihydroxy-2,2,6,6-tetramethylpiperidines by reduction of nitroxyls with L-ascorbic acid. *Synthesis* 619–622.
134. Sosnovsky G., Rao N. U. M., Li S. W. and Swartz H. M. (1989) Synthesis of nitroxyl (aminoxyl) labeled probes for studies of intracellular environment by EPR and MRI. *J. Org. Chem.* **54**: 3667–3674.
135. Sosnovsky G. and Li S. W. (1985) In the search for new anticancer drugs. XII. Synthesis and biological evaluation of spin-labeled nitrosoureas. *Life Sci.* **36**: 1479–1483.
136. Korytowski W., Sarna T., Kalyanaraman B. and Sealy R. C. (1987) Tyrosinase-catalyzed oxidation of dopa and related catechol(amine)s: a kinetic electron spin resonance investigation using spin-stabilization and spin label oximetry. *Biochim. Biophys. Acta* **924**: 383–392.
137. Hu H., Sosnovsky G. and Swartz H. (1992) Simultaneous measurements of intra- and extra-cellular oxygen concentration in viable cells. *Biochem. Biophys. Acta* **1112**: 161–166.
138. Eriksson U. G., Tozer T. N., Sosnovsky G., Lukszo J. and Brasch R. C. (1986) Human erythrocyte membrane permeability and nitroxyl spin-label reduction. *J. Pharm. Sci.* **75**: 334–337.
139. Hu H., Sosnovsky G., Li S. W., Rao N. U. M., Morse II P. D. and Swartz H. M. (1989) Development of nitroxides for selective localization inside cells. *Biochem. Biophys. Acta* **1014**: 211–218.
140. Sosnovsky G. and Bell P. (1998) In the search for new anticancer drugs. 29. A study on the correlation of lipophilicities, ionization constants and anticancer activities of aminoxyl labeled TEPA congeners. *Life Sci.* **62**: 639–648.
141. Raikov Z., Demirov G., Todorov D. and Ilarionova M. (1980) Spin-labeled derivatives of 1-(2-chloroethyl)urea, method of synthesis and their application. *Bulg. Patent* 31409.
142. Raikov Z., Todorov D., Ilarionova M., Demirov G., Tsanova T. and Kafalieva D. (1985) Synthesis and study of spin-labeled nitrosourea. *Cancer Biochem. Biophys.* **7**: 343.

143. Raikov Z., Zheleva A. and Raikova E. (1990) Activation of the anticancer drug CCNU into a free radical intermediate via UV irradiation – an ESR study. *Free Radical Biol. Med.* **9**: 423.
144. Raikov Z., Gadsheva V., Koch M. and Lolar G. (1993) Synthesis of spin-labeled triazenes. *Org. Prep. Proced. Int.* **25**: 473.
145. Raikov Z., Todorov D., Ilarionova M., Demirov G., Tsanova T. and Kafalieva D. (1985) Synthesis and study of spin-labeled nitrosourea. *Cancer Biochem. Biophys.* **7**: 343.
146. Raikov Z., Zheleva A., Raikova E., Ilarionova M. and Todorov D. (1990) *N*-[*N*'-(2-chloroethyl)-*N*'-nitrosocarbamoyl]-Δ-(2,2,6,6-tetramethyl-1-oxyl-amidopiperidine-4), method of synthesis and application. *Bulg. Patent* 52013A, 14.3.
147. Gadzheva V., Ichimori K., Nakazawa H. and Raikov Z. (1994) Superoxide scavenging activity of spin labeled nitrosourea and triazene derivatives. *Free Radical Res.* **21**: 197.
148. Konovalova N. P., Diatchkovskaya R. F., Volkova L. M. and Varfolomeev V. N. (1996) Modulatory effect of tempol on toxicity and antitumor activity of 6-mercaptopurine and on P450 cytochrome level. *Neoplasia* **43**: 341–346, and *Vopr. Onkol. (Problems in Oncology)* **42**: 57–63.
149. Raikov Z. D., Raikova E. T. and Atanasov A. T. (2001) Nitric oxide and free stable nitroxyl radicals in the mechanism of biological action of the spin-labeled compounds. *Med. Hypotheses* **57**: 302–305.
150. Feldman P. L., Griffith O. W. and Stuehr D. J. (1993) The surprising life of nitric oxide. *Chem. Eng. News* **71**(51): 26–38.
151. Griffith O. W. and Kilbourn R. G. (1997) Design of nitric oxide synthase inhibitors and their use to reverse hypotension associated with cancer immunotherapy. *Adv. Enzyme Regul.* **37**: 171–194.
152. Stuehr D. J., Wei C. C., Santolini J., Wang Z., Aoyagi M. and Getzoff E. D. 2004) Radical reactions of nitric oxide synthases. *Biochem. Soc. Symp.* 39–49.
153. Chiang T. M., Sayre R. M., Dowdy J. C., Wilkin N. K. and Rosenberg E. W. (2005) Sunscreen ingredients inhibit inducible nitric oxide synthase (iNOS): a possible biochemical explanation for the sunscreen melanoma controversy. *Melanoma Res.* **15**: 3–6.
154. Russo P. A. and Halliday G. M. (2006) Inhibition of nitric oxide and reactive oxygen species production improves the ability of a sunscreen to protect from sunburn, immunosuppression and photocarcinogenesis. *Br. J. Dermatol.* **155**: 408–415.
155. Konovalova N. P., Goncharova S. A., Volkova L. M., Raevskaia T. A., Eremenko L. T. and Korolev A. M. (2003) Nitric oxide donor in-

creases the effectiveness of cytostatic therapy and inhibits the development of drug resistance. *Vopr. Onkol. (Problems in Oncology)* **49**: 71–75.

156. Qiu H., Orr F. W., Jensen D., Wang H. H., McIntosh A. R., Hasinoff B. B., Nance D. M., Pylypas S., Qi K., Song C., Muschel R. J. and Al-Mehdi A. B. (2003) Arrest of B16 melanoma cells in the mouse pulmonary microcirculation induces endothelial nitric oxide synthase-dependent nitric oxide release that is cytotoxic to the tumor cells. *Am. J. Pathol.* **162**: 403–412.
157. Postovit L. M., Adams M. A., Lash G. E., Heaton J. P. and Graham C. H. (2004) Nitric oxide-mediated regulation of hypoxia-induced B16F10 melanoma metastasis. *Int. J. Cancer* **108**: 47–53.
158. Perrotta C., Falcone S., Capobianco A., Camporeale A., Sciorati C., De Palma C., Pisconti A., Rovere-Querini P., Bellone M., Manfredi A. A. and Clementi E. (2004) Nitric oxide confers therapeutic activity to dendritic cells in a mouse model of melanoma. *Cancer Res.* **64**: 3767–3771.
159. Fukuzawa K., Kogure K., Morita M., Hama S., Manabe S. and Tokumura A. (2004) Enhancement of nitric oxide and superoxide generations by alpha-tocopheryl succinate and its apoptotic and anticancer effects. *Biochemistry (Moscow)* **69**: 50–57.
160. Masri F. A., Comhair S. A., Koeck T., Xu W., Janocha A., Ghosh S., Dweik R. A, Golish J., Kinter M., Stuehr D. J., Erzurum S. C. and Aulak K. S. (2005) Abnormalities in nitric oxide and its derivatives in lung cancer. *Am. J. Respir. Crit. Care Med.* **172**: 597– 605.
161. Campos A. C., Molognoni F., Melo F. H., Galdieri L. C., Carneiro C. R., D'Almeida V., Correa M. and Jasiulionis M. G. (2007) Oxidative stress modulates DNA methylation during melanocyte anchorage blockade associated with malignant transformation. *Neoplasia* **9**: 1111–1121.
162. Madhunapantula S. V., Desai D., Sharma A., Huh S. J., Amin S. and Robertson G. P. (2008) PBISe, a novel selenium-containing drug for the treatment of malignant melanoma. *Mol. Cancer Ther.* **7**: 1297–1308.
163. Mijatovic S., Maksimovic-Ivanic D., Mojic M., Malaponte G., Libra M., Cardile C., Miljkovic D., Harhaji L., Dabideen D., Cheng K. F., Bevelacqua Y., Donia M., Garotta G., Al-Abed Y., Stosic-Grujicic S. and Nicoletti F. (2008) Novel nitric oxide-donating compound (*S,R*)-3-phenyl-4,5-dihydro-5-isoxazole acetic acid-nitric oxide (GIT-27NO) induces p53 mediated apoptosis in human A375 melanoma cells. *Nitric Oxide* **19**: 177–183.

164. Afanasev I. B. (2007) Signaling functions of free radicals superoxide & nitric oxide under physiological & pathological conditions. *Mol. Biotechnol.* **37**: 2–4.
165. Konovalova N. P., Goncharova S. A., Volkova L. M., Rayevskaya T. A., Eremenko L. T. and Korolev A. M. (2003) Nitric oxide donor increases the effectiveness of cytostatic therapy and inhibits drug resistance development. *Vopr. Onkol. (Problems in Oncology)* **49**: 71–75.
166. Gadzheva V., Raikova E., Raikov Z. and Vlaikova T. (1991) Syntheses and study of tyrosine nitrosoureas as potential anticancer agents. *Eur. J. Cancer* **27**: S3 852.
167. Raikov Z., Blagoeva P. M. and Yordanov N. D. (1976) Activating effect of 2,2,6,6-tetramethyl-4-oxopiperidine-1-oxyl on tyrosinase ex mushroom. *Compt. Rend. Acad. Bulg. Sci.* **29**: 709.
168. Blagoeva P. M., Raikov Z. D. and Yordanov N. D. (1976) EPR study of 2,2,6,6-tetramethyl-4-oxopiperidine-1-oxyl in hamsters with transplanted pigmental melanoma. *Compt. Rend. Acad. Bulg. Sci.* **29**: 881.
169. Rachkova M., Raikova E. and Raikov Z. (1991) New nitrosoureas and their spin-labeled derivatives influence DOPA-oxidase activity of tyrosinase. *Cancer Biochem. Biophys.* **12**: 593.

CHAPTER THREE

MECHANISMS OF EXCITATION AND ENERGY DISSIPATION WITH RELEVANCE TO THE PHOTOCHEMISTRY OF SUNSCREENS

A. General Aspects

The mechanisms of light-induced excitations and energy dissipations of organic molecules have been extensively studied, and there exists an enormous amount of literature on these subjects. Now, an attempt is made to delineate the most important aspects of physical and chemical photoreactions with relevance to the fate of the UV energy absorbing substances that are used for the protection of human skin against solar radiation.

A photochemical reaction, whether it is a synthesis or a degradation of the molecule involved, can only proceed if the energy of light is absorbed by the molecule. This recognition by Grotthus in 1817 is known as the first law of photochemistry. The second law of photochemistry was formulated by Stark in 1908 and Einstein in 1912 that one quantum of light is absorbed per molecule of absorbing and reacting substance that disappears. This law is valid only for the primary photochemical event, i.e., for the formation of excited species immediately on absorption. In photochemistry, the unit of radiation is called a photon or the quantum. The absorption of UV light and visible light of the electromagnetic spectrum results in an excitation of the outer electrons of the molecules, i.e., electrons participating in chemical bonds. Hence, such excitations can cause chemical changes in the molecules [1–6].

The emission of light from a material under the influence of an exciting agent, such as various types of radiation, is termed fluorescence. When the emission of light persists after the cessation of the exciting agent, it is termed phosphorescence. The two processes are practically identical, except for the duration of the light emission. The term luminescence is used for both phenomena. The emission can be affected by the purity of the fluorescent substance, by particle size, water content, solvents, polarity of solvent, hydrogen bonding, and concentrations of the solute [1, 4, 6, 7]. A fluorescent molecule is characterized by two spectra, i.e., the excitation and the emission spectrum. Generally, for analytical purposes, the longest wavelength absorption band is chosen as the excitation wavelength in order to avoid degradation of the chosen compounds that may occur with shorter wavelengths. However, when sunscreen agents on the human skin are exposed to solar UVA and UVB radiation, the wavelengths have been predetermined by evolutionary events. A molecule in an excited state differs from that in the ground state in chemical and physical properties, and can be viewed as a metastable isomer of the ground state molecule. Hence, it may undergo a series of chemical reactions not available to the molecule in the ground state. For example, while a ground state sunscreen molecule is a stable compound that does not react with molecular oxygen of the air, upon solar irradiation, it may fragment and/or react with molecular oxygen and other compounds. Thus, if the irradiated and absorbed energies exceed the bond dissociation energy of the compound, the compound will undergo photolysis, i.e., a photodecomposition process [2]. However, in some cases, the photodecomposition of a compound can occur on absorption of a radiant energy that is below the bond dissociation energy of the compound. In such cases, the compound on irradiation absorbs a photon and is raised to a stable excited state without undergoing decomposition. This species in the stable excited state then undergoes a radiationless transition to an unstable excited state, and the absorbed energy is then dissipated by bond breaking [1–3]. This type of a predissociation process involving a radiationless transition is an important mechanism, e.g., for the dissipation of excitation energy of some saturated compounds, and many aliphatic compounds which exhibit luminescence by this process. In polar solvents, the excited state is more polar than the ground state. Therefore, a shift of both absorbance and fluorescence spectra to lower energy, i.e., longer wavelength is observed (red shift) as the dielectric constant of a solvent is increased [1, 6]. The fluorescence intensity and wavelength shift can vary with changes in the pH [1, 5]. Hence, the fluorescence can be used as a colored titration indicator, and various classes of fluorescent compounds are available as fluorescent indicators to cover the pH ranges from zero to fourteen [1].

The nature of the solvent can affect the fluorescence spectra in various ways [1, 6, 7].

1. The polarization shift, i.e., the energy of the fluorescence maximum can shift either to higher or to lower energy as a function of either the polarity or polarizability of the solvent.

2. The hydrogen bonding can affect the fluorescence, if the solute and solvent can interact to form hydrogen bonds.
3. The fluorescence of the solute can be quenched, i.e., inhibited by certain solvents, and the efficiency and energy of the fluorescence can be affected by changes in temperature, since the dielectric constant values decrease with raising temperature.
4. The changes of the fluorescence energy with solvent are called the polarization shifts, and are attributable to the polarization of solvent molecules, induced by dipoles of the solute. Many organic molecules are more polar when electronically excited.

The hydrogen bonding of a fluorescent solute to the solvent can result in changes of the emission frequency of the solute, whereby shifts to shorter (blue shift) or longer (red shift) wavelengths can occur. The red shift of the fluorescence emissions to longer wavelength depends on the type of solute–solvent interactions. Thus, there could be:

i. a permanent dipole–dipole interaction
ii. a permanent dipole–induced dipole interaction
iii. a transition dipole–induced dipole interaction

5. The fluorescence spectrum can be influenced by one or more of these interactions. In general, as the dielectric constant of the solvent is increased, the hydrogen bonding will result in lowering of the energy and an increase of the wavelengths of absorbance and fluorescence. Thus, the all-important water, the principle component of the human body and life, has been predestined by evolution to have a dielectric constant of 80, while other polar liquids like alcohols have dielectric constants between 20 and 30, and many other organic liquids have lower dielectric constants of 2–10 [1]. Some aromatic ketones, which have no fluorescent properties in nonpolar solvents, can acquire fluorescent properties in very polar hydrogen-bonding solvents. Similarly, nonfluorescent ketones on substitution with hydrogen-bonding groups, such as a hydroxyl group, will exhibit fluorescence because of hydrogen bonding to the carbonyl oxygen atom [1, 4].

The hydrogen bonding can also produce quenching effects, i.e., inhibition of the luminescence, if the hydrogen bonds involve π electrons of the proton donor, and if the π electrons of both the donor and acceptor are conjugated. In the case where the hydrogen bond is isolated from the π-

electron system of the proton donor by a sigma bond, the fluorescence is enhanced by the hydrogen bonding [1].

Compounds with a total quantum spin number of one have all electrons paired, i.e., the sum of the individual spins is zero, and, hence, the ground state is a singlet according to the equation: $2\,S + 1 = 1$, where $S = +\frac{1}{2} + -\frac{1}{2} = 0$.

Molecular oxygen, in contrast, is a triplet in the ground state with a spin quantum number of three: $2\,S + 1 = 3$, where $S = \frac{1}{2} + \frac{1}{2} = 1$.

A compound with a ground state singlet, on irradiation with light of a suitable wavelength, can be promoted either to the excited singlet or triplet state [1, 2].

The luminescence of the singlet excited state species can be specifically quenched by many compounds, e.g., by diacetyl [1, 2].

The excited triplet state species can be quenched by various substances, such as alkenes, dienes, and, most importantly, by molecular oxygen, which is the most efficient quenching agent [1]. In the following discussions, the superscript numbers one (1) and three (3) denote the singlet excited state S_1 and the triplet excited state T_1, respectively.

B. Various Quenching Processes

There are several processes that can cause quenching of either the excited singlet or triplet state [1,2]. Thus, the quenching can occur by absorption of the excited energy of radiation, by high concentrations of impurities, and by absorbance of the emitted light.

Another process of quenching occurs by transfer of the irradiated energy. Thus, compound Cpd1, on absorption of a photon, is elevated to the species Cpd1*, which is either in a singlet or a triplet excited state. The species Cpd1* could then interact with a molecule of Cpd2, which is still in the ground state, by transferring the irradiated energy to the ground state molecule of Cpd2, which is promoted to the excited state, Cpd2*, while the species Cpd1* returns to the ground state Cpd1.

$$\text{Cpd1} \xrightarrow{h\nu} \text{Cpd1}^* \xrightarrow{\textit{Cpd2}} \text{Cpd1} + \text{Cpd2}^*$$

The conditions for energy transfer would be particularly favorable if compound Cpd1 would have been promoted to the excited triplet state ^{3}Cpd1*, because a species in the triplet state has a longer lifetime than a species in the excited singlet state. Hence, there would be a better chance for ^{3}Cpd1* to interact with compound Cpd2. In such a case, compound Cpd2 would be promoted to the triplet state, ^{3}Cpd2*, via an energy-transfer mechanism. In such transactions, compound Cpd1 is the sensitizer and compound Cpd2 is a quencher. The ground state sensitizer Cpd1 can also react with the triplet state of the quencher ^{3}Cpd2 to give a new compound, Cpd3.

$$\text{Cpd1} \xrightarrow{h\nu} {}^3\text{Cpd1*} \longrightarrow \text{Cpd1} + {}^3\text{Cpd2*} \longrightarrow \text{Cpd3}$$

This type of energy transfer is only possible if the triplet state energy of the sensitizer, ^{3}Cpd1*, is higher than the triplet state energy of the quencher, ^{3}Cpd2*.

Some quenchers, Cpd2, can quench the reactions while the sensitizer, Cpd1, is still in the excited singlet state, 1Cpd1*, resulting in a different type of compound, Cpd4.

$$\text{Cpd1} \xrightarrow{h\nu} {}^1\text{Cpd1*} \xrightarrow{Cpd2} \text{Cpd4}$$

In the case where a quencher (Q) is used to quench the triplet state, another type of product can be obtained, involving intersystem crossing.

$$\text{Cpd1} \xrightarrow{h\nu} {}^1\text{Cpd1*} \xrightarrow{ISC} {}^3\text{Cpd1*} \xrightarrow{\text{Q}} \text{Cpd5}$$

ISC = intersystem crossing Q = quencher of triplet states

Molecular oxygen quenches equally well the singlet and triplet states. The rates of oxygen quenching of many compounds are often diffusion-controlled, i.e., almost all collisions of oxygen with the photoexcited species are effective. Since the diffusion coefficient of oxygen is large [1], the quenching by oxygen is efficient and effective. This fact may be the reason for the inhibition of phosphorescence and fluorescence of many organic compounds by molecular oxygen. Several mechanisms have been invoked [1] to explain this efficiency of oxygen quenching. Thus, in one explanation, it may involve the transfer of the electronic energy from the excited states of solutes to the oxygen molecule, which is a triplet in the ground state. However, a more likely explanation is that oxygen as a paramagnetic species may increase the spin-orbit coupling in many electronically excited molecules in solution, and, thereby, increase the rates of the singlet-to-triplet and the triplet-to-singlet transitions. Hence, an effective quenching of both fluorescence and phosphorescence can occur. In contrast, most diamagnetic compounds are inefficient quenching agents of luminescence. Certain aromatic and heteroaromatic compounds and ketones are very sensitive to oxygen quenching [1].

Another excellent quencher is the ground state triplet nitric oxide (NO) [1]. In the past decades, the significance of some biological events involving nitric oxide has been extensively evaluated [8–20]. It is significant that nitric oxide can participate in quenching of the triplet state species. Nitric oxide can also undergo reactions with reactive oxygen species (ROS). Thus, the reaction of nitric oxide with superoxide anion radical ($O_2\cdot^-$) produces the very toxic peroxynitrite species ($ONOO^-$ H^+). Conceivably, this type of reaction can occur exogenously and endogenously, i.e., on the human skin and deeper in the skin tissues [21]. Thus, it was shown that the oxidative reaction of peroxynitrite with DNA causes mutagenic lesions, with formation of 8-oxoguanidine nucleotide [22].

Furthermore, the reaction of molecular oxygen ($\cdot O_2\cdot$) with nitric oxide produces the nitrosoperoxy radical and its degradation products, the nitro radicals [18, 19].

$$\cdot NO + \cdot O_2\cdot \rightarrow ON\text{—}O\text{—}O\cdot \xrightarrow{\cdot NO} [ON\text{—}O\text{—}O\text{—}NO] \rightarrow 2\,\cdot NO_2$$

The reactions of these species with biologically important molecules result in the formation of nitro derivatives, such as nitrotyrosine [18, 19].

Since the atmosphere worldwide contains nitric oxide, caused by industrial and automobile pollutions, one could hypothesize that the formation of peroxynitrite species and related compounds would inadvertently occur on the human skin.

C. Chemical Reactions of Photoexcited Molecules

Photoexcited molecular species in the singlet and triplet states can undergo various reactions, including chemical reactions [2]. Chemical reactions are much more common with the triplet species than with the singlet species, because the triplets have much longer lifetimes than the singlets; the latter can preferentially undergo physical processes before chemical reactions. Hence, the photochemistry is essentially a chemistry of molecular species in the triplet state. There are a number of photochemical processes that are relevant to topics of this review. The primary photochemical reactions often result in unstable intermediates, such as free radicals [2]. The primary products are, with few exceptions, in their ground states. The energies of the solar UVA and UVB radiations are of the same order as, or exceed those of, common covalent bonds [**Fig. 1B-1**]. Thus, these energies between 280 and 380 nm correspond to 107–75 kcal/mol. The energy requirement for the homolytic cleavage of selected important covalent bonds is as follows: 95 kcal/mol for C–H bonds at 300 nm, 88 kcal/mol for C–O bonds at 325 nm, 83 kcal/mol at 345 nm for C–C bonds, and 72 kcal/mol for C–N bonds [2]. Thus, theoretically, photolytic cleavage of most bonds in organic compounds, including those of sunscreen agents, is feasible. The photolysis usually results in the homolytic breaking of covalent bonds producing free radical species. The heterolytic cleavage into two ions is much less likely and more difficult to achieve because of higher energy requirements. The radicals that are produced in photolytic cleavages have the same properties as those formed in other processes such as thermolysis. The manifold reactivities and properties of free radicals have been extensively explored by photophysical, photochemical, chemical, and biological methods over the past fifty years, and many monographs and books have been published. Specifically, the fundamental aspects of free radical chemistry have been discussed in detail in several books [2, 25–27]. In the present section, the discussion is limited to photoinduced reactions of several types of sunscreens. The full details are treated in Sections 3F and 3G.

D. Excited States of Sunscreens and Their Reactions

There are about fifty compounds that have been used worldwide in commercial sunscreen formulations [23, 24]. (See **Table 3F-1** below.) These compounds can be classified into the following groups based on their chemical structures: ten benzophenone analogs, one dibenzoylmethane derivative, nine cinnamates, eight salicylates, eight 4-aminobenzoic acid derivatives, one 2-aminobenzoic acid derivative (anthranilate), six camphor derivatives containing aromatic moieties, ten miscellaneous heterocyclic compounds, and two inorganics (titanium dioxide and zinc oxide). Despite their structural diversity, these compounds have in common only a small number of simple, conjugated chromophores, e.g. **1–7** [**Fig. 3D-1**]. These chromophores contain bonding π electrons and nonbonding n electrons that are conjugated to the chromophoric aromatic ring systems; they also often contain the auxochromic hydroxyl and amino groups and their derivatives. In most cases, the syntheses of these compounds have been achieved by well-established methodologies, and many of the sunscreen compounds had been known for years before their utilization in sunscreen formulations.

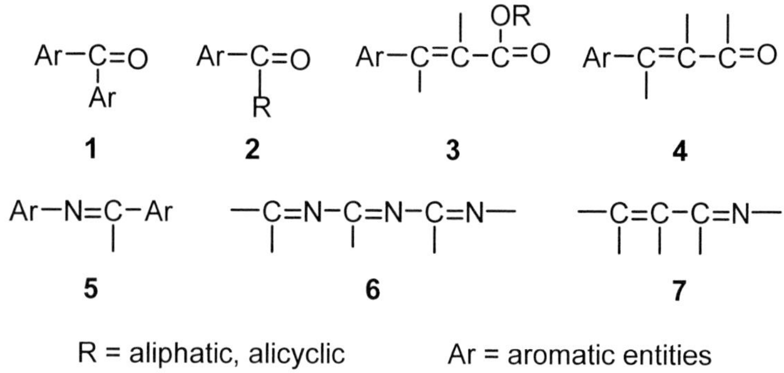

Fig. 3D-1. Structures of chromophores 1–7.

The term chromophore has been frequently used quite liberally to describe ill-defined chromophoric properties of large molecules like DNA, melanins, and other compounds utilized in photochemical reactions. Instead of the ill-defined terms, it is possible to recognize in the energy of light-absorbing compounds well-defined structural elements that were predestined by evolutionary events to act as chromophores. A chromophore is that part in a molecule which absorbs the energy of light, such as that of solar radiation, resulting in “promotion” of the molecule to an energetically higher level, i.e., to an excited state. The chromophore to be effective must be composed of at least two atoms linked together by covalent bonds. Thus, the groups >C=C<, >C=O, >C=N–, and $–CO_2R$ are “simple” chromophores, which absorb in the far UV region. This type of chromophore would not be sufficient to elevate the parent molecule to an excited state by solar radiations in the ranges of UVB radiations at 280–320 nm, and UVA radiations at 320–380 nm. However, in conjugation, these chromophoric systems absorb the energy of UVA and UVB radiations. The bathochromic (red shift) to longer wavelengths can be further enhanced by conjugation with the phenyl and aryl chromophores, and by auxochromes, such as hydroxy, amino, and sulfhydryl groups and their derivatives [2].

The absorption of a photon of ultraviolet light by the sunscreen compounds would be expected to result in a “promotion” of chromophoric electrons in the n and π orbitals from the ground state to higher energy levels. These higher energy states are molecular orbitals that are vacant in the ground state or unexcited state. The electrons that participate in bonding, like in olefinic π bonds, are elevated to antibonding orbitals, and are denoted as π*. The electrons that are not involved in bonding are the nonbonding n electrons, such as those of the molecular orbitals of oxygen and nitrogen atoms in sunscreen compounds. Thus, the electronic transitions of sunscreen compounds in the ultraviolet A and B regions would be the π,π* transitions involving the unsaturated functions and n,π* transitions of the nonbonding electrons. Hence, the olefinic functions in sunscreen compounds will undergo on UV radiation only the π,π* transitions, while the carbonyl groups will be involved in n,π* transitions [**Sch. 3D-1**].

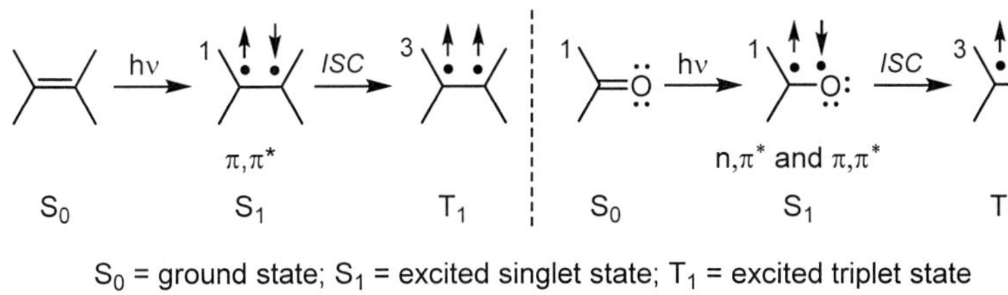

Sch. 3D-1. Photolysis to give excited states of olefinic and carbonyl chromophores.

The difference in energy of the singlet and triplet states, the so-called singlet–triplet split and rates of intersystem crossing (ISC) can be used to determine whether the transition state is a n,π* or π,π* [1]. Intersystem crossing occurs when the photoexcited species is changing from a singlet state, with all electrons paired, to a triplet state, with electrons unpaired. This intersystem crossing, involving a change of spins, is theoretically a forbidden transition because of the angular momentum. However, this difficulty can be overcome. Since the ISC occurs without loss of energy and the singlet state has usually a higher energy than the triplet state, this energy must be dissipated by the molecules by crossing from S_1 to T_1 at high vibrational levels, and the energy of T_1 must then "cascade" down at 10^{-12} s to its lowest vibrational level. Solvent polarity has a pronounced influence on the transitions, i.e., as the polarity of the solvent is increased, the π,π* transition occurs at longer wavelengths, while the n,π* transition takes place at shorter wavelengths. Thus, the properties of the species after excitation will depend on the nature of the lowest excited singlet state [1]. Since, in general, the n,π* transitions are less intense than the π,π* transitions, the n,π* excited states have longer lifetimes, and, as a result, intersystem crossing from the n,π* state will be enhanced. Molecules containing heteroatoms with n,π* and π,π* states that are energetically close together often undergo a change of relative energies of these states on changing solvents from nonpolar to polar. In such cases, an inversion occurs, as the nonbonding electrons of the heteroatoms interact with the polar moieties of the solvent, such as the hydroxyl groups, thereby raising the energy levels of the n,π^* transitions and lowering the energy levels of the π,π^* transitions. As a result, the π,π^* transition becomes the lower-energy transition.

The UV light induced photoisomerization of cis (*Z*) and trans (*E*) isomers of cinnamic acid derivatives involve π,π^* transitions of the olefinic double bonds, whereby the cis isomer is more sterically hindered and less stable than the trans isomer. The π,π^* transition of the trans isomer would be expected to occur at somewhat longer wavelength than that of the cis isomer. The condensation of species with photoexcited double bonds results in the formation of cyclobutane dimers and analogous cyclobutane derivatives [**Sch. 3D-2**].

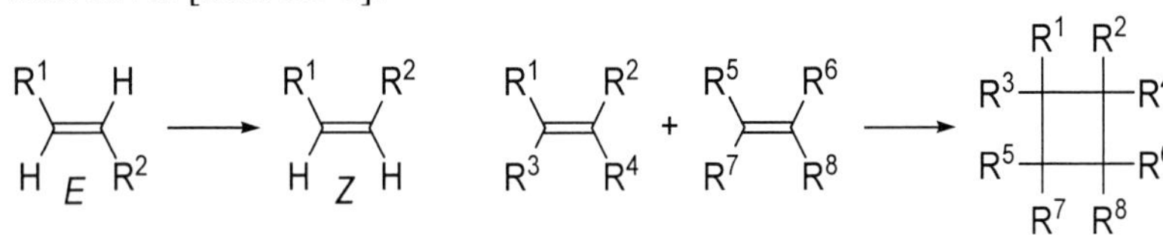

Sch. 3D-2. UV Light induced isomerizations of alkenes and their condensations to cyclobutane derivatives.

Furthermore, reactions of alkenes are also feasible with photoexcited species that are capable of n,π^* transitions to give oxetane and azetidine derivatives. (See **Sections 2D** and **2E**.)

Essentially, all sunscreen compounds shown in Section 3F and containing the listed chromophores **1–7** [**Fig. 3D-1**] would be considered as photosensitizers that could undergo the already mentioned reactions. Specifically, the benzophenone analogues, on irradiation with UV light, would be elevated to the excited state species, which then could either transfer the energy from the excited singlet to another molecule or it may, by intersystem crossing, move to the excited triplet energy level [**Sch. 3D-3**].

The excited triplet state can also transfer energy to another molecule, e.g., a solvent molecule, resulting in the formation of aldehydes and carbon monoxide [**Sch. 3D-4**].

In the case of benzophenone, about 100% of molecules in the excited state S_1 undergo crossover to the triplet state T_1. Benzophenone and analogues are known to abstract a hydrogen atom from many solvents, such as isopropyl alcohol and cyclohexane, resulting in the formation of pinacols, bicyclohexyl, and either ketones or aldehydes, depending on the alcohol solvent used. In the case of aldehydes, further degradations to carbon monoxide occur [2, 27] [**Sch. 3D-4**].

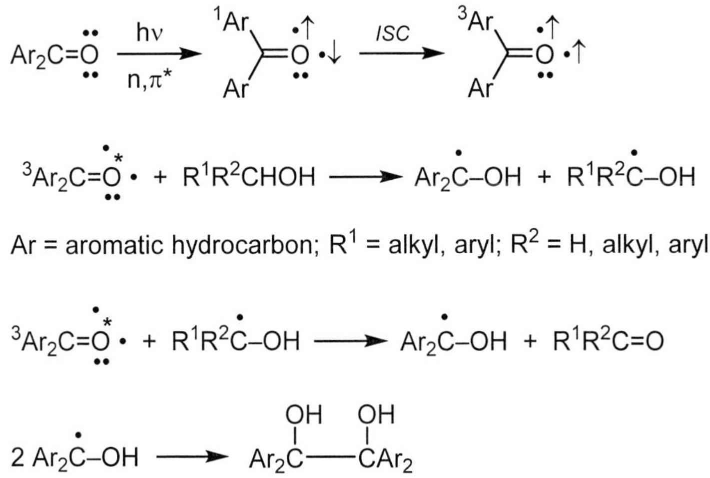

Sch. 3D-3. Behavior of sunscreen compounds containing the benzophenone chromophore upon irradiation with UV light.

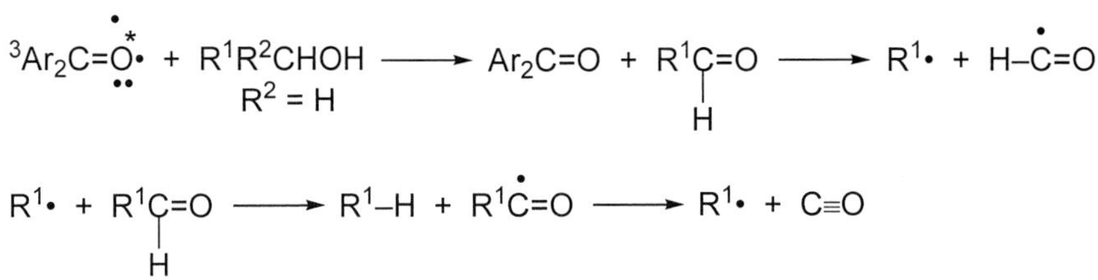

Sch. 3D-4. Photoreactions of benzophenones with organic solvents.

Single-bond cleavage into radicals can readily occur with ketones. Ketones usually absorb in the region of 230–330 nm resulting in a n,π* transition causing a cleavage of the photoexcited ketone into carbon centered radicals. This type of reaction of ketones is called the Norrish Type I reaction [**Sch. 3D-5**]. This type of degradation occurs with the frequently employed sunscreen agent 4-*tert*-butyl-4'-methoxybenzoylmethane [2, 28]. (For details, see **Section 3E**.)

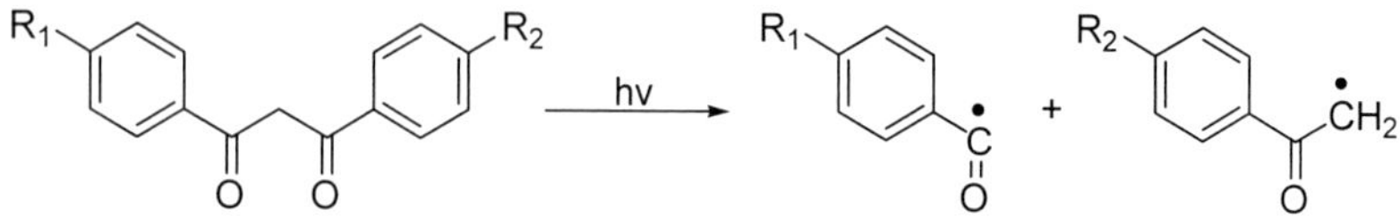

$R_1 = OCH_3$, $R_2 = C(CH_3)_3$

Sch. 3D-5. Photodegradation of the frequently employed sunscreen agent 4-*tert*-butyl-4'-methoxybenzoylmethane by the Norrish Type I reaction.

The singlet and triplet species can also interact very efficiently with molecular oxygen to produce reactive oxygen species by mechanisms I and II [29, 30]. It is important to be aware that commercial sunscreen formulations contain a multitude of ingredients that seldom receive a careful scrutiny. A casual perusal of commercial sunscreen products, which are freely available in the USA and Europe, reveals that ten randomly selected products contain 80 different additives in various combinations, besides the actual sunscreen agents. Each product formulation usually contains about 25 different ingredients composed, in part, of well-defined, mostly organic compounds, and, in part, chemically ill-defined ingredients, such as plant oils, plant extracts, and others. The following classes of organic compounds can be discerned among these formulation ingredients: alcohols (~15), esters (~15), acids (3), aldehydes (3), vegetable oils (~10), polymers (~11), and an assortment of other organic and inorganic ingredients (~15), not including dyes and fragrances which are known to cause often allergic and photoallergic responses. Furthermore, the Food and Drug Administration in the USA estimates, in the *Federal Register* of 1999 [31], that there are approximately 2800 over-the-counter sunscreen ingredients, not including the coloring matters. Thus, it would not be surprising that many of these ingredients are, inadvertently, preprogrammed for chemical, biochemical, and photochemical reactions on and in the skin.

The bewildering complexity of the formulations of sunscreen agents can be even further augmented by the fact that there are many organic compounds, which when administered to humans, can cause adverse biological effects at the skin upon exposure to solar radiations. These include a number of products that are available, without prescription, for topical applications, such as cosmetic formulations, antifungal agents, antiseptics, disinfectants, essential oils, fragrances and dyestuffs, just to mention a few [31]. Many of these ingredients have been shown to cause cutaneous photosensitivity responses. Another large group of organic compounds with photosensitizing properties are various drugs which are orally administered to patients, such as diuretic agents, systemic dermatological agents, oral contraceptive agents, nonsteroidal anti-inflammatory drugs, antimalarials, antidepressants, antimicrobials, antihistamines, antipsychotic drugs, anticonvulsants, hypoglycemics, cardiovascular drugs, anticancer drugs, hormones, and miscellaneous other agents. These drugs are used by large populations of various ages, entirely unaware that these substances can readily undergo photophysical and photochemical reactions at the skin upon exposure to solar radiations, resulting in biological defects [32–35].

The reason that these topically and orally administered compounds, although structurally diverse, elicit similar biological responses upon solar irradiation of the skin can be attributed to the following common properties. All such compounds are either entirely, or in part, composed of aromatic and/or heteroaromatic ring systems, often linked to alicyclic ring systems containing oxygen, nitrogen, or sulfur atoms and having molecular weights usually below 600, and seldom exceeding 1000. All compounds contain, as was shown with sunscreen agents, analogous, well-recognizable chromophores and auxochromes that absorb the energy of solar UVA and UVB radiations, resulting in π,π^* and n,π^* transitions to give excited singlet and triplet states. These transitions result in chemical changes—such as degradations, cyclizations, decarboxylations, carbon–halogen cleavage, and photodynamic reactions—that result in interactions with molecular oxygen to give ROS, which further interact with biological entities and cause defects. (See **Sections 2D**, **2E**, and **3F**.)

E. Photoinduced Electron-Transfer Processes of Excited Triplet States of Organic Substances in Reactions with Molecular Oxygen

The photooxidations and oxygenations of organic biomolecules are of immense biological significance in many areas such as inflammation processes in various diseases, including cancers.

The photoinduced reactions in aqueous media of excited triplet states of biomolecules with molecular oxygen, which is a triplet diradical ($^3{\cdot}O_2{\cdot}$) in the ground state with unpaired electrons, produce a cascade of reactive oxygen species (ROS). The first step in these photoinduced reactions has been iconically depicted as a direct transfer of one electron from the excited triplet species to molecular oxygen with the formation of superoxide radical species $O_2{\cdot}^-$. However, actually, these initiation reactions proceed first with formation of a contact charge-transfer complex (CCT) between the organic substance acting as an electron donor and molecular oxygen acting as an electron acceptor. Although these are energetically very weak charge-transfer (CT) interactions between the organic substances and oxygen, the CT can be observed and measured by UV spectroscopy [2, 25, 27, 35]. The photoinduced electron transfer (PET) occurs on photoexcitations of the CCT complex. The electron-donor sites of the organic substances are composed of electron pairs on the nitrogen functions, as in amines, the oxygen functions, as in ethers, and the π electrons of the carbon double bonds, as in [2 + 2] dimerizations of the heterobases of DNA [36] [**Sch. 3E-1**].

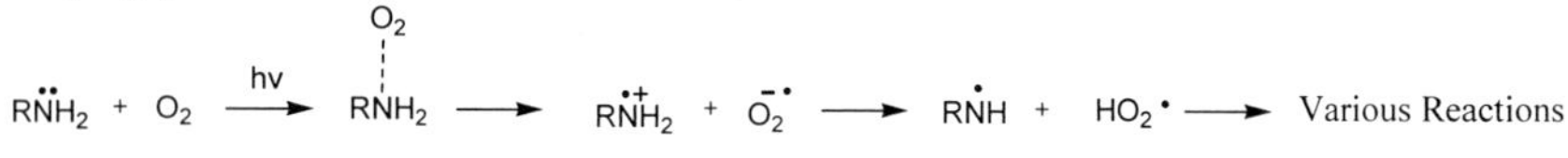

Photooxidation of Amines

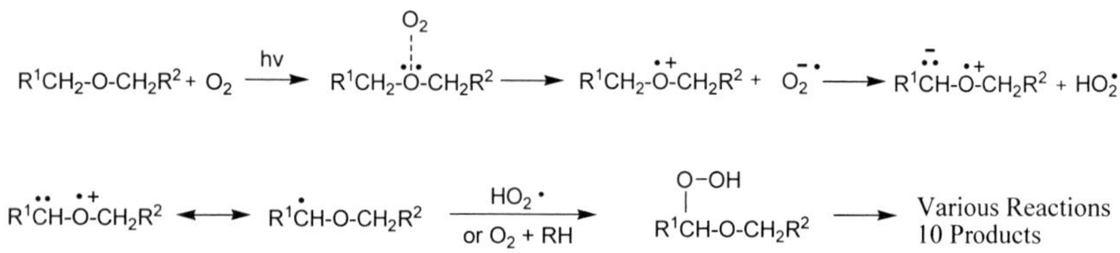

Photooxidation of Ethers

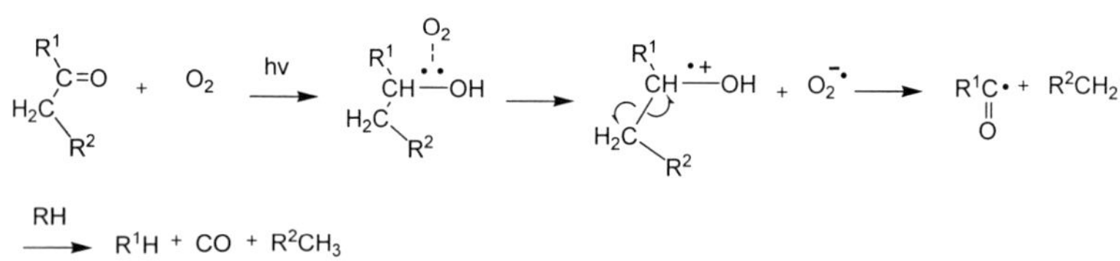

Photodegradation of Ketones by the Norrish Type 1 Cleavage

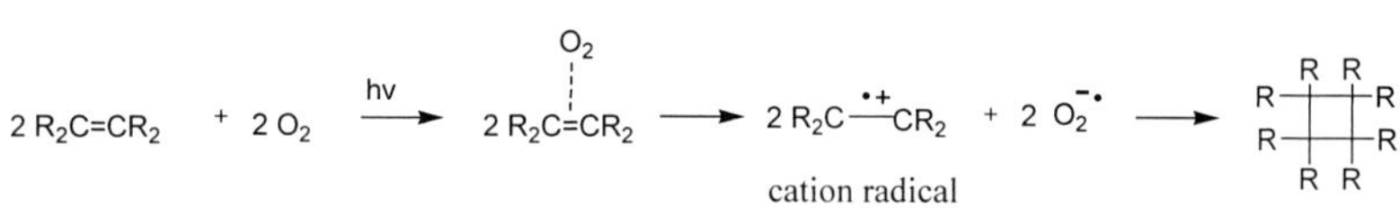

Formation of Cyclobutene Type Dimers by the [2+2] Cycloaddition Reactions of Double Bonds, e.g. Cyclobutane Pyrimidine Dimers by the Photoinduced reaction of DNA

Sch. 3E-1. Photoinduced reactions of electron-donor substances with molecular oxygen as electron acceptor. R, R^1, R^2 = various groups; RH = hydrogen-donor compounds.

References

1. Gillespie A. M. (1985) *A Manual of Fluorometric and Spectrophotometric Experiments*, Gordon and Breach Science Publishers, New York.
2. Smith M. B. and March J. (2001) *March's Advanced Organic Chemistry. Reactions Mechanisms, and Structure,* 5th ed., John Wiley & Sons, New York.
3. Martincigh B. S., Allen J. M. and Allen K. (1997) Sunscreens: the molecules and their photochemistry. In: *Sunscreen Photochemistry*, pp 11–46, Gasparro F. P. (ed.), Springer Verlag, Berlin.
4. Kauzmann W. (1957) *Quantum Chemistry*, pp 542–544, Academic Press, New York.
5. Hercules D. (ed.) (1967) *Fluorescence and Phosphorescence Analysis*, pp 136–137, Interscience, New York.
6. Underfriend S. (1962) *Fluorescence Assay in Biology and Medicine*, p 402, Academic Press, New York.
7. Williams R. T. and Bridges J. W. (1964) Fluorescence of solutions: a review. *J. Clin. Pathol.* **17**: 371–394.
8. Raikov Z. D., Raikova E. T. and Atanasov A. T. (2001) Nitric oxide and free stable nitroxyl radicals in the mechanism of biological action of the spin-labeled compounds. *Med. Hypothesis* **57**: 302–305.
9. Raikov Z., Raikova E., Zheleva A. and Gadzheva V. G. (1999) Nitric oxide and nitroxyls in the mechanism of biological action of the spin labeled compounds. *Bulg. Med.* **V11**: 3–4, 60.
10. Mellion B. T., Ignarro L. J., Ohlstein E. H., Pontecorvo E. G., Hyman A. L. and Kadowitz P. J. (1981) Evidence for the inhibitory role of guanosine 3',5'-monophosphate in ADP-induced human platelet aggregation in the presence of nitric oxide and related vasodilators. *Blood* **57**: 946–955.
11. Samama C. M., Diaby M., Fellahi J. L., Mdhafar A., Eyraud D., Arock M., Guillosson J. J., Coriat P. and Rouby J. J. (1995) Inhibition of platelet aggregation by inhaled nitric oxide in patients with acute respiratory distress syndrome. *Anesthesiology* **83**: 56–65.
12. Rubbo H., Darley-Usmar V. and Freeman B. (1996) Nitric oxide regulation of tissue free radical injury. *Chem. Res. Toxicol.* **9**: 809–820.
13. Williams R. (1996) Nitric oxide in biology: its role as a ligand. *Chem. Soc. Rev.* **25**: 77–83.
14. Tamir S., Burney S. and Tannenbaum R. (1996) DNA damage by nitric oxide. *Chem. Res. Toxicol.* **9**: 821–827.

15. Hensley K., Tabatabaie T., Stewart C. A., Pye O. and Floyd R. A. (1997) Nitric oxide and derived species as toxic agents in stroke, AIDS, dementia, and chronic neurodegenerative disorders. *Chem. Res. Toxicol.* **10**: 527–532.
16. Zoellner S., Haseloff R., Kirilyuk I., Blasig I. E. and Rubanyi G. B. (1997) Nitroxides increase the detectable amount of nitric oxide released from endothelial cells. *J. Biol. Chem.* **272**: 23076.
17. Konovalova N. P., Goncharova S. A., Volkova L. M., Rayevskaya T. A., Yeremenko L. T. and Korolev A. M. (2003) Nitric oxide increases the effectiveness of cytostatic therapy and inhibits drug resistance development. *Probl. Oncol.* (*Vopr. Onkol.*) **49**: 71–75.
18. Giorgini E., Petrucci R., Astolfi, P., Mason R. P. and Greci L. (2002) On the role of nitrogen monoxide (nitric oxide) in the nitration of a tyrosine derivative and model compounds *Eur. J. Org. Chem.* 4011–4017, and references therein.
19. Astolfi P., Panagiotaki M., Rizzoli C. and Greci L. (2006) Reactions of indoles with nitrogen dioxide and nitrous acid in an aprotic solvent. *Org. Biomol. Chem.* **4**: 3282–3290.
20. Damiani E., Greci L. and Rizzoli C. (2001) Reaction of indolinonic aminoxyls with nitric oxide. *J. Chem. Soc., Perkin Trans.* **2**: 1139–1144.
21. Halliwell B. (1993) Reactive oxygen species in pathology with special reference to the skin. In: *Oxidative stress in dermatology*, pp 3–11, Fuchs J. and Packer L. (eds.), Marcel Dekker, New York.
22. Henderson P. T., Delaney J. C., Muller J. G., Neeley W. L., Tannenbaum S. R., Burrows C. J. and Essigmann J. M. (2005) The hydantoin lesions formed from oxidation of 7,8-dihydro-8-oxoguanine are potent sources of replication errors in vivo. *Biochemistry* **42**: 9257–9262.
23. Vainio H. and Branchini F. (2001) Sunscreens. In: *IARC Handbooks on Cancer Prevention,* Vol. 5, International Agency for Research on Cancer, Lyon.
24. Osterwalder U. and Herzog B. (2009) Chemistry and properties of organic and inorganic UV filters. In: *Clinical Guide to Sunscreens and Photoprotection*, pp 11–38, Lim H. W. and Draelos Z. D. (eds.), Informa Healthcare, New York.
25. Walling C. (1957) *Free Radicals in Solution*, John Wiley & Sons, New York.
26. Sosnovsky G. (1964) *Free Radical Reactions in Preparative Organic Chemistry,* The MacMillan Company, New York.

27. Nonhebel D. C. and Walton J. C. (1974) *Free Radical Chemistry Structure and Mechanism*, Cambridge University Press, Cambridge.
28. Schwack W. and Rudolph T. (1995) Photochemistry of dibenzoylmethane UVA filters: Part 1. *J. Photochem. Photobiol., B* **28**: 229–234.
29. Foote C. S. (1991) Definition of Type I and Type II photosensitized oxidation. *Photochem. Photobiol.* **54**: 659.
30. Foote C. S. (1981) Photooxidation of biological model compounds. In: *Oxygen and oxy-radicals in Chemistry and Biology,* pp 425–428, Rodgers M. A. and Powers E. L. (eds.), Academic Press, New York.
31. Federal Drug Administration (1999) Rules and Regulations. *Fed. Register* **64** (98): 27666–27693.
32. Gibbs N. K. (2001) Drug-induced skin phototoxicity: Lessons from the fluoroquinolones. In: *Sun Protection in Man*, pp 337–356, Giacomoni, P. U. (ed.), Elsevier Science, Amsterdam.
33. Moore D. E. (2002) Drug-induced cutaneous photosensitivity. Incidence, mechanism, prevention and management. *Drug Saf.* **25**: 345–372.
34. Orentreich D., Leone A.-S., Arpino G. and Burack H. (2001) Sunscreens: practical applications. In: *Sun protection in Man*, pp 535–559, Giacomoni, P. U. (ed.), Elsevier Science, Amsterdam.
35. Marrot L. and Meunier J. R. (2008) Skin DNA photodamage and its biological consequences. *J. Am. Acad. Dermatol.* **57** (5 Suppl 2): S139–148.
36. Kojima M. (2003) Photoinduced Electron Transfer Reactions of Organic Substances with Oxygen in Solutions and Zeolite Nanocavities. In: *Handbook of Photochemistry and Photobiology*, Vol. 2: Organic Photochemistry, pp 501–521, Nalwa H. S. (ed.), American Scientific Publishers.

F. Photophysical and Photochemical Reactions of Organic Sunscreen Agents

Various formulations—applied directly to the human skin with the intention of preventing sunburn—have been used since ancient times; however, only in the past 80 years, has selection of sunrays-absorbing ingredients been based on scientific principles.

These ingredients have been used in complex compositions collectively called sunscreens, ultraviolet filters, sunblocks, suntan lotions, and others. The vast realm of issues related to sunscreens has been covered in over 2000 pages of three editions of monographs published in 1990 [1],

1997 [2], and 2005 [3]. In addition, the subject was extensively discussed in recent books dealing with dermatology [4–12]. Considering the importance of the issue and the volume of effort around the world devoted to discovery of effective protection against the harmful consequences of exposure of human skin to ultraviolet radiation, the conclusions are still controversial, confusing and the accomplishments are questionable. A recent summary of the search toward the ideal sunscreen has been presented in a review article [13].

The evaluation of commercial sunscreen products was summarized in the fourth annual *Sunscreen Guide*, published on May 21, 2010, by the Environmental Working Group (EWG). It led to the conclusion that only a small fraction, 39 out of 500 beach and sport sunscreens offered on the market during that season, could be recommended for a relatively safe use. This report was supported by several hundred references. A more recent edition, the fifth annual *Sunscreen Guide*, was released on May 23, 2011, and included evaluation of 1700 sunscreen products. It contains equally negative conclusions about the efficacy of these commercial products.

An ideal sunscreen should have a strong absorption band in the entire UV region of the spectrum and, on absorption of UV radiation, should revert quickly to its ground state without producing decomposition products. The formulation applied to the skin should also be nontoxic, nonphototoxic, and must be photostable over a reasonable exposure time. It should be chemically inert in contact with water and oxygen. It turns out that satisfying these criteria is very difficult. All sunscreens are intended to shield the skin from intense ultraviolet radiation. At the same time, it is known that every organic molecule in the presence of oxygen, water, and light undergoes degradation. Many of these light-promoted chemical transformations, known as photochemical reactions, are desirable and can be utilized in preparative chemistry. The main aim of photochemistry is to investigate the physicochemical processes taking place during the interaction of photons with molecules, predict the outcome of these interactions, and employ them for synthetic purposes [14–24].

The objectives of research involving sunscreens are exactly the opposite. The goal is to create molecules that are highly resistant to any chemical transformation caused by exposure to ultraviolet and visible radiation for a prolonged period of time. It turns out that this goal remains elusive. Practically every UV absorber subjected to irradiation undergoes certain degradation. Unfortunately, only in very few studies, the researchers were able to elucidate the structures of the decomposition products. In most cases, the structures and fragments resulting from photodegradation remain unknown. Photochemical reactivity applies to active pharmaceutical ingredients the same way it does to common molecules; therefore, the International Conference on Harmonisation of Technical Requirements for Registration of Pharmaceuticals for Human Use (ICH) requires assessment of the photostability of new drugs [25, 26]. The regulations involving sunscreens are much less stringent.

The number of chemical entities selected as sun-protecting agents and approved for human use worldwide is relatively small. A special report [7], prepared by the working group on the evaluation of cancer-preventing agents invited by the International Agency of Research on Cancer, includes 53 chemical agents divided into UVB absorbers, UVA absorbers, both UVA and UVB absorbers, and inorganic absorbers. Fifty-one organic absorbers belong to the following structural groups: 7 are derivatives of *para*-aminobenzoic acid (PABA), 8 are esters of cinnamic acid (cinnamates), 8 are derivatives of salicylic acid, 6 are camphor derivatives, 9 are benzophenones, and the remaining 13 compounds belong to a variety of chemical classes. There are only two inorganic absorbers: zinc oxide and titanium dioxide [**Table 3F-1**].

The organic ingredients of sunscreens are known in commerce under a variety of trade names and generally more than one correct or incorrect chemical name. For example, several UV-absorbing esters contain the 2-ethylhexyl moiety. In a majority of publications, these esters are called octyl esters, and commercial names for commonly used ingredients such as Padimate O, Octisalate, Octocrylen, Octinoxate, were given to 2-ethylhexyl esters of 4-diaminobenzoic, salicylic, 2-cyano-3,3-diphenylacrylic, and 4-methoxycinnamic acids, respectively. The only reliable "Ariadne's clew of thread" in this labyrinth of confusing chemical and trade names is the CAS Registry Number^{SM}, a unique numerical identifier assigned by Chemical Abstracts Service (CAS), a division of the American Chemical Society, to every chemical that has been described in the literature. As of June 26, 2013, there were over 72.4 million organic and inorganic substances (and over 117 million as of July 31, 2016), just 18 months after reaching the 60-million milestone, and more than 64 million sequences in the CAS Registry. Around 50,000 new numbers are added each week. For example, the ethyl ester of 4-aminobenzoic acid has in the CAS Registry 14 chemical names and over 20 commercial names.

These substances are not uniformly accepted around the world. Individual countries or regions have introduced their own regulations classifying them as either over-the-counter drugs or as cosmetics. The most recent and comprehensive source [27] provides the lists of permitted UV filters in the United States, European Union, Canada, Australia and New Zealand, China, India, Japan, Korea, South Africa, Association of Southeast Asian

Nations (ASEAN), and Mercado Común del Sur, Southern Common Market (MERCOSUR). The chemical names corresponding to the most commonly used commercial names are listed in **Table 3F-1**. Among them, the United States has the most restrictive regulations, and only 16 of them were accepted in the United States in 1999 by the Food and Drug Administration (FDA) [28]. None of them has been used as an individual, chemically pure entity. Commercial sunscreens contain several UV absorbers dissolved or suspended in complex formulations containing solvents, emulsifiers, stabilizers, and other excipients. (See **Section 3D**.) On July 24, 2006, the FDA approved a new over-the-counter sunscreen product from L'Oreal called Anthelios® SX for the prevention of sunburn and for protection against ultraviolet B (UVB) and ultraviolet A (UVA) radiation.

This product with a sun protection factor (SPF) of 15 contains a combination of three UV filters. One of these ingredients, Ecamsule, a well-known compound since 1983, was introduced and approved in the United States as the seventeenth chemical entity that had been marketed as Mexoryl® SX in Europe and Canada since 1993. The CAS Registry file lists two chemical names for Ecamsule (Mexoryl® SX): 3,3'-(1,4-phenylenedimethylidene) bis(7,7-dimethyl-2-oxobicyclo[2.2.1]heptane-1-methanesulfonic acid and teraphthalidene-3,3'-dicamphor-10,10'-sulfonic acid. The complete IUPAC chemical name that includes the stereochemistry of the molecule is [(3*Z*)-3-[[4-[(*Z*)-[7,7-dimethyl-2-oxo-1-(sulfomethyl)-3-bicyclo[2.2.1]heptanylidene]methyl]phenyl]methylidene]-7,7-dimethyl-2-oxo-1-bicyclo-[2.2.1]heptanyl]methanesulfonic acid. This example illustrates the complexity of the nomenclature and potential problems in communication, taking into consideration that there are similar commercial names such as Mexoryl® XL.

Table 3F-1. Organic UV absorbers approved in various countries for sunscreens [7, 27].

para-Aminobenzoic Acid (PABA) and Derivatives

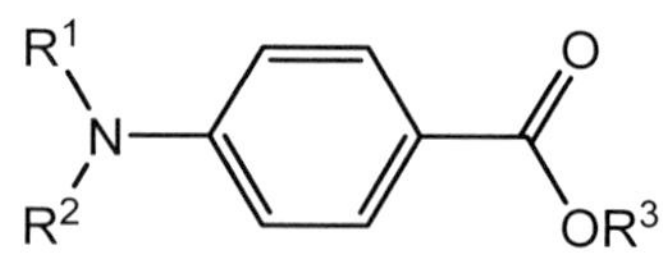

1. 4-Aminobenzoic acid, PABA, CAS 150-13-0, $R^1 = R^2 = R^3 = H$
2. Ethyl 4-[bis(2-hydroxypropyl)amino]benzoate, Roxadimate, CAS 58882-17-0, $R^1 = R^2 = CH_2CH(OH)CH_3$, $R^3 = CH_2CH_3$

3. *n*-Pentyl 4-(dimethylamino)benzoate, Padimate, CAS 14779-78-3, $R^1 = R^2 = CH_3$, $R^3 = (CH_2)_4CH_3$
4. 2-Ethylhexyl 4-(dimethylamino)benzoate, Padimate O, CAS 21245-02-3, $R^1 = R^2 = CH_3$, $R^3 = CH_2CH(CH_2CH_3)(CH_2)_3CH_3$
5. Ethyl 4-aminobenzoate, Benzocaine, Anesthesine, CAS 94-09-7, $R^1 = R^2 = H$, $R^3 = CH_2CH_3$
6. 4-Aminobenzoic acid monoglyceryl ester, Glyceryl PABA, Escalol® 106, CAS 136-44-7, $R^1 = R^2 = H$, $R^3 = CH_2CH(OH)CH_2OH$
7. PEG-25 PABA, Uvinul® P25, CAS 116242-27-4, $R^1 = H(OCH_2CH_2)_m$, $R^2 = H(OCH_2CH_2)_n$, $R^3 = CH_3CH_2(OCH_2CH_2)_l$ $m + n + l = 25$

Cinnamates

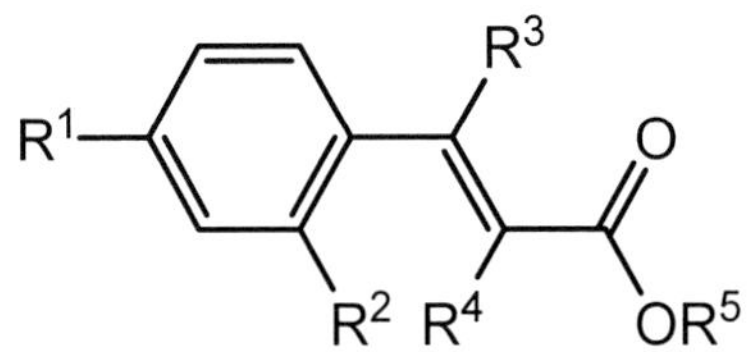

8. 2-Ethoxyethyl 4-methoxycinnamate, Cinoxate, CAS 104-28-9, $R^1 = OCH_3$, $R^2 = R^3 = R^4 = H$, $R^5 = CH_2CH_2OCH_2CH_3$
9. 4-Methoxycinnamic acid diethanolamine salt, CAS 56265-46-4, $R^1 = OCH_3$, $R^2 = R^3 = R^4 = H$, $R^5 = (CH_2CH_2OH)_2NH_2^+$
10. Methyl 2,4-di-isopropyl cinnamate, CAS 32580-71-5, $R^1 = R^2 = CH(CH_3)_2$, $R^3 = R^4 = H$, $R^5 = CH_3$
11. 2-Ethylhexyl 4-methoxycinnamate, Octinoxate, CAS 5466-77-3, $R^1 = OCH_3$, $R^2 = R^3 = R^4 = H$, $R^5 = CH_2CH(CH_2CH_3)(CH_2)_3CH_3$
12. Ethyl 4-methoxycinnamate, CAS 99880-64-5, $R^1 = OCH_3$, $R^2 = R^3 = R^4 = H$, $R^5 = CH_2CH_3$
13. 3-Methylbutyl 4-methoxycinnamate, Amiloxate, CAS 71617-10-2, $R^1 = OCH_3$, $R^2 = R^3 = R^4 = H$, $R^5 = (CH_2)_2CH(CH_3)_2$
14. 2-Ethylhexyl 2-cyano-3-phenylcinnamate, Octocrylene, CAS 6197-30-4, $R^1 = R^2 = H$, $R^3 = C_6H_5$, $R^4 = CN$, $R^5 = CH_2CH(CH_2CH_3)(CH_2)_3CH_3$
15. Ethyl 2-cyano-3,3-diphenylprop-2-enoate, Etocrylene, CAS 5232-99-5, $R^1 = R^2 = H$, $R^3 = C_6H_5$, $R^4 = CN$, $R^5 = CH_2CH_3$

Salicylates

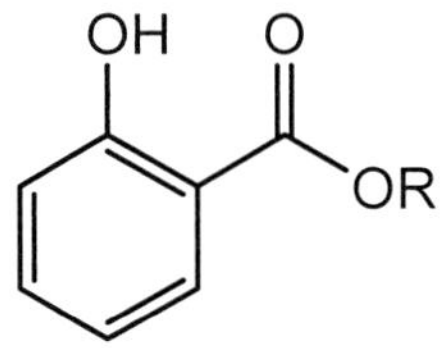

16. Methyl salicylate, CAS 119-36-8, R = CH_3
17. Phenyl salicylate, CAS 118-55-8, R = C_6H_5
18. 4-Isopropylbenzyl salicylate, CAS 94134-93-7, R = 4-$(CH_3)_2CHC_6H_4CH_2$
19. 2-Ethylhexyl salicylate, Octisalate, Escalol® 587, CAS 118-60-5, R = $CH_2CH(CH_2CH_3)(CH_2)_3CH_3$
20. 3,3,5-Trimethylcyclohexyl salicylate, Homosalate, CAS 118-56-9,

R =

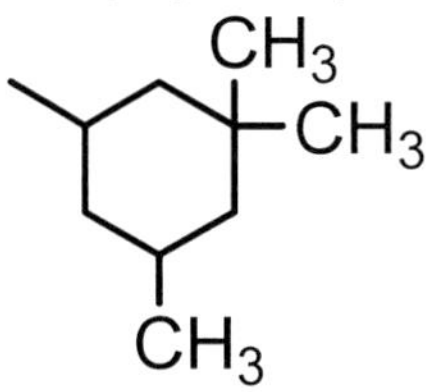

21. 2-Hydroxyethyl salicylate, CAS 87-28-5, R = CH_2CH_2OH
22. Salicylic acid triethanolamine salt, CAS 2174-16-5, R = $(CH_2CH_2OH)_3N^+$
23. Ester of salicylic acid with 1,1'-oxydi-2-propanol, CAS 7491-14-7, R = $CH_2(CH_3)CH_2OCH_2CH(OH)CH_3$

Camphor Derivatives

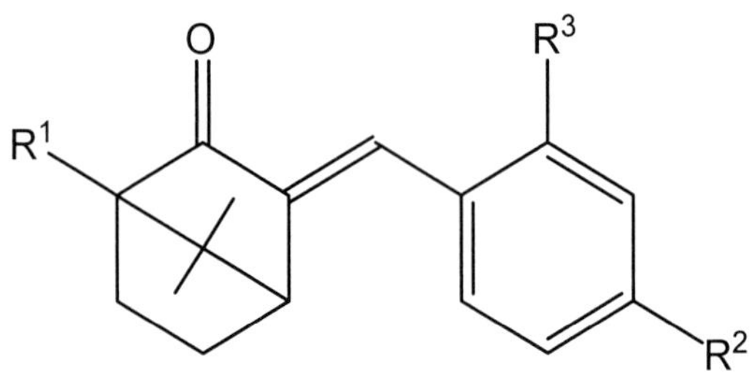

24. 3-Benzylidenecamphor, Mexoryl® SD, Eusolex® 6900, CAS 15087-24-8, $R^1 = CH_3$, $R^2 = R^3 = H$
25. (4'-Sulfo-3-benzylidene) camphor, Mexoryl® SL, CAS 56039-58-8, $R^1 = CH_3$, $R^2 = SO_3H$, $R^3 = H$
26. 3-[(*N,N,N*-Trimethylammonium)benzylidene]camphor methyl sulfate, Camphor benzalkonium methosulfate, Mexoryl® SO, CAS 52793-97-2, $R^1 = CH_3$, $R^2 = (CH_3)_3N^+$, $R^3 = CH_3OSO_3$
27. 3-(4'-Methylbenzylidene)camphor, Eusolex® 6300, Parsol® 500, CAS 38102-62-4, $R^1 = R^2 = CH_3$, $R^3 = H$
28. Polyacrylamidomethyl benzylidene camphor, Mexoryl® SW, CAS 113783-61-2, $R^1 = CH_3$, $R^2 = R^3 = CH_2NHC(O)CH{=}CH_2$
29. Terephthalidene 3,3'-dicamphor-10,10'-disulfonic acid, Mexoryl® SX, Ecamsule, CAS 90457-82-2

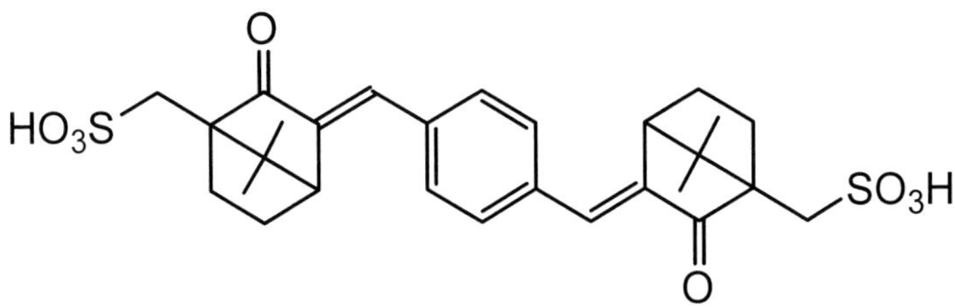

Benzophenones

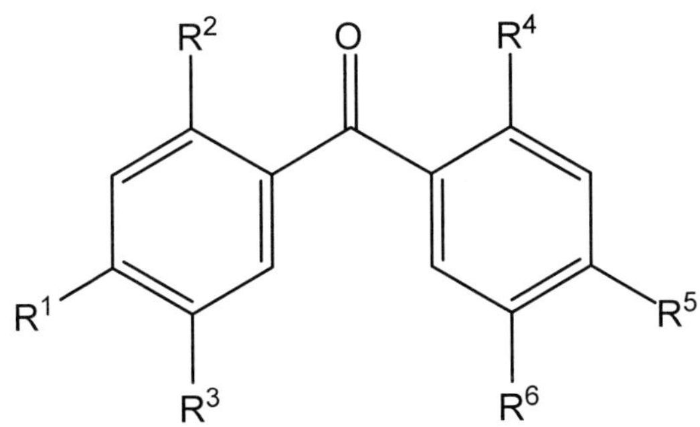

30. 2,4-Dihydroxybenzophenone, Benzophenone-1, CAS 131-56-6, $R^1 = R^2 = OH$, $R^3 = R^4 = R^5 = R^6 = H$
31. 2,2',4,4'-Tetrahydroxybenzophenone, Benzophenone-2, CAS 131-55-5, $R^1 = R^2 = R^4 = R^5 = OH$, $R^3 = R^6 = H$

32. 2-Hydroxy-4-methoxybenzophenone, Benzophenone-3, Oxybenzone, Eusolex® 4360, Escalol® 567, CAS 131-57-7, $R^1 = OCH_3$, $R^2 = OH$, $R^3 = R^4 = R^5 = R^6 = H$
33. 2-Hydroxy-4-methoxybenzophenone-5-sulfonic acid, Sulisobenzone, Benzophenone-4, CAS 4065-45-6, $R^1 = OCH_3$, $R^2 = OH$, $R^3 = SO_3H$, $R^4 = R^5 = R^6 = H$
34. 2-Hydroxy-4-methoxybenzophenone-5-sulfonic acid monosodium salt, Benzophenone-5, CAS 6628-37-1, $R^1 = OCH_3$, $R^2 = OH$, $R^3 = SO_3Na$, $R^4 = R^5 = R^6 = H$
35. 2,2'-Dihydroxy-4,4'-dimethoxybenzophenone, Benzophenone-6, CAS 131-54-4, $R^1 = R^5 = OCH_3$, $R^2 = R^4 = OH$, $R^3 = R^6 = H$
36. 2,2'-Dihydroxy-4'-methoxybenzophenone, Benzophenone-8, CAS 131-53-3, $R^1 = OCH_3$, $R^2 = R^4 = OH$, $R^3 = R^5 = R^6 = H$
37. 2,2'-Dihydroxy-4,4'-dimethoxybenzophenone-5,5'-disulfonic acid disodium salt, Benzophenone-9, Univul® 3048, CAS 76656-36-5, $R^1 = R^5 = OCH_3$, $R^2 = R^4 = OH$, $R^3 = R^6 = SO_3Na$
38. 2-Hydroxy-4-methoxy-4'-methylbenzophenone, Benzophenone-10, CAS 1641-17-4, $R^1 = OCH_3$, $R^2 = OH$, $R^5 = CH_3$, $R^3 = R^4 = R^6 = H$
39. Hexyl 2-[4-(diethylamino)-2-hydroxybenzoyl)benzoate, (4-diethylamino-2-hydroxybenzoyl-2'-hexyl benzoate, DHHB), Uvinul® A Plus, CAS 302776-68-7, $R^1 = (C_2H_5)_2N$, $R^2 = OH$, $R^3 = R^5 = R^6 = H$, $R^4 = (CH_2)_5CH_3$

Dibenzoylmethane

40. 4-*tert*-Butyl-4'-methoxydibenzoylmethane, Avobenzone, Eusolex® 9020, Parsol® 1789, Escalol® 51, CAS 70356-09-1

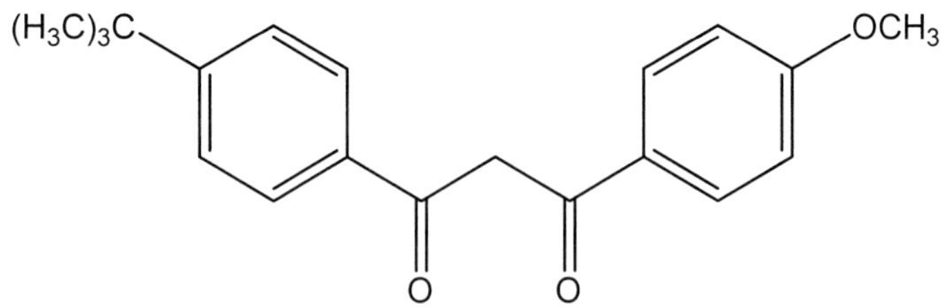

Triazines

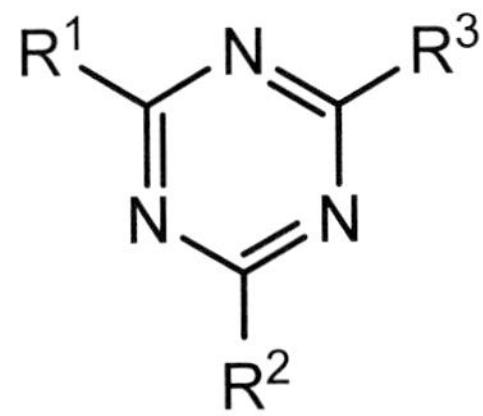

41. Di(2-ethylhexyl)-*tert*-butamidotriazone, CAS 154702-15-5,

$R^1 = R^2 =$

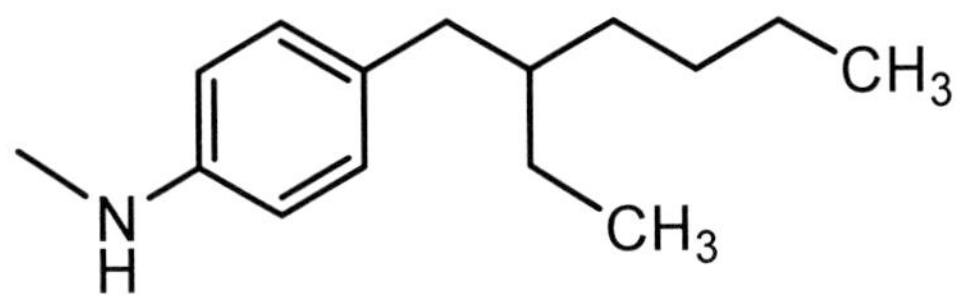

$R^3 =$

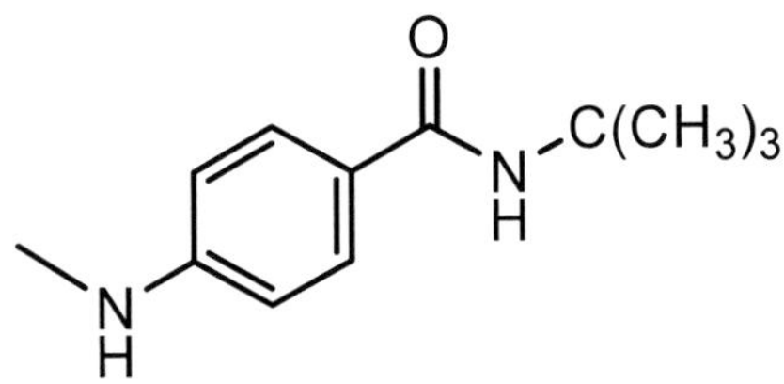

42. 2-Ethylhexyl triazone, Octyltriazone, EHT, CAS 88122-00-0,

$R^1 = R^2 = R^3 =$

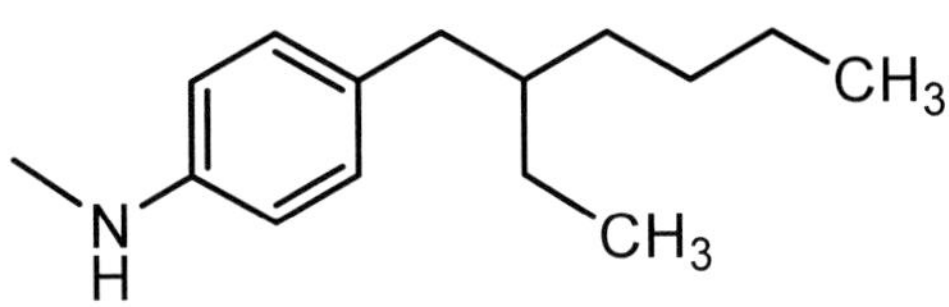

43. 2,4-[2-Hydroxy-4-(2-ethylhexyloxy)phenyl]-6-(4-methoxyphenyl)-1,3,5-triazine; Bemotrizinol, Tinosorb®, Escalol® S, CAS 187393-00-6,

$R^1 = R^2 =$

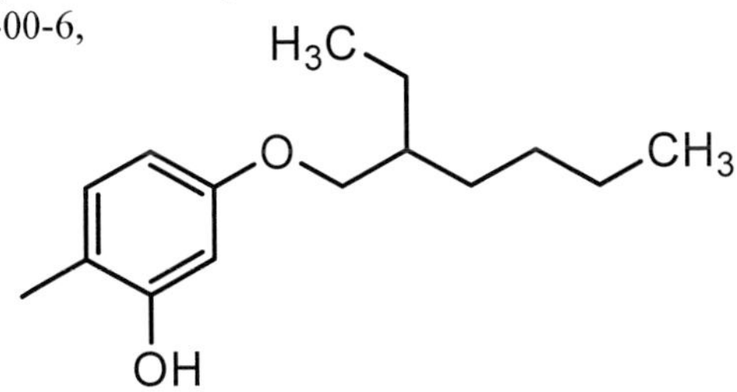

R^3 =

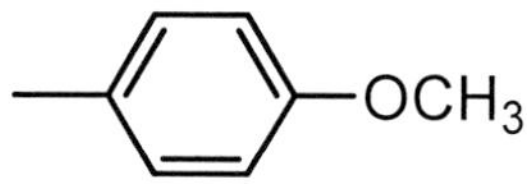

Miscellaneous

44. 5-Methyl-2-phenylbenzoxazole, CAS 7420-86-2

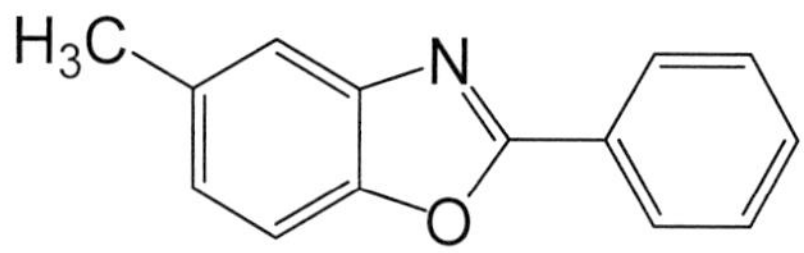

45. Menthyl anthranilate, Meradimate, CAS 134-09-8

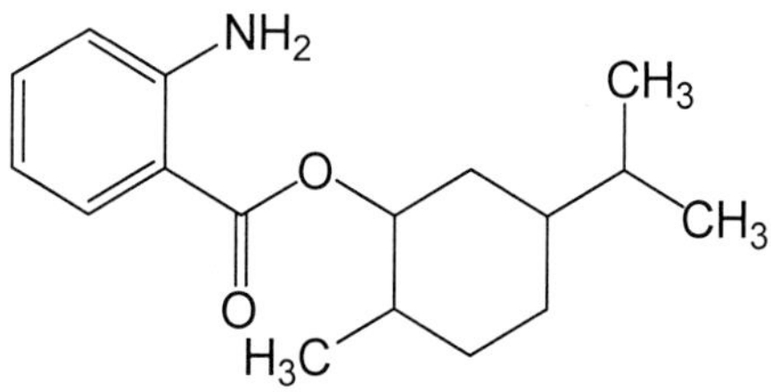

46. 2-Phenyl benzimidazole-5-sulfonic acid, Ensulizole, Eusolex® 232, PBSA, Parsol® HS, CAS 27503-81-7

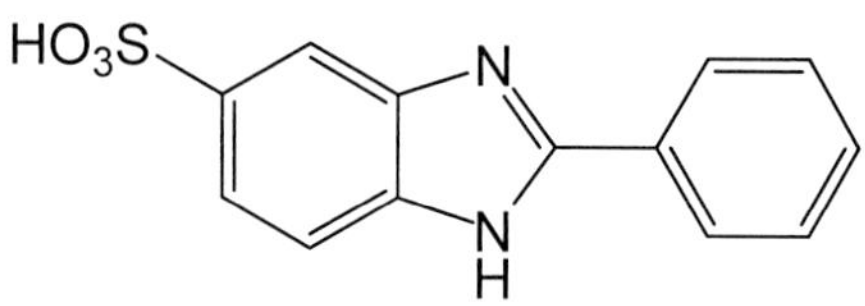

47. 1,4-Phenylenedibenzimidazoletetrasulfonic acid, Bisimidazylate, CAS 180898-37-7

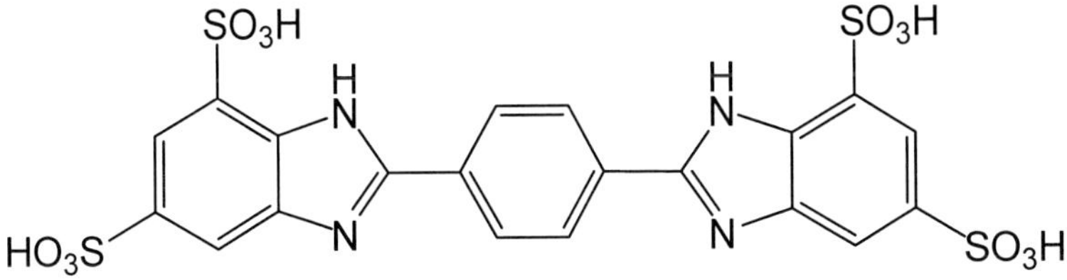

48. Drometrizole trisiloxane, Mexoryl® XL, CAS 155 633-54-8

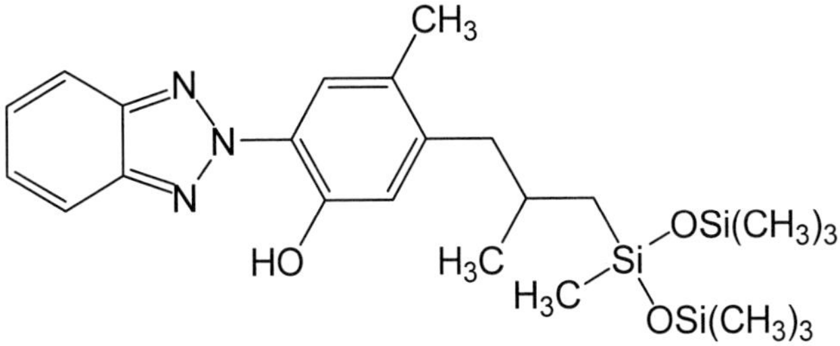

50. Methylene bis(benzotriazoyl (tetramethylbutyl)phenol) (MBBT), Tinosorb® M, Tinuvin® 360, Bisoctrizole, CAS 103597-45-1

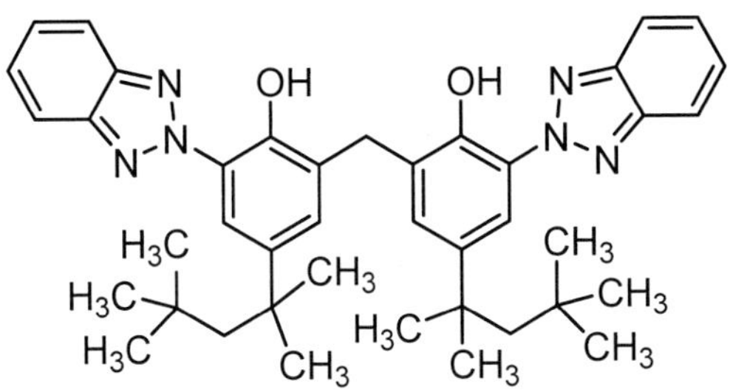

i. Photodegradation of *para*-Aminobenzoic acid (PABA) and Esters

Among the main groups of sunscreen absorbers listed in **Table 3F-1**, the derivatives of *para*-aminobenzoic acid (PABA) used to be very popular in commercial cosmetic and pharmaceutical products [**Table 3F-1**, **1**–**7**].

In spite of its poor photostability, reported as early as 1935 [29] and in 1943 [30], PABA was selected as one of the first UV absorbers employed in UVB sunscreens because of its low oral toxicity. It was widely used in the 1950s and 1960s, until later studies identified multiple problems [31]. Initially, PABA was recommended as a remedy for the prevention of skin cancers, including melanoma [32–36]. Although PABA itself has no toxicity [36, 37], and mutagenic activity in the Ames bacterial test [38], a likelihood of DNA damage was found in UV irradiations of repair-deficient strain of *Escherichia coli* in the presence of PABA [39–41].

Systematic investigations of PABA derivatives that showed their poor photostability alarmed the public and producers about potential hazards such as phototoxicity [42], allergic contact photodermatitis [43, 44], systemic immunologic alterations [45], and sensitization of near-UV radiations killing of mammalian cells [46]. (See **Sections 2A** and **2F**.) The photodecomposition of PABA has been studied by electron paramagnetic resonance spectroscopy (EPR) using 2-methyl-2-nitrosopropane as a spin trap [47]. Irradiation of an aqueous solution of *para*-aminobenzoic acid in the presence of 2-methyl-2-nitrosopropane resulted in the formation of free-radical photolysis products confirmed by a very strong EPR signal of the stable di-*tert*-butyl nitroxyl (DTBN) radical [47], as well as the spectrum of *tert*-butyl 4-carboxyphenyl nitroxyl radical. The primary radical, resulting from the irradiation of PABA, was believed to be the benzoic acid radical $\cdot C_6H_4CO_2H$ formed by the photolytic deamination of PABA [47]. Further studies [48] indicated that this radical was not the main intermediate in the chemical transformations of PABA, and that some additional photodegradation mechanisms are more significant. The decomposition pattern and the resulting products depend on the solvents and the presence or absence of oxygen.

Irradiation of aerated aqueous solutions of PABA in a photochemical reactor with UV monochromatic light at 254 or 313 nm led to the formation of two photoproducts, *cis*- and *trans*-azodibenzene-4,4'-dicarboxylic acids, which were isolated by ion exchange chromatography and characterized on the basis of their UV and mass spectral data [49]. Their formation was explained as the result of air oxidation of the PABA radical cation leading to 4-hydroxylaminobenzoic acid. Hydroxylamines are known to disproportionate to the corresponding nitroso and amino compounds. The reaction between the nitroso and amino groups may lead to the symmetric azodibenzoic acid; however a different mechanism is shown in **Sch. 3F.i-1**. The photoexcited PABA was reported to combine with other nitrogen atoms in proteins to form azobenzoic acid–protein derivatives that could account for its photoallergic responses [43, 44]. Furthermore, the PABA radical cation was shown to react directly with an amino group of a nucleic acid base, leading to the alteration of genetic information and possible mutagenic and carcinogenic effects [49, 50].

The formation of photodegradation products by the mechanism involving the intermediate benzoic acid radical [47] was disputed [51]. There is strong evidence that the key intermediate seems to be the 4-carboxyanilino radical formed by interaction of the photoexcited molecules of PABA with reactive oxygen species. Experiments on the photodegradation of PABA, carried out in the presence and absence of oxygen in aqueous solutions, led to the identification of several decomposition products. In the deoxygenated solution between pH 7.5 and 11.0, two photoproducts were identified by ^{1}H and ^{13}C NMR and by mass spectroscopy: 4-(2'-amino-5'-carboxyphenyl)aminobenzoic acid (**2**) and 4-(4'-aminophenyl)aminobenzoic acid (**3**) [51]. To confirm their identity, both compounds were also synthesized by independent routes. It appears that both photoproducts are formed by dimerization of intermediate radicals. The authors have not explained the mechanism of the initial deprotonation step leading to the 4-carboxyanilino radical. It is very unlikely that this radical can be formed without the presence of an oxidizing agent. The anaerobic solutions were prepared by bubbling pure nitrogen for 15 minutes; however, this procedure seems to be ineffective in removing every trace of oxygen, since it is known that it is very difficult to remove oxygen from the surface of glass and the solution itself without a series of freezing and thawing of solutions under high vacuum. Interestingly, azodibenzene-4,4'-dicarboxylic acid (**8**) was not detected as a significant photoproduct.

When PABA was photolyzed in aerated solutions, three major products were obtained: 4-amino-3-hydroxybenzoic acid (**4**), 4-aminophenol (**5**), and 4-(4'-hydroxyphenyl)aminobenzoic acid. The latter was also prepared by independent synthesis. Subsequently, the photochemistry of *para*-aminobenzoic acid in a 0.1% solution of 0.05 M phosphate buffer (pH = 7.0) was investigated using two validated reversed-phase HPLC methods [52]. The photolysis was carried out in a photoreactor with an output from 303 to 400 nm, with the maximum at 366 nm. The UV irradiation experiments were carried out up to 120 hours and produced a complex mixture of photochemical degradation molecules containing up to nine photoproducts such as 4-nitrobenzoic acid, 4-nitrosobenzoic acid, azoxybenzene-4,4'-dicarboxylic acid, 4,4'-hydrazobenzenedicarboxylic acid (**7**), azobenzene-4,4'-dicarboxylic acid (**8**), and several unidentified photoproducts. The composition of the resulting mixture of photodegradation products depends on the pH and the presence or absence of molecular oxygen. The interaction of photoexcited species with water and oxygen can lead to the formation of the superoxide anion radical, singlet oxygen, hydrogen peroxide, and hydroxyl radicals, as well as secondary products [**Sch. 3F.i-1**].

The physical properties of PABA, such as its poor solubility in commercial formulations and its moderate extinction coefficient of 13,600 [53], led to the introduction of several liquid ester derivatives, in which the chemically labile amino and carboxylic groups are shielded by aliphatic substituents, such as *n*-pentyl or 2-ethylhexyl. These two esters of 4-(*N,N*-dimethylamino)benzoic acid are known commercially as Padimate and Padimate O [**Table 3F-1**, **4**]. The latter is a liquid with a higher extinction coefficient of about 28,400 in polar solvents [53].

Although the development and application of the liquid esters successfully solved the issue of poor solubility in cosmetic media, the problem of poor photostability remained. Initial studies were carried out on a simple model compound, methyl 4-(*N,N*-dimethylamino)benzoate, that is not approved as a sunscreen. However, its simplicity allowed the isolation and identification of the decomposition products and the understanding of the degradation processes better than in the case of more complex molecules. Thus, this ester was irradiated for 48 hours in a 1,4-dioxane solution with a UV light source in the presence of oxygen to give methyl 4-(mono-*N*-methylamino)benzoate, methyl 4-(*N*-methyl-*N*-formyl)benzoate, methyl 4-(*N*-formylamino)benzoate, methyl 4-(formylamino)benzoate, and methyl 4-aminobenzoate. All five photoproducts were isolated and identified by comparisons of their IR, NMR, and mass spectra with synthesized reference samples. Although the degradation mechanisms were not discussed, one can assume that the formation of the demethylation products involved free radical species [54, 55]. Several sunscreen active ingredients, including PABA (**1**) [56] and Padimate O (**4**) [57], when irradiated in air-saturated aqueous solutions with sunlight-range artificial light, produced singlet molecular oxygen. Singlet oxygen is known to be cytotoxic [56, 57].

Although the remaining six PABA derivatives [**Table 3F-1, 2-7**] are better photostable than the parent PABA, the entire group bears similar problems. [58–60]. Half-life times of PABA (**1**), 1-glyceryl 4-aminobenzoate (Escalol® 106) (**6**) and 2-ethylhexyl 4-(*N,N*-dimethyl)aminobenzoate (Escalol® 507, Padimate O) (**4**) in 5 x 10^{-5} M dilute ethanolic solutions were 177, 155, and 253 minutes, respectively [61]. 4-(*N,N*-Dimethyl) aminobenzoic acid also undergoes partial photodecomposition [49, 50]. The isopentyl ester of *N,N*-dimethyl-PABA (Padimate A) was found to cause a phototoxic and allergic contact response in humans [43, 44]. After comparing the results of this elaborate research spanning over 20 years, the only conclusion that can be drawn is that PABA and its derivatives decompose when irradiated with UV light. One wonders how these results obtained in various media, using artificial light sources applied for up to 96 hours, can be related to the fate of PABA and its derivatives in formulations containing several other UV absorbers, emulsifiers, fragrances, polymers, and other ingredients, when applied to the surface of human skin exposed to a few hours of natural sunlight. For example, 2-ethylhexyl 4-(*N,N*-dimethylamino)benzoate (Padimate O) was irradiated for 70, 100, and 140 hours in cyclohexane [62]. After irradiation, the solution was analyzed by GC, GC/MS, and HPLC. After 70 h of irradiation, the monomethyl ester, 2-ethylhexyl 4-(*N*-methylamino)benzoate, was observed with no detectable additional products. However, after 140 h of irradiation, the resulting mixture contained 21% of a mono-demethylation product, 5% of 2-ethylhexyl 4-dimethylamino-(*ortho/meta*)-methylbenzoic acid (monomethylation of the ring), and less than 1% of 2-ethylhexyl 4-aminobenzoate containing a double demethylated *N,N*-dimethylamino group [62]. The monodemethylation product was identified by GC/MS in another study [63]. In addition, the second photodegradation product was identified as 2-ethylhexyl 4-(formylmethylamino)benzoate. It has been reported that Padimate O, or impurities present in the commercial product, can undergo nitrosation to carcinogenic nitrosamines. [64, 65]. A systematic spectroscopic examination of PABA and Padimate O irradiated by simulated sunlight proved that both compounds are highly photounstable [66]. After 60 minutes of UV illumination, the absorption of the air-equilibrated solution of PABA in hexane, water, methanol, and acetonitrile in the region between 250 and 300 nm was decreased by 87%, 65%, 60%, and 45%, respectively. The photodegradation of Padimate O was even faster. In *n*-hexane and acetonitrile solution, photodegradation, 97% and 94%, respectively, was almost complete in 20 minutes. The decomposition in water and methanol was somewhat slower, 75% and 15% [**Table 3F.i-1**] [66].

Two compounds from this group, PEG-25 PABA and 2-ethylhexyl 4-(*N,N*-dimethylamino)benzoic acid were irradiated in an oil–water emulsion prepared from 13 ingredients. The half-life times of these UV filters were 115 and 85 minutes, respectively. They lost 10% of their effectiveness after 20 minutes [67].

As discussed in Section 2D, the components of nucleic acids undergo UV-light-induced damage by various mechanisms. The major effect is attributed to the [2 + 2] cycloaddition of the C_5–C_6 double bonds of adjacent pyrimidines [68]. PABA acts as photosensitizer in the formation of thymine dimers in DNA [69–75]. Furthermore, PABA photoproducts were

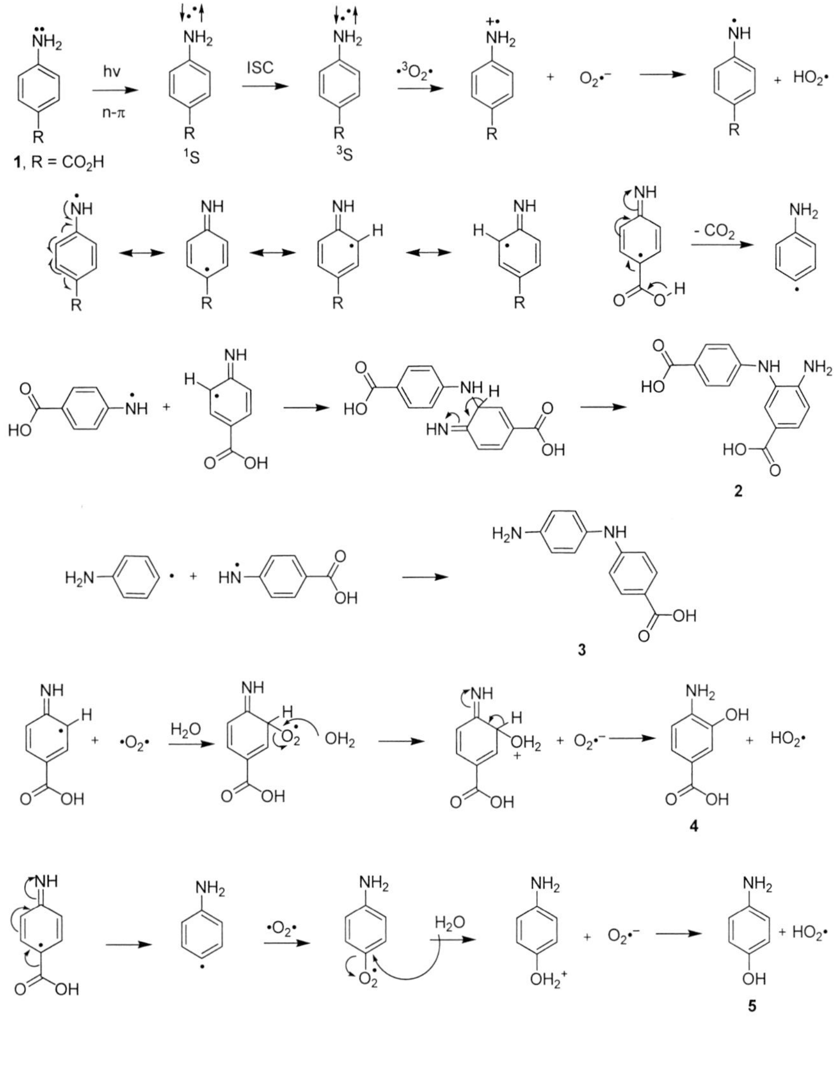
hv
n-π
1, R = CO2H
1S
ISC
3S
•3O2•
O2•−
HO2•
- CO2
2
3
H2O
4
5

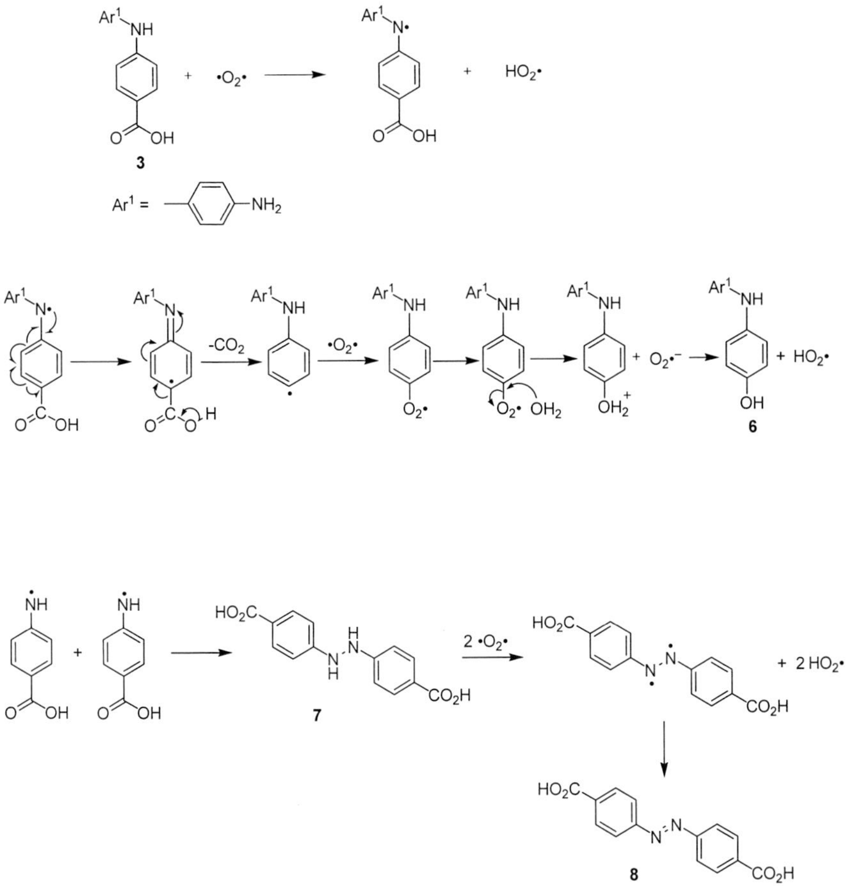

Sch. 3F.i-1. Mechanisms for the UV radiation induced degradation of PABA.

found to interact with DNA to form covalent bonds with various nucleobases [73].

Thus, the irradiation of an aqueous solution of PABA and thymine [**Sch. 3F.i-2**, **9**, R = H] in water for 72 h at $\lambda = 254$ nm resulted in the formation of the 1:1 thymine–PABA adduct, 5-(2-amino-5-carboxyphenyl)-5,6-dihydrothymine (**11**, R=H). A similar reaction takes place between PABA and thymidine with the formation of **11** (R = **10**).

Table 3F.i-1. UV Radiation Induced Degradations of Sunscreens at Wavelengths Longer than 290 nm. Of Significance Are the Results Obtained with Aqueous Solutions [66].

Sunscreen Agent	Solvent	Time	Percent Degradation
para-Aminobenzoic Acid (PABA)	Water	1 h	>65
	Methanol	1 h	>60
	n-Hexane	1 h	87
	Acetonitrile	1 h	45
2-Ethylhexyl 4-(*N,N*-dimethylamino)benzoate (Padimate O)	Water	20 min	>75
	Methanol	20 min	>15
	n-Hexane	20 min	97
	Acetonitrile	20 min	94
2-Ethylhexyl 4-methoxycinnamate (Octinoxate)	Water	30 min	90
	Methanol	30 min	40
	n-Hexane	30 min	40
	Acetonitrile	30 min	45
2-Hydroxy-4-methoxybenzophenone (Oxybenzone, Benzophenone-3)	Water	2 h	20
	Methanol	2 h	90
	n-Hexane	2 h	15
	Acetonitrile	2 h	5–10
2-Phenyl-1*H*-benzimidazole-5-sulfonic acid	Water	10 min	90
	Acetonitrile	20 min	50
	Acetonitrile	2 h	70

Both photoexcited molecules can form diradical intermediates as a result of n,π^* and π,π^* transitions. A photoexcited molecule of PABA that forms, by interaction with oxygen, the 4-carboxyanilino radical attacks position 5 of the thymidine diradical. However, the results of in vivo studies on photogenotoxicity and photomutagenicity of PABA derivatives did not support concerns raised on the basis of in vitro studies. Despite the exaggerated UV radiation exposure resulting in tumorogenesis in most animals, PABA derivatives seem to protect against UV-induced skin tumor formation in rodents [76].

It has been demonstrated that PABA readily penetrates human skin and undergoes further metabolism in the blood stream. HPLC analyses of urine samples collected from volunteers, whose skin was treated with PABA sunscreen formulations, allowed the detection of PABA and its metabolites, such as 4-aminohippuric, 4-acetamidobenzoic, and 4-acetamidohippuric acids [77]. In order to prevent skin penetration, most of the newly added sunscreen molecules have molecular weights compliant with "the 500 Dalton rule" [78]. 2,4,6-Trianilino(4-carbo-2-ethylhexyloxy)-1,3,5-triazine (EHT) with a molecular weight of 823 is definitely too large to penetrate the skin; nevertheless, the molecule contains three PABA chromophores, that are also present in Padimate O, attached to the triazine ring that manifest the same photolytic instability and can cause the same phototoxic injuries as low-molecular-weight PABA derivatives [79].

The materials in most of the photodegradation studies have been exposed to various forms of UV radiation under unnatural conditions remotely resembling the actual environment of organic UV filters either dispersed or dissolved in a commercial formulation interacting with human skin covered with sweat or water in recreational waters such as swimming pools or salty sea water. In a recent study of the photochemical behavior of 2-ethylhexyl 4-(*N,N*-dimethylamino)benzoate (**4**) in different aqueous media, such as distilled water, chlorinated swimming pool water, and seawater, it was demonstrated that the ester degrades photochemically in the aquatic environment leading to formation of several photoproducts, including monochloro- and dichloro-substitution products [80].

Although all seven PABA derivatives still appear on the lists of UV absorbers approved in the U.S.A., the European Union, Japan, and Australia, the overwhelming evidence of their deficiencies resulted in the gradual withdrawal of these products from current formulations. Several producers began to label commercial products as "PABA-free" a few decades ago. A recent inspection of over 200 products on the shelves of a drugstore in the U.S.A. revealed that none of them contained any PABA

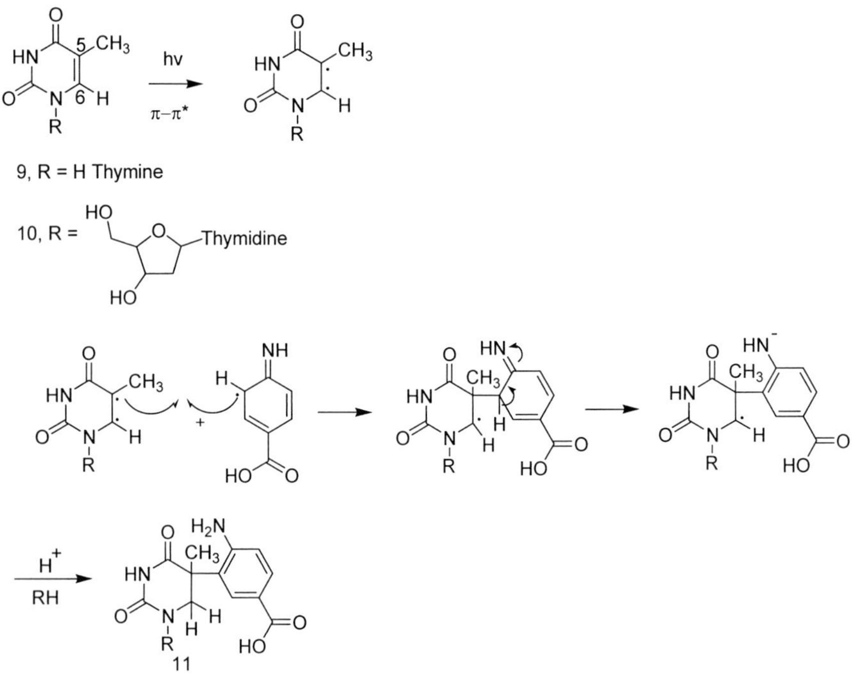

Sch. 3F.i-2. Photochemical reactions of thymine and thymidine with *para*-aminobenzoic acid (PABA).

derived compound. All products with SPF values between 4 and 60 contained more than one UV absorber, usually 4 to 6, and over 20 so-called inactive ingredients, such as alcohols and glycols, benzyl alcohol, phenoxyethanol, various esters, such as alkylparabens, i.e., methyl, ethyl, propyl, and butyl esters of 4-hydroxybenzoic acid, and esters of fatty acids, vegetable oils, and extracts, polymers, such as acrylamide/sodium acrylate copolymer, polyethylene glycol 40 acrylate, fragrances, barium sulfate, urea, and others. (See **Section 3D**.) At the same time, Aubrey Organics, a U.S.A. company with more than 4500 retailers around the world, proudly promotes "Green Tea Natural Sun Screen SPF 25 for Children" containing 8% Padimate O and 10% titanium dioxide suspended in *Simmondsia chinensis* (jojoba) oil, *Simmondsia chinensis* (jojoba butter), alcohol denaturated, *Helianthus annuus* (sunflower) oil, *Camellia japonica* (camellia) oil, lecithin, glycerin, *Epilobium angustifolium* (willowherb) extract, *Butyrospermum parkii* (shea butter), *Aloe barbadensis* (aloe) leaf juice, *Camellia sinensis* (green tea) leaf, glyceryl linoleate and glyceryl linolenate (vitamin E), silica, *Citrus grandis* (grapefruit) seed extract, tocopheryl acetate (vitamin E), *Hamamelis virginiana* (witch hazel) extract, ascorbic acid (vitamin C), *Glycine soja* (soybean) oil, *Daucus carota sativa* (carrot) root extract, β-carotene, *Jasminum officinale* (jasmine) oil, and *Tanacetum annuum* (Moroccan blue chamomile) oil. Although PABA itself and other herbal extracts possess a very low oral toxicity, it does not mean that they are safe when they are exposed to solar radiation. Every herbal extract consists of a complex mixture of organic compounds. It was proven a long time ago that bergamot oil, a common component of food products, perfumes, and sunscreen formulations, has phototoxic and photosensitizing properties [81–83].

ii. Cinnamates

Esters of cinnamic acid such as methyl, ethyl, and benzyl cinnamates are used as components in food flavoring compositions, perfumes, and pharmaceuticals. Cosmetic grades of substituted cinnamic esters have been utilized as sunscreen agents to reduce skin damage by blocking UV radiations [**Table 3F-1**, **8**–**15**]. Benzyl cinnamate is used today as a common flavoring agent. It was introduced in 1928 as one of the earliest sunscreens [84]. This ester is not employed in currently approved ultraviolet (UV) filters. There are 17 derivatives of cinnamic acid listed by the European Cosmetics Association (COLIPA), however, only eight of them have been permitted by various international regulations as components of sunscreens [**Table 3F-1**, **8**–**15**] [7, 85]. Cinnamates have high molar extinction coefficients (>23000) [1] and are present in over 90% of suncare products [86]. They absorb UV light corresponding to a wavelength of about 305 nm, i.e., UVB radiation [84]. Among them two, 2-ethylhexyl 4-methoxycinnamate (EHMC), commonly and incorrectly called octyl methoxycinnamate (OMC, or octinoxate, **11**) and 2-ethylhexyl 2-cyano-3-phenylcinnamate, known as octocrylene (OCR, **14**) are still ubiquitous in commercial formulations, in spite of inadequate stability. Unfortunately, both of them are relatively unstable, and, when irradiated in air-saturated aqueous solutions with sunlight-range artificial light, produce cytotoxic singlet molecular oxygen [57].

Cinnamic acid derivatives undergo photochemical [2 + 2] cycloadditions and trans–cis (*E*–*Z*) photoisomerization [87–89]. The *E*–*Z* photoisomerization of cinnamates used in sunscreens was studied by steady-state and laser flash photolysis in aqueous and organic solutions. 2-Ethylhexyl 4-methoxycinnamate undergoes reversible trans–cis photoisomerization with a considerable loss of absorbance at 310 nm [90].

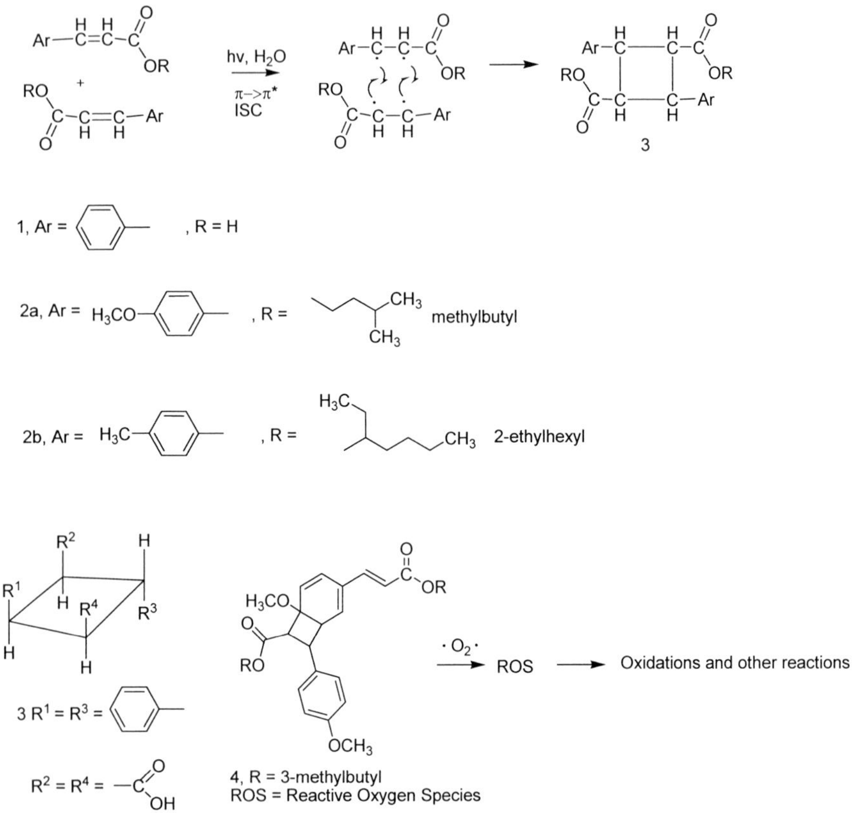

Sch. 3F.ii-1. The UV radiation induced reactions of cinnamic acid and its esters proceed by a [2 + 2] cycloaddition to form cyclobutane derivatives **3**. In nature, five steroisomers of 2,4-diphenyl-1,3-cyclobutanedicarboxylic acid (**3**, truxillic acid) are found in cocaine. The gamma isomer is called cocaic acid. Analogous reactions occur with sunscreen agents **2a** and **2b**, whereby a more complex condensation by the [2 + 2] addition involves the aromatic rings.

The quantum yields were fairly high (~0.5–1); however, no photoproducts were isolated. It was assumed, therefore, that the reversible *E–Z* photoisomerization is the only transformation. Nevertheless, it was reported earlier that the photoinduced dimerizations of derivatives of cinnamic acid [**Sch. 3F.ii-1, 1**] result in the formation of stereoisomeric truxinic/truxilic acid derivatives **3** [91]. This kind of photochemical transformation was observed when a 10% solution of 3-methylbutyl 4-methoxycinnamate, an analog of EHMC (OMC, **2a**), in *n*-hexane or isopropanol, was irradiated in a solar simulator to give **4** [92, 93]. Similar results were obtained with cinnamates **2b**. Initially, the cinnamic ester produced an equilibrium of the cis and trans forms. The ratio between the trans and cis isomers was 25:1.

These isomers underwent further complex transformation to give [2 + 2] and [2 + 4] cycloadducts. Interestingly, the cycloaddition did not take place between two aliphatic double bonds but between one trans double bond of the cinnamic ester and the 3–4 double bond of the aromatic ring in the second molecule of the cinnamic ester. The reaction of the resulting adduct with molecular oxygen formed an epoxide. The epoxide, in turn, was rearranged to the lactone. The dimerization of the [2 + 2] cycloadduct led to a small amount of a tetramer. Eight individual compounds were isolated by column chromatography and preparative TLC. The isolated fractions were analyzed by ^{1}H and ^{13}C NMR [**Sch. 3F.ii-1**]. These transformations lead to a significant loss of absorbance [92, 93].

Several research groups have studied the photostability of cinnamates under various conditions. In most cases, the measurements were carried out on commercial products containing several ingredients. A composition containing 4% of 2-ethylhexyl 4-methoxycinnamate was exposed to a solar simulator. After one hour, the degradation did not exceed 4.5% [94, 95]; therefore, the conclusion was reached that the ester has a satisfactory stability in a medium close to those used in cosmetics. Dilute solutions of 2-ethylhexyl 4-methoxycinnamate in mineral oil, isopropyl myristate, and a 70:30 mixture of ethanol and water were irradiated in quartz cells with a solar simulator equipped with filters eliminating radiation between <290 nm and >400 nm. After exposure of the ester to 5 minimal erythemal doses (MED), the absorbance in these three solvents decreased by 18.7%, 18.7%, and 39.1%, respectively [96]. The same ester and 3-methylbutyl 4-methoxycinnamate were studied in vitro by a modified method. Both cinnamate esters suffered very significant protection efficacy losses up to 50–60% of their initial values [97, 98]. A poor photostability of cinnamates was also reported in more recent papers [67, 69, 99–113]. Some of these publications were devoted to stabilization of unstable active ingredients used in commercial formulations. For example, addition of 2,4-[2-hydroxy-4-(2-ethylhexyloxy)phenyl]-6-(4-methoxyphenyl)-1,3,5-triazine, bis-ethylhexyl-oxyphenol methoxyphenyl triazine (Tinosorb® S, **Table 3F-1**, **43**), significantly improves the photostability of 2-ethylhexyl 4-methoxycinnamate (EHMC) [102]. EHMC kept in the dark at 4, 20, 32, and 60 °C for one month remains stable; however, it degrades to a new product when exposed to sunlight. The photodegradation product was isolated by semi-preparative HPLC. NMR spectra of this product indicated a change from the trans (*E*) isomer to the cis (*Z*) isomer [103, 104]. The extinction coefficient of the cis isomer is around 15,000; therefore, without any further structural degradation, the photoprotection of this form is much lower than that of the trans isomer (23,000) [86]. A photostability assessment of five UV filters, including EHMC, by recovering the emulsions from human volunteers' forearms after 40-MED irradiation confirmed a significant loss of stability (–42.3%) [105]. A similar result was obtained in an in vivo study of three solar-simulated and actual sun-exposed marketed sunscreen products with SPF 23–30 containing EHMC and octocrylene (OC). Two products containing 7.5% of EHMC, in combination with other active ingredients, were found to be photounstable, and one containing OC was found to be photostable [106]. The trans–cis isomerization of EHMC (OMC) can be decreased by grafting the molecule onto a silicone polymer. The resulting poly[3-(*p*-methoxycinnamido) (propyl)(methyl)siloxane copolymer was shown to have a lower degree of isomerization when exposed to UVB light [107]. Another attempt at stabilizing EHMC involves encapsulation of the compound in solid lipid nanoparticles (SLN) [108, 109]. However, it has been shown in a number of studies that nanosize materials with 1–20 nm size can have a range of detrimental biological properties and, hence, should be carefully investigated in new applications. (See **Section 3G**.)

Since the behavior of sunscreens is not predictable based on the photostabilities of their individual components, several studies were conducted using various analytical methods with artificial and commercial formulations [110–117]. Recent experiments have shown that the presence of antioxidants and free-radical scavengers such as α-tocopherol (vitamin E), vitamin E acetate, or the stable free radical bis(2,2,6,6-tetramethyl-1-oxyl-piperidine-4-yl)sebacate, may improve the performance of sunscreens [113]. A more radical approach involves incorporation of free-radical moieties into the molecules of UV absorbers. For example, 2-ethylhexyl 4-methoxycinnamate was combined with 4-hydroxy-2,2,6,6-tetramethyl-piperidinol (TEMPOL) to form a novel sunscreen antioxidant [114]. Similarly, the same ester was modified by replacing one hydrogen atom in the methoxy group with a moiety of the stable free radical 3-hydroxymethyl-2,2,5,5-tetramethylpyrrolidine [115]. The new substances absorb the UV radiations, and, at the same time, can function as free-radical scavengers with antioxidant activities comparable to those of vitamin E and butylated hydroxytoluene (BHT), and hence can effectively reduce the sunlight-induced lipid peroxidation in liposomes [114, 115]. These two molecules may be excellent photostable additions to the present list of UV filters. (See **Section 5**.)

The UV-induced changes in the UV transmittance of sunscreen products depend on the composition and concentrations of sunscreen agents. The concomitant photolysis of EHMC and avobenzone predominates the expected trans–cis isomerization. Moreover, irradiation of a film containing both products in a cavity of an electron spin resonance (ESR) spectrometer produced free radicals which were detected by ESR spectroscopy. The ESR signal of free radicals appears after 3 minutes of exposure. These radicals persisted even after shutting down the light source [118].

Recently, the photochemistry of 2-ethylhexyl 4-methoxycinnamate was studied in the presence of another widely used photounstable UV absorber, 4-*tert*-butyl-4'-methoxydibenzoylmethane (Avobenzone, **Table 3F-1**, **40**). These two active sunscreen agents were irradiated by a solar simulator in pure solvents separately and together in solution and in neat form. Irradiation of the cinnamate and diketone together led to the [2 + 2] photocycloaddition products **7** and **8** shown in **Sch. 3F.ii-2**. Chromatographic separations of the resulting mixtures revealed the presence of cinnamate dimers and cross-adducts identified by distortionless enhancement polarization transfer (DEPT) and two-dimensional NMR experiments [119].

iii. Salicylates

This group is represented by eight compounds [**Table 3F-1**, **16–23**]. Three of them are approved by the FDA for use in the U.S.A. (**19**, **20**, and **22**). Although benzyl salicylate was introduced in the United States as the first commercial sunscreen in 1928, then successfully launched in France in 1936, it is not approved anymore as a sunscreen. In spite of several problems, such as being a well-recognized consumer allergen and estrogen [120], it is still being used in fragrances for women, shampoos, bar soaps, hair sprays, hand creams, and other products. Benzyl salicylate was shown to have estrogenic activity by increasing the proliferation of breast cancer cells in vitro [117].

Otherwise, the salicylate esters, as a group, are very versatile. They can be used for dissolving other solid sunscreens, such as benzophenones. The ortho-substituted structures are able to form intramolecular hydrogen bonds, thus stabilizing the molecules against external interactions with other ingredients. Until now, no information is available about any photodegradation products of salicylate esters. Only one of them, 3,3,5-trimethylcyclohexyl salicylate (homosalate, HS, **20**), undergoes cis–trans isomerization of the cyclohexane ring [84]. Film layers of homosalate and phenyl salicylate were spectrophotometrically monitored on stratum corneum sheets before and after solar irradiation. From the changes in the absorption spectra, it was determined that the spectral stability of homosalate was good and the photostability of phenyl salicylate was poor [121]. The stability of salicylate esters depends on the medium. Dilute solutions (200 ppm) of homosalate and 2-ethylhexyl salicylate (octisalate, EHS) in mineral oil, isopropyl myristate (IPM), and a 70:30 mixture of ethanol and water were irradiated with a solar simulator. After 5 MED, the absorbance of homosalate declined by 4.0, 4.7, and 1.6%, while the absorbance of octisalate was not changed in mineral oil; however it was reduced by 9.8% in IPM and 1.5% in ethanol–water [121]. Both homosalate and octisalate were studied in vivo on twelve healthy men and women by diffuse reflectance spectroscopy as components of three marketed products with SPF of 23–30 [106]. One product was found to be photostable and two products were photounstable. It is difficult to judge what positive or negative role salicylate ingredients have in these mixtures of four or five sunscreens, since the two unstable products contained components with well-documented instability.

Representatives from both groups, PABA derivatives and cinnamates, when irradiated in air-saturated solutions with artificial sunlight, produced cytotoxic singlet oxygen; however, octisalate subjected to the same treatment was stable [57]. This result indicates that octisalate is a better choice for sunscreen formulations with regard to the formation of undesirable reactive oxygen species than other classes of compounds. Photostability of salicylates was also measured in two independent studies including 14 substances [111] and 18 substances [67]. While in the first case octisalate was found to be stable, in the second study conducted under different conditions both octisalate and homosalate had a moderate stability. The half-life times for octisalate and homosalate were 85 min and 300 min, respectively.

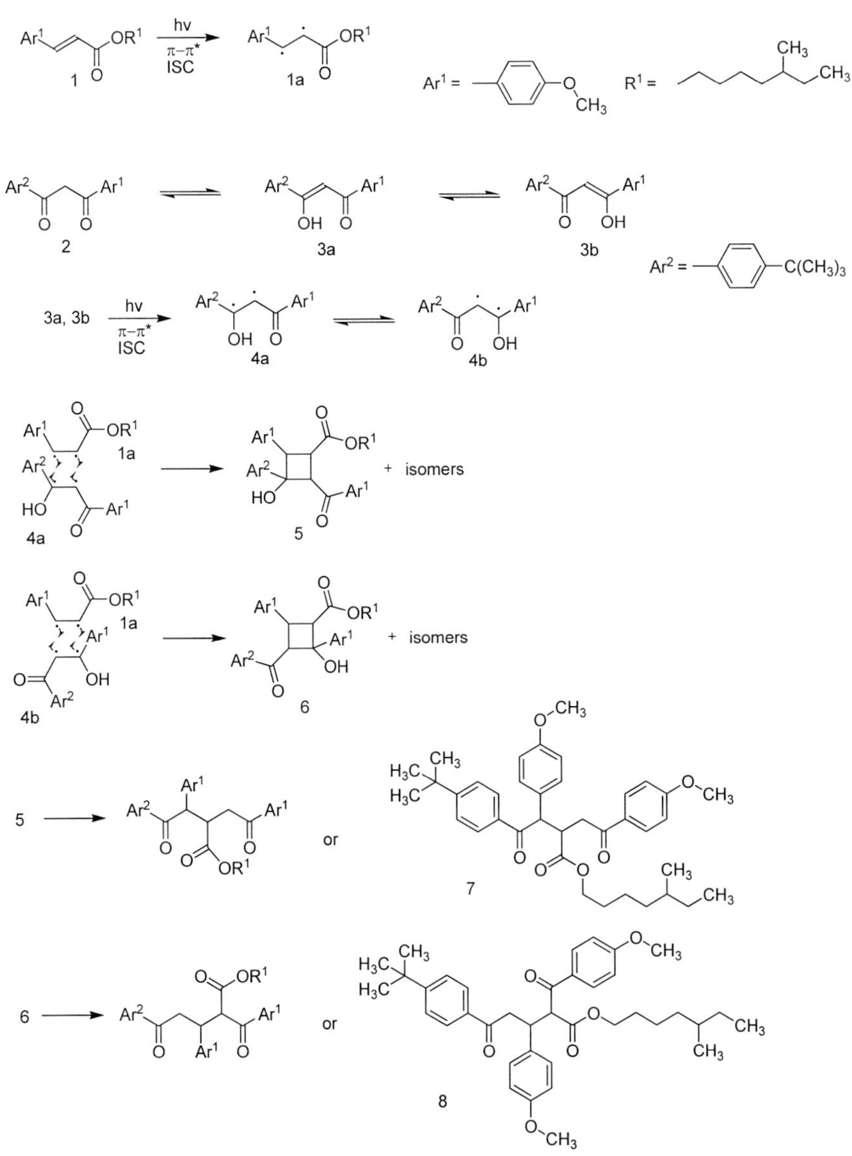

Sch. 3F.ii-2. The UV radiation induced reactions of 4-*tert*-butyl-4-methoxy-dibenzoylmethane and 2-ethylhexyl 4-methoxycinnamate.

iv. Camphor Derivatives

From compounds **14–29** [**Table 3F-1**], only Ecamsule (Mexoryl® SX, **29**) was approved in the United States in 2006. Camphor derivatives have high molar extinction coefficients and good photostability. The entire group of camphor derivatives was developed and introduced in a series of patents by the French company L'Oréal in the 1970s to 1980s. Application of Mexoryl® SX to the skin of hairless mice either reduced or prevented damages, such as sagging and wrinkling of unprotected skin, induced by UVA irradiation [122]. Similar results were observed in experiments with human skin [123]. Several older [124, 125] and newer studies [63, 94, 95] have shown that benzylidene camphor derivatives undergo reversible cis–trans (*E–Z*) isomerization leading to photostationary equilibria; however, these transformations cause no destructive changes. This general conclusion was confirmed in meticulous studies with 14 UV filters, including 3-(4'-methylbenzylidene)camphor (**27**) and Mexoryl® SX (**29**) [110, 111]. Percutaneous absorption of Mexoryl® SX was measured in human volunteers using a compound labeled at two benzyl carbon atoms with the ^{14}C isotope [126]. The radioactivity in urine samples slightly exceeded background levels and corresponded maximally to 0.014% of the topically applied dose. No radioactivity could be detected in the blood samples drawn at 0, 2, 3, 4, 6, 8, 10, 12, 14, 24, 34, 48, 72, 96, and 168 hours after application. Formulations containing Mexoryl® SX have a dose-dependent level of protection against pigmentation, pyrimidine dimer formation, and accumulation of p53, the tumor suppressing gene [127]

v. Benzophenones

This group includes 10 aromatic ketones with a variety of functional groups [**Table 3F-1**, **30–39**]. All of them contain at least one hydroxyl group, which, as a phenolic function, may contribute to their vulnerability to oxidation. Nevertheless, those that were subjected to UV irradiation have shown remarkable photostability. Apparently, the ortho hydroxyl groups form strong intramolecular hydrogen bonds with the carbonyl group that stabilize the molecule. One of them, 2-hydroxy-4-methoxybenzophenone, (oxybenzone, benzophenone-3, BP-3, **32**) is frequently included in sunscreens and various skin cosmetic products [128]. Several studies have shown that it has a relatively high photostability. For example, a cyclohexane solution of oxybenzone (0.01 M) was irradiated for 100 h with a mercury vapor immersion lamp [62]. After this treatment, the dissolved material was completely recovered with no evidence of any degradation. Two benzophenones, oxybenzone (**32**) and 2-hydroxy-4-methoxy-4'-methylbenzophenone (benzophenone-10, **38**), were irradiated with 20 MED of UVB, followed by irradiation with 100 J/cm^2 of UVA. Absorption spectra for both compounds before and after irradiation were not significantly changed [63]. The half-life times for benzophenone-3 and benzophenone-5 in oil–water emulsions were determined as 1500 and 1150 minutes, respectively. More recent investigations have shown that the photostability of oxybenzone depends on the medium [66]. After 2 hours of exposure to UV irradiation, it was degraded in acetonitrile by 5–10%, in *n*-hexane by 15%, and in water by 20%. The photodegradation in methanol was almost complete, around 90%. The degradation rate was influenced by oxygen. The decomposition in air-equilibrated aerobic solutions occurs much faster than under anaerobic conditions. It was also found that oxybenzone undergoes significant photodegradation in the presence of the light-scattering filter titanium dioxide [66]. Oxybenzone has also been found to readily penetrate the human skin and is then excreted in urine as derivatives [128]. In hepatocytes (liver cells), BP-3 is converted into a number of derivatives. (See **Section 2F**.) Oxybenzone was studied by Fourier transform Raman spectroscopy after topical application to the skin. It was rapidly photo-oxidized yielding intermediates that react with the thiol groups of antioxidant enzymes, such as thioredoxin reductase and reduced glutathione. These results indicate that oxybenzone may be harmful to the epidermal antioxidant system [129].

The photoexcitation of diarylbenzophenones involves S_1 (n,π*) to T_1 (n,π*) and T_1 (π,π*) transitions with a rapid 10^{-10} to 10^{-12} s^{-1} intersystem crossing (ISC), which is, theoretically according to the El-Sayed rule, a forbidden transition (**Section 1C**), followed by degradations that, in the case of BP-3, can result in ortho- and para-semiquinones [**Sch. 3F.v-1]** [23].

vi. Dibenzoylmethanes

The dibenzoylmethane derivatives have high molar extinction coefficients at long UVA wavelengths [53, 130]. The keto–enol tautomerization between the methylene group and the carbonyl moiety results in the shift of λ_{max} from 260 nm to 355 nm. This property puts dibenzomethane derivatives in a group of highly desirable UVA sun filters; however, after thorough evaluation of several candidates, only one controversial compound, 4-*tert*-butyl-4'-methoxydibenzoylmethane (avobenzone, Parsol® 1789, **40**) remains on the market. A typical absorption of avobenzone appears near 355 nm with a specific molar extinction of 35,000 $M^{-1}cm^{-1}$. The irradiation of a dilute solution of **40** in acetonitrile in a quartz cell using a filtered xenon lamp (290–450 nm) gave after 20 seconds an absorption near 280 nm. This photoreaction took place without photochemical degradation. After a certain time, the diketone form reverted slowly to its enol form [131]. Five dibenzoylmethane derivatives, including avobenzone, were suspended in a non-ionic emulsion and irradiated during one hour with a solar simulator between quartz plates.

The compounds containing a hydroxyl group ortho to the carbonyl group were more stable than the non-hydroxylated derivatives; however, the interaction of the hydroxyl group with the carbonyl oxygen shifts λ_{max} to 370 nm, which is too high to provide a significant protection from UVA irradiation (320–350 nm). All three non-hydroxylated derivatives lost 25 to > 40% of their initial absorptivity. Irradiation of avobenzone in cyclohexane produced *tert*-butylbenzene, 4-*tert*-butylbenzoic acid, 4-methoxybenzoic acid, and products formed by reaction of degradation intermediates with cyclohexane, such as cyclohexyl esters of 4-*tert*-butyl- and 4-methoxybenzoic acids [62]. The photochemistry of 4-isopropyldibenzoylmethane and 4-*tert*-butyl-4'-methoxydibenzoylmethane was investigated in 3.5 mmolar solutions of non-deaerated cyclohexane, isooctane, isopropanol, and methanol. The progress of photodegradation was monitored by HPLC and GC-MS. The compounds were quite stable in the polar solvents, whereas in hydrocarbon solvents, both compounds produced about a dozen protodegradation products identified by GC-MS, such as substituted benzaldehydes, benzoic acids, phenylglyoxals, acetophenones, benzyls, dibenzoylmethanes, dibenzoylethanes, perbenzoic acids, α-hydroperoxyacetophenones, and α-hydroxyacetophenones. The degradation mechanism is illustrated in **Sch. 3F.vi-1**. Avobenzone (**1**) decomposed to 4-*tert*-butylphenyl glyoxal (**2**), 4,4'-di-*tert*-butylbenzyl (**3**), 4-*tert*-butyl-4'methoxydibenzoylmethane (**4**), *tert*-butylbenzaldehyde (**5**), 4-methoxybenzaldehyde, 4-*tert*-butylbenzoic acid (**6**), 4-methoxybenzoic acid, 4-*tert*-butylacetophenone, 4-methoxyacetophenone (**7**), 4-methoxyphenyl-α-hydroxyacetophenone (**8**), 4-methoxyphenyl glyoxal (**9**), 4-*tert*-butyl-4'-methoxybenzil, 4,4'-dimethoxydibenzoylmethane, and 4-*tert*-butyl-4'-methoxydibenzoylethane [132]. The same two compounds were suspended in petroleum jelly and exposed to 20 minimal erythema doses (MED) of UVA irradiation followed by 100 J/cm^2 of UVA irradiation [63]. Both compounds rapidly decomposed to form a variety of degradation products. Photochemical studies by nanosecond laser flash photolysis have shown that irradiation of avobenzone with the 266 nm laser leads to formation of the triplet state of the keto form with a lifetime of approximately 500 ns. Under these conditions, the keto form is quenched by oxygen [133].

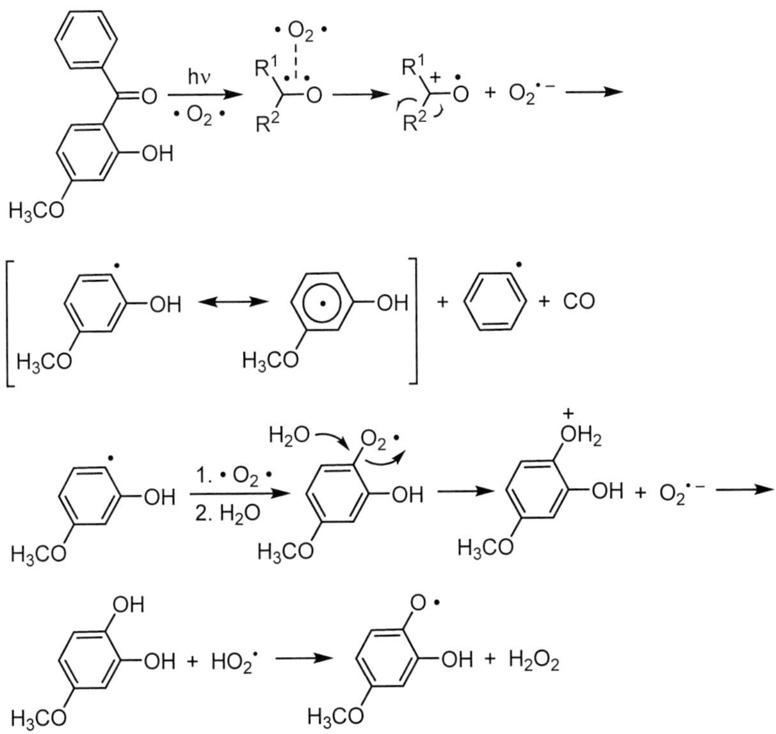

Sch. 3F.v-1. The Norrish Type I oxidative photochemical degradation of 2-hydroxy-4-methoxybenzophenone, (BP-3 = oxybenzone), resulting in the formation of ortho- and para-semiquinones. In nature, the ortho-semiquinones are prevalent. (See **Section 1C**.)

Molecular oxygen ($\cdot{}^3O_2\cdot$) is a diradical in the ground state, and is known to readily react with carbon radicals to yield peroxy radicals. These radicals in aqueous media undergo elimination reactions to give a hydroxyl derivative and either a superoxide anion radical $O_2\cdot^-$, or the more stable hydroperoxy radical HOO· ($HO_2\cdot$). In all such reactions in various schemes, the spontaneous heterolysis of the carbon–peroxyl bonds produce the corresponding carbon cations and the superoxide radical anion

($O_2\cdot^{-}$). This heterolysis proceeds at a high rate $k \geq 10^6$ s^{-1}. The reactions of carbon cations with water (H_2O) produce hydroxyl derivatives [134–136].

4-Isopropyldibenzoylmethane was a common cause of sunscreen allergies and was removed from the market in 1993. 4-*tert*-Butyl-4'-methoxydibenzoylmethane remains in use and is still considered one of the most frequently observed photoallergens [137]. In a study concerned with the photocontact allergy of this compound, 2 mM solutions in cyclohexane and in ethanol were irradiated in a falling film photoreactor. The photodegradation in ethanol was much slower than in cyclohexanol; thus, irradiation in cyclohexane was carried out for 90 min and in ethanol for 210 min. The degradation products were quantitatively analyzed by HPLC and GC-MS then tested as potential contact photoallergens. The individual degradation products arylglyoxals and benzyls were synthesized, and their allergenic potential was tested in the murine local lymph node assay. Their cytotoxic properties were tested in a cell proliferation assay. The study has shown that the photocontact allergy is caused by arylglyoxals, while benzyls were found to be cytotoxic [137].

vii. Heterocyclic Compounds

Numerous deficiencies of traditional sunscreens described in the preceding sections require further research toward the development of more stable, efficient, and safer molecules. Most of the newer additions include various heterocyclic moieties (**Table 3F-1**, **41–44**, **46–50**). During the last decade, the main effort has been devoted to derivatives of triazine (**41–43**) with molecular weights above 500 Daltons. These compounds are covered in depth in review articles [13, 78, 138]. It has been shown that they do not penetrate the skin; however, until now, there has been little systematic research regarding their photostability. Bemotrizinol (**43**) seems to be very stable; however, 2-ethylhexyltriazone (octyltriazone, ETH, **42**), which contains three Padimate O moieties undergoes significant degradation [79].

The remaining molecules require more time and scrutiny. One of them, water-soluble 2-phenylbenzimidazole-5-sulfonic acid (ensulizole, PBSA, **46**) appears on the list of sunscreens approved by the FDA for use in the U.S.A., and has been widely utilized in sunscreen formulations and cosmetics. PBSA and the parent compound 2-phenyl-1*H*-benzimidazole (PBI), upon UV irradiation, readily undergo reactions with various compounds including DNA, causing damages by the Type I and Type II mechanisms, whereby PBI and PBSA are rapidly degraded [**Sch. 3F.vii-1**]. PBSA in neutral aqueous solutions at pH 7.4 has strongly oxidizing properties

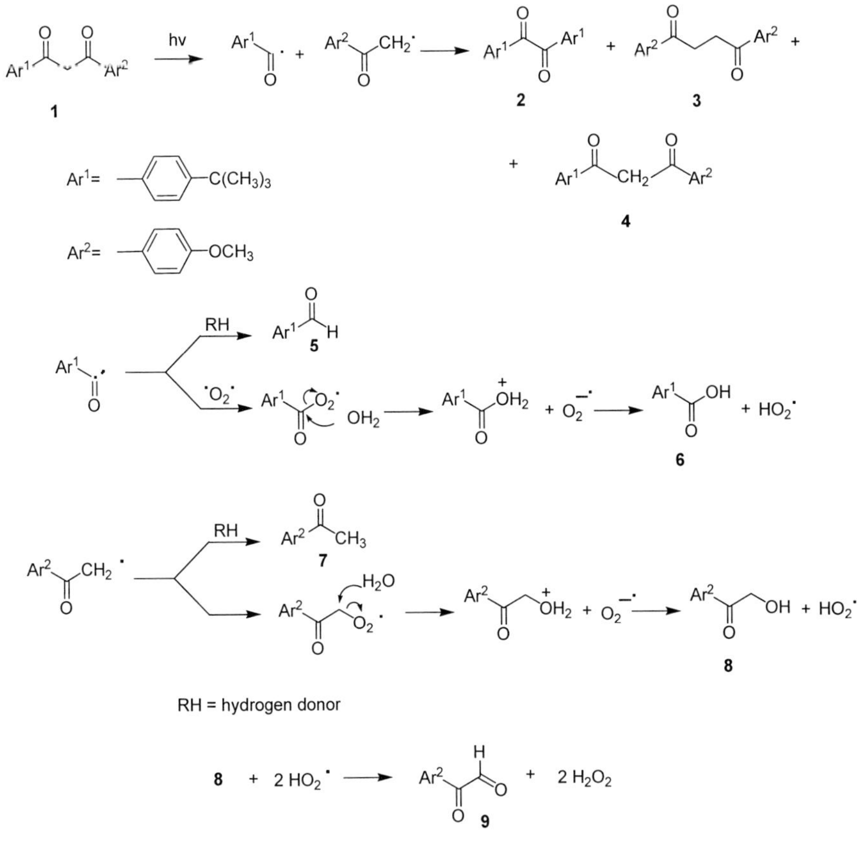

Sch. 3F.vi-1. Photodegradation of 4-*tert*-butyl-4'-methoxydibenzoylmethane by the Norrish Type I cleavage reaction.

[139]. Thus, for example, glutathienyl and *S*-cysteinyl radicals are formed from the corresponding anions GS^- and ^-S-Cys involving direct oxidations by the exciting state **46A** via electron transfer [139]. In the presence of molecular oxygen, the photoexcited triplet of PBSA (**46B**) has reducing properties resulting in the formation of a peroxy anion-radical $O_2\cdot^-$, followed by a cascade of radicals and reactive oxygen species. Since the triplet of PBSA has a higher energy than 22.7 kcal/mol, triplet $^3O_2$ is also converted into singlet oxygen $^1O_2$ [139]. The irradiation-induced degradation of PBSA was markedly reduced by complexation with hydroxypropyl-β-cyclodextrin (HP-beta-CD). In addition, electron paramagnetic reso-

nance (EPR) spin-trapping studies showed that the inclusion of PBSA into HP-beta-CD cavity completely inhibited the formation of free radicals generated by PBSA on exposure to simulated sunlight [140]. Nevertheless, recent studies of PBSA in vitro and in cellulo involving the formation of oxidatively generated DNA damage upon UV exposure still undermine its suitability for sunscreen applications [141, 142].

viii. Commercial Formulations

While photostability studies of individual ingredients are complex enough to understand and interpret their physical and chemical changes, understanding the fate of multiple components in commercial products is even more difficult [96–103]. In spite of all efforts to produce photostable formulations, the commercial products undergo degradations. A set of 16 commercial sunscreen products with Sun Protection Factor (SPF) values between 16 and 26, advertised by their producers as formulations offering a broad-spectrum protection against UVA and UVB radiation, was subjected to irradiation from a solar simulator, corresponding to solar radiation at midsummer noon and cloudless sky in central Europe [101]. Nine of these products were recommended for use for infants and children. Seven suncare products were exposed to 50 SED (Standard Erythema Dose), while the remaining nine products recommended for children were exposed to 25 SED. In the UVB range, all 16 products maintained above 98% of their initial absorbance; however, in the UVA range, 5 products lost 5 to 18% of their absorbance after exposure of 5 SED. After exposure corresponding to 12.5 SED, 7 products lost 12 to 36% of their effectiveness, and after 25 SED the same 7 products lost 12 to 48% of their absorbance. The first set of seven products was then irradiated with 50 SED, corresponding to about 4 hours of the mean biologically effective irradiance [**Table 3F-2**]. Four products out of seven lost 27 to 52 % of their initial absorbance. None of the examined compositions contained the unstable *para*-aminobenzoic acid (PABA) derivatives of isopropyldibenzoylmethane; however, 14 out of 16 products contained 4-butyl-4'-methoxydibenzoylmethane (avobenzone). On the basis of these results, it can be concluded that, even after 4 hours of UV irradiation, all prevalent sunscreens are expected to retain about 50% of their effectiveness. However, the fate of their degradation products, such as generation of reactive oxygen species, their facility to penetrate the human skin, their capacity to function as carriers of xenobiotics through the human skin, and their estrogenic effects on mammals and the environment are as yet not fully explored. (See **Section 2F**.)

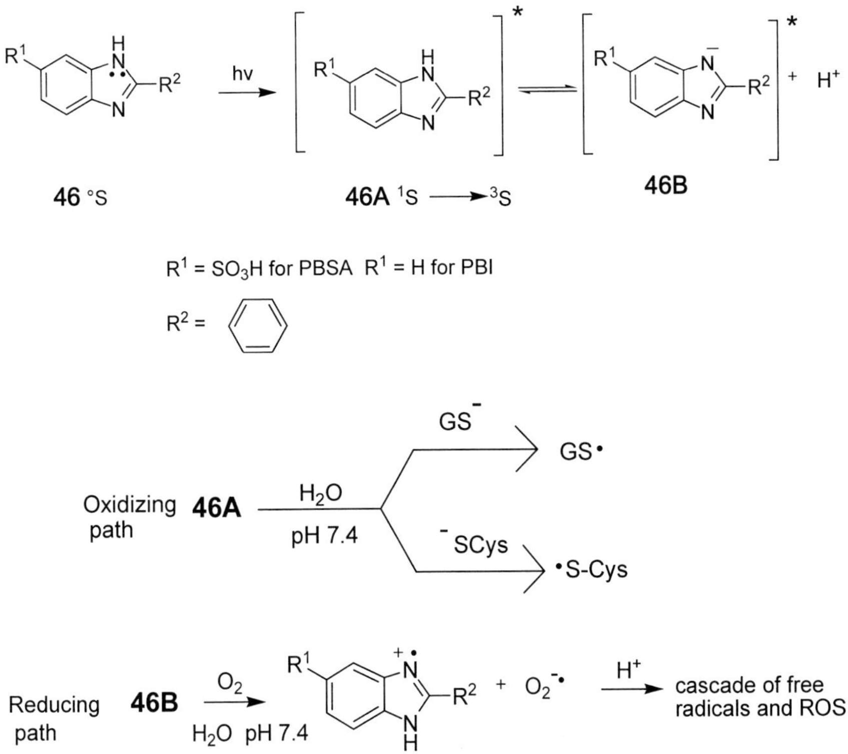

Sch. 3F.vii-1. UV Irradiation of 2-phenyl-1*H*-benzimidazole (PBI) and sunscreen agent 2-phenyl-1*H*-benzimidazole-5-sulfonic acid (PBSA).

Table 3F-2. Photoinactivation of Commercial Sunscreen Mixtures Using UVB (280–320 nm) and UVA (320–380 nm) Radiations [101].

Sunscreen Product	**Ingredients**	**Mean % Photoinactivation after Exposures of**	
		25 SED	**50 SED**
B	TiO_2, 4-*tert*-butyl-4-methoxy-dibenzoylmethane, 2-ethylhexyl 4-methoxycinnamate, 3-benzylidenecamphor	28	30
C	2-Phenylbenzimidazole-5-sulfonic acid, 4-*tert*-butyl-4-methoxy-dibenzoylmethane, 2-ethylhexyl 4-methoxycinnamate, 2-ethylhexyl-triazone	48	52
E	TiO_2, 4-*tert*-butyl-4-methoxy-dibenzoylmethane, 2-ethylhexyl 4-methoxycinnamate, 2-ethylhexyltriazone, 3-benzylidenecamphor	27	33
F	4-*tert*-Butyl-4-methoxydibenzoyl-methane, 3-methylbutyl 4-methoxycinnamate, 2-ethylhexyl 4-methoxycinnamate, 2-ethylhexyl-triazone	12	27
I	TiO_2, 4-*tert*-butyl-4-methoxy-dibenzoylmethane, 2-ethylhexyl 4-methoxycinnamate, 3-benzylide-necamphor	24	
P	TiO_2, 4-*tert*-butyl-4-methoxy-dibenzoylmethane, 2-ethylhexyl 4-methoxycinnamate, 3-methylbutyl 4-methoxycinnamate, 2-ethyl-hexyltriazone	23	
Q	TiO_2, 4-*tert*-butyl-4-methoxy-dibenzoylmethane, 2-ethylhexyl 4-methoxycinnamate, 3-benzyl-idenecamphor	32	

References

1. Lowe N. J. and Shaath N. A. (eds.) (1990) *Sunscreens, Development, Evaluation and Regulatory Aspects*, 1st ed., Marcel Dekker, New York.
2. Lowe N. J., Shaath N. A. and Pathak M. A. (eds.) (1997) *Sunscreens, Development, Evaluation and Regulatory Aspects*, 2nd ed., Marcel Dekker, New York.
3. Shaath N. A. (ed.) (2005) *Sunscreens, Regulations and Commercial Development*, 3rd ed., Taylor & Francis, Boca Raton.
4. Gasparro F. P. (ed.) (1997) *Sunscreen Photobiology: Molecular, Cellular and Physiological Aspects*, Springer-Verlag, Heidelberg and New York.
5. Lowe N. J. (ed.) (1991) *Physician's Guide to Sunscreens*, Marcel Dekker, New York.
6. Thiers B. H. (consult. ed.) and Draelos Z. D. (ed.) (2006) Dermatologic Clinics, Vol. 24, No. 1: *Sunscreens*, W. B. Saunders Company, Philadelphia.
7. Vainio H. and Bianchini F. (eds.) (2001) IARC Handbooks of Cancer Prevention, Vol. 5: *Sunscreens*, International Agency for Research on Cancer, Lyon.
8. Demas C. (2006) *Sunscreens*, Lulu, Inc., self-published.
9. Bens G. (2008) Sunscreens. In: *Sunlight, Vitamin D and Skin Cancer*, 137–161, Reichrath J. (ed.), Springer Verlag, Berlin.
10. Giacomoni P. U. (ed.) (2001) *Sun Protection in Man*, Elsevier Science, Amsterdam.
11. Giacomoni P. U. (ed.) (2001) *Biophysical and Physiological Effects of Solar Radiation on Human Skin*, RSC Publishing, Cambridge.
12. Lim H. W. and Draelos Z. D. (eds.) (2009) *Clinical Guide to Sunscreens and Photoprotection*, Informa Healthcare USA, Inc., New York.
13. Osterwalder U., Herzog B. (2010) The long way towards the ideal sunscreen--where we stand and what still needs to be done. *Photochem. Photobiol. Sci.* **9**: 470–81.
14. Arnold D. R., Baird N. C., Bolton J. R., Brand J. C. D., Jacobs P. C. D., de Mayo P. and Ware W. R. (1974) *Photochemistry*, Academic Press, New York and London.
15. Cowan D. O. and Drisko R. L. (1976) *Elements of Organic Photochemistry*, Plenum Press, New York and London.
16. Horspool W. M. (1976) *Photochemistry*, Academic Press, New York.

17. Coyle J. D. (1986) *Introduction to Organic Photochemistry*, John Wiley & Sons, Chichester.
18. Wayne R. P. (1988) *Principles and Applications of Photochemistry*, Oxford University Press, Oxford.
19. Michl J. and Bonačic'-Koutecky' V. (1990) *Electronic Aspects of Organic Photochemistry*, John Wiley & Sons, Chichester.
20. Kopecky' J. (1992) *Organic Photochemistry, A Visual Approach*, VCH Verlagsgesellschaft, Weinheim.
21. Murov S. L., Carmichael L. and Hug G. L. (eds.) (1993) *Handbook of Photochemistry*, Marcel Dekker, New York.
22. Turro N. J. (1991) *Modern Molecular Photochemistry*, University Science Books, Mill Valley, CA.
23. Turro N. J., Ramamurthy V. and Scaiano J. C. (2009) *Principles of Molecular Photochemistry. An Introduction*, University Science Books, Sausalito, CA.
24. Turro N. J., Ramamurthy V. and Scaiano J. C. (2010) *Modern Molecular Photochemistry of Organic Molecules*, University Science Books, Sausalito, CA.
25. ICH Stability testing: Photostability Testing on New Drug Substances and Products. (1997), ICH, Geneva. *Fed. Register* **62**: 271175–27122.
26. Albini A. and Fasani E. (2003) Photochemistry of drugs. In: *Handbook of Photochemistry and Photobiology*, Nalwa H. S. (ed.), American Scientific Publishers, Stevenson Ranch, CA.
27. Ahmed K. F. (2009) Worldwide regulation of UV filters: current status and future trends. In: *Clinical Guide to Sunscreens and Photoprotection*, Lim H. W. and Draelos Z. D. (eds.), Informa Healthcare USA, Inc., New York.
28. The final over-the-counter drug products monograph on sunscreens, (1999) *Fed. Register* **64**: 27666–27963. Sunscreen drug products for over-the-counter human use; proposed amendment of final monograph (2007) *Fed. Register* **72**, No. 165: 49069–49122. Labeling and effectiveness testing; sunscreen drug products for over-the-counter human use (2011) *Fed. Register* **76**: 35620–35665.
29. Malaviya B. K. and Dutt S. (1935) Photoreaction in tropic sunlight. *Proc. Acad. Sci., United Provinces Agra Oudh, India* **4**: 319–329.
30. Rothman S. and Rubin J. (1942) Sunburn and *para*-aminobenzoic acid. *J. Invest. Dermatol.* **5**: 445–457.
31. Mackie B. S. and Mackie L. E. (1999) The PABA story. *Australasian J. Dermatol.* **40**: 51–53.

32. Snyder D. S. and May M. (1975) Ability of PABA to protect mammalian skin from ultraviolet light-induced skin tumors and actinic damage. *J. Invest. Dermatol.* **65**: 543–49.
33. Kligman L. H., Akin F. J. and Kligman A. M. (1980) Sunscreens prevent ultraviolet photocarcinogenesis. *J. Am. Acad. Dermatol.* **3**(a): 30–35.
34. Kligman L. H., Akin F. J. and Kligman A. M. (1982) Prevention of ultraviolet damage to the dermis of hairless mice by sunscreens. *J. Invest. Dermatol.* **78**: 181–89.
35. Kligman L. H., Akin F. J. and Kligman A. M. (1983) Sunscreens promote repair of ultraviolet radiation-induced dermal damage. *J. Invest. Dermatol.* **81**: 98–102.
36. Flindt-Hansen H., Thune P. and Nielsen C. J. (1989) Photocarcinogenesis is retarded by a partly photodegraded solution of *para*-aminobenzoic acid. *Photodermatol.* **6**: 263–267.
37. Pathak M. A., Fitzpatrick T. B. and Frenk E. (1969) Evaluation of topical agents that prevent sunburn-superiority of *para*-aminobenzoic acid and its ester in ethyl alcohol. *N. Engl. J. Med.* **280**: 1459–63.
38. Stenback F. and Shubik P. (1974) Lack of toxicity and carcinogenicity of some commonly used cutaneous agents. *Toxic Appl. Pharmacol.* **30**: 7–13.
39. Hodges N. D. M., Moss S. H. and Davies D. J. G. (1977) The sensitizing effect of a sunscreening agent, *p*-aminobenzoic acid, on near UV-induced damage in a repair deficient strain of *Escherichia coli. Photochem. Photobiol.* **26**: 493–498.
40. Hodges N. D. M., Moss S. H. and Davies D. J. G. (1976) Evidence for increased genetic damage due to the presence of a sunscreen agent *para*-aminobenzoic acid during irradiation with near ultraviolet light (proceedings). *J. Pharm. Pharmacol.* **28** (Suppl.): 53p.
41. Hodges N. D. M., Moss S. H. and Davies D. J. G. (1977) Elucidation of the nature of genetic damage formed in the presence of the sunscreen agent *para*-aminobenzoic acid during irradiation with near ultraviolet light (proceedings). *J. Pharm. Pharmacol.* **29** (Suppl. S1): 72P.
42. Kaidbey K. H. and Kligman A. M. (1978) Phototoxicity to a sunscreen ingredient. *Arch. Dermatol.* **114**: 547–549.
43. Mathias C. G. T., Maibach H. I. and Epstein J. (1978) Allergic contact photodermatitis to *para*-aminobenzoic acid. *Arch. Dermatol.* **114**: 1665–1666.

44. Thune P. (1984) Contact and photocontact allergy to sunscreens. *Photodermatol.* **1**: 5–9.
45. Morison W. L. (1984) The effect of a sunscreen containing *para*-aminobenzoic acid on the systemic immunologic alterations induced in mice by exposure to UV-B radiation. *J. Invest. Dermatol.* **83**: 404–8.
46. Osgood P. J., Moss S. H. and Davies D. J. (1982) The sensitization of near-ultraviolet radiation killing of mammalian cells by the sunscreen agent *para*-aminobenzoic acid. *J. Invest. Dermatol.* **79**: 354–357.
47. Chignell C. F., Kalyanaraman B., Mason R. P. and Sik R. H. (1980) Spectroscopic studies of cutaneous photosensitizing agents. I. Spin-trapping of photolysis products from sulfanilamide, 4-aminobenzoic acid and related compounds. *Photochem. Photobiol.* **32**: 563–571.
48. Motten A. G. and Chignell C. F. (1983) Spectroscopic studies of cutaneous photosensitizing agents--III. Spin trapping of photolysis products from sulfanilamide analogs. *Photochem Photobiol.* **37**: 17–26.
49. Gasparro F. P. (1985) UV-induced photoproducts of *para*-aminobenzoic acid. *Photodermatol.* **2**: 151–157.
50. Gasparro F. P. and Battista J. (1987) Characterization of *para*-aminobenzoic acid DNA-photoadducts. *Photochem. Photobiol.* **45**: 49S.
51. Shaw A. A., Wainschel L. A. and Shetlar M. D. (1992) The photochemistry of *p*-aminobenzoic acid. *Photochem. Photobiol.* **55**: 647–656.
52. Langford S. A., Sugden J. K. and Fitzpatrick R. W. (1996) Detection and determination of the hydrazo and azo photoproducts of 4-aminobenzoic acid by high-performance liquid chromatography. *J. Pharm. Biomed. Anal.* **14**: 1615–1623.
53. Shaath N. A. (1997) Evolution of modern sunscreen chemicals. In: *Sunscreens, Development, Evaluation and Regulatory Aspects*, 2nd ed., pp 3–33, Lowe N. J., Shaath N. A. and Pathak M. A. (eds.), Marcel Dekker, New York.
54. Ten Berge C. D. M., Bruins C. H. P. and Faber J. S. (1972) Die Photochemie von Sonnenschutzmitteln. I. Über die Photochemie von Methyl-*p*-dimethylaminobenzoat. *J. Soc. Cosmet. Chem.* **23**: 289–299.
55. Ten Berge C. D. M. and Bruins C. H. P. (1974) Die Photochemie von Sonnenschutzmitteln. II. Über die Photochemie von Methyl-*p*-dimethylaminobenzoat. *J. Soc. Cosmet. Chem.* **25**: 263–269.

56. Allen, J. M., Gosset C. J. and Allen S. F. (1996) Photochemical formation of singlet molecular oxygen ($^1O_2$) in illuminated aqueous solutions of *p*-aminobenzoic acid (PABA). *J. Photochem. Photobiol., B* **32**: 33–37.
57. Allen, J. M., Gossett C. J. and Allen S. F. (1996) Photochemical formation of singlet molecular oxygen in illuminated aqueous solutions of several commercially available sunscreen active ingredients. *Chem. Res. Toxicol.* **9**: 605–609.
58. Knowland J., McKenzie E. A., McHugh P. J. and Cridland N. A. (1993) Sunlight-induced mutagenicity of a common sunscreen ingredient. *FEBS Lett.* **324**: 309–313.
59. McHugh P. J. and Knowland J. (1997) Characterization of DNA damage inflicted by free radicals from a mutagenic sunscreen ingredient and its location using an in vitro genetic reversion assay. *Photochem. Photobiol.* **66**: 276–281.
60. Xu C., Green A., Parisi A. and Parsons P. G. (2001) Photosensitization of the sunscreen octyl *p*-dimethylaminobenzoate by UVA in human melanocytes but not in keratinocytes. *Photochem. Photobiol.* **73**: 600–604.
61. Flindt-Hansen H., Nielsen C. J. and Thune P. (1988) Measurements of the photodegradation of PABA and some PABA derivatives. *Photodermatol.* **5**: 257–260.
62. Roscher N. M., Lindemann M. K. O., Kong S. B., Cho C. G. and Jiang P. (1994) Photodecompositon of several compounds commonly used as sunscreen agents. *J. Photochem. Photobiol., A* **80**: 417–421.
63. Tarras-Wahlberg N., Stenhagen G., Larkö O., Rosén A., Wennberg A.-M. and Wennerström O. (1999) Changes in ultraviolet absorption of sunscreens after ultraviolet irradiation. *J. Invest. Dermat.* **113**: 547–553.
64. Loeppky R. N., Hastings R., Sandbothe J., Heller D., Bao Y. and Nagel D. (1991) Nitrosation of tertiary aromatic amines related to sunscreen ingredients. In: *Relevance to Human Cancer of N-Nitroso Compounds. Tobacco Smoke and Mycotoxins*, pp 244–252, O'Neill, I. K., Chen J. and Bartsch H. (eds.), IARC, Lyon.
65. Kenney G. E., Sakr A., Lichtin J. L., Chou H. and Bronangh R. L. (1995) In vitro skin absorption and metabolism of Padimate-O and a nitrosamine formed in Padimate-O containing cosmetic products. *J. Soc. Cosmet. Chem.* **46**: 117–127.
66. Serpone N., Salinaro A., Emeline A. V., Horikoshi S., Hidaka H. and Zhao J. (2002) An in vitro systematic spectroscopic examination of

the photostabilities of a random set of commercial sunscreen lotions and their chemical UVB/UVA active agents. *Photochem. Photobiol. Sci.* **1**: 970–981.
67. Couteau C., Faure A., Fortin J., Paparis E. and Coiffard L. J. M. (2007) Study of photostability of 18 sunscreens in cream by measuring the SPF in vitro. *J. Pharm. Biomed. Anal.* **44**: 270–273.
68. Ravanat J.-L., Douki T. and Cadet J. (2001) UV damage to nucleic acid components. In: *Sun Protection in Man*, pp 207–230, Giacomoni P. U. (ed.), Elsevier Science, Amsterdam.
69. Sutherland B. M. (1982) *p*-Aminobenzoic acid-sunlamp sensitization of pyrimidine dimer formation and transformation in human cells. *Photochem. Photobiol.* **36**: 95–97.
70. Sutherland, J. C. and Griffin K. P. (1984) *p*-Aminobenzoic acid can sensitize the formation of pyrimidine dimers in DNA: direct chemical evidence. *Photochem. Photobiol.* **40**: 391–394.
71. Premachamdra B. R. (1989) Interaction of *p*-aminobenzoic acid with erythrocyte membrane; photoaffinity labeling of the binding sites. *Biochem. Med. Metab. Biol.* **262**: 1261–1267.
72. Rutherford C. E., Salter L. F. and Thomas R. C. (1990) pH effects on *p*-aminobenzoic acid photosensitized dimer formation from the free thymine base. *J. Photochem. Photobiol., A* **52**: 337–343.
73. Shaw A. A., Wainschel L. A. and Shetlar M. D. (1992) Photoaddition of *p*-aminobenzoic acid to thymine and thymidine. *Photochem. Photobiol.* **55**: 657–663.
74. Gasparro F. P., Mitchnick M. and Nash J. F. (1998) A review of sunscreen safety and efficacy. *Photochem. Photobiol.* **68**: 243–256.
75. Aliwell S. R., Martincigh B. S. and Salter L. F. (1993) *p*-Aminobenzoic acid-photosensitized dimerization of thymine. 1. In DNA-related model systems. *J. Photochem. Photobiol., A* **71**: 137–146.
76. Aliwell, S. R., Martincigh B. S. and Salter L. F. (1993) *p*-Aminobenzoic acid-photosensitized dimerization of thymine. II. In pUC19 plasmid DNA. *J. Photochem. Photobiol., A* **71**: 147–153.
77. Wang L. H., Huang W. S. and Tai H. M. (2007) Simultaneous determination of *p*-aminobenzoic acid and its metabolites in the urine of volunteers, treated with *p*-aminobenzoic acid sunscreen formulation. *J. Pharm. Biomed. Anal.* **43**: 1430–1436.
78. Osterwalder U. and Herzog B. (2009) Chemistry and properties of organic and inorganic UV filters. In: *Clinical Guide to Sunscreens and Photoprotection*, pp 11–38, Lim H. W. and Draelos Z. D. (eds.), Informa Healthcare USA, Inc., New York.

79. Damiani E., Baschong W. and Greci L. (2007) UV-Filter combinations under UV-A exposure: Concomitant quantification of overall spectral stability and molecular integrity. *J. Photochem. Photobiol., B* **87**: 95–104.
80. Sakkas V. A., Giokas D. L., Lambropoulou D. A. and Albanis T. A. (2003) Aqueous photolysis of the sunscreen agent octyl-dimethyl-*p*-aminobenzoic acid. Formation of disinfection byproducts in chlorinated swimming pool water. *J. Chromatogr. A* **1016**: 211–222.
81. Molière P., Hüppe G., Averbeck D., Young A. R., Santus R. and Dubertret L. (1990) *In vitro* photostability and photosensitizing of bergamot oil. Effects of a cinnamate sunscreen. *J. Photochem. Photobiol., B* **7**: 199–208.
82. Dubertret L., Serraf-Tircazes D., Jeanmougin M., Molière P., Averbeck D. and Young A. R. (1990) Phototoxic properties of perfumes containing bergamot oil on human skin: photoprotective effect of UVA and UVB sunscreens. *J. Photochem. Photobiol., B* **7**: 251–259.
83. Young A. R., Walker S. L., Kinley J. S., Plastow S. R., Averbeck D., Molière P. and Dubertret L. (1990) Phototumorigenesis studies of 5-methoxypsoralen in bergamot oil: evaluation and modification of risk on human use in an albino mouse skin model. *J. Photochem. Photobiol., B* **7**: 231–250.
84. Shaath N. A. (2005) Evolution of modern sunscreens. In: *Sunscreens, Regulations and Commercial Development*, 3rd ed., pp 3–33, Shaath N. A. (ed.), Taylor & Francis, Boca Raton.
85. Ahmed K. F. (2009) Worldwide regulations of UV filters: Current status and future trends. In: *Clinical Guide to Sunscreens and Photoprotection*, pp 65–88, Lim H. W. and Draelos Z. D. (eds.), Informa Healthcare USA, Inc., New York.
86. Cantrell A., McGarvey D. J. and Truscott T. G. (2001) Photochemical and photophysical properties of sunscreens. In: *Biophysical and Physiological Effects of Solar Radiation on Human Skin*, pp 495–519, Giacomoni P. U. (ed.), RSC Publishing, Cambridge.
87. Montaudo G., Caccamese S. and Librando V. (1974) Photodimers of Cinnamic Acids and Related Compounds. A Stereochemical Study by NMR. *Org. Magn. Reson.* **6**: 534–536.
88. Paolillo L., Ziffer H. and Buchardt O. (1970) Nuclear magnetic resonance analysis of several photodimers containing a cyclobutane ring. *J. Org. Chem.* **35**: 38–42.
89. Ziffer H., Bax A., Highet R. J. and Green B. (1988) Investigation by two-dimensional NMR of the structure and stereochemistry of a methyl *p*-nitrocinnamate photodimer. *J. Org. Chem.* **53**: 895–896.

90. Morliere P., Avice O., Sa'e Melo T., Dubertret, L., Giraud M. and Santus R. (1982) A study of the photochemical properties of some cinnamate sunscreens by steady state and flash photolysis. *Photochem. Photobiol.* **36**: 395–399.
91. Meier H. (1975) Cis-trans Isomerisierung der C=C Doppelbindung. In: *Methoden der Organischen Chemie*, 4, 5a: Photochemie, pp189–221, Müller G. and Houben J. (eds.), George Thieme Verlag, Stuttgart.
92. Schrader, A., Jakupovic J. and Baltes W. (1994) Photochemical studies on *trans*-3-methylbutyl 4-methoxycinnamate. *J. Soc. Cosmet. Chem.* **45**: 43–52.
93. Schrader, A., Jakupovic J. and Baltes W. (1994) Photochemical reaction products of 4-methoxycinnamic acid 3'-methylbutyl ester. *Tetrahedron Lett.* **35**: 1169–1172.
94. Deflandre A. and Lang G. (1988) Photostability assessment of sunscreens: benzylidene camphor and dibenzoylmethane derivatives. *Int. J. Cosmet. Sci.* **10**: 53–63.
95. Deflandre A. and Lang G. (1988) Photoisomerization of benzylidene camphor and derivatives. *Cosmet. Toiletries* **103**: 69–75.
96. Shaath N. A., Fares H. M. and Klein K. (1990) Photodegradation of sunscreen chemicals, solvent considerations. *Cosmet. Toiletries* **105**: 41–44.
97. Diffey B. L., Stokes R. P., Forestier S., Mazilier C. and Rougier A. (1997) Suncare product photostability: a key parameter for a more realistic *in vitro* efficacy evaluation. *Eur. J. Dermatol.* **7**: 226–228.
98. Diffey B., Stokes R., Forestier S., Mazilier C., Richard A. and Rougier A. (1998) Suncare product photostability: a key parameter for a more realistic *in vitro* efficacy evaluation. Part I: *in vitro* efficacy assessment. In: *Protection of the Skin Against Ultraviolet Radiations*, pp 137–142, Rougier A. and Schaefer H. (eds.), John Libbey Eurotext, Paris.
99. Bredholt K., Christensen B., Hannevik M., Johnsen B., Seim J. and Reitan J. B. (1998) Effects of sunscreening agents and reactions with ultraviolet radiation. *Tidsskr. Nor. Laegeforen.* **118**: 2640–2645.
100. Smith J. G. and Miller I. J. (1998) The effect of molecular environment on the photochemistry of *p*-methoxycinnamic acid and its esters. *J. Photochem. Photobiol., A* **118**: 93–97.
101. Maier H., Schauberger G., Brunnhofer K. and Hönigsman H. (2001) Change in ultraviolet absorbance of sunscreens by exposure to solar-simulated radiation. *J. Invest. Dermatol.* **117**: 256–262.

102. Chatelain E. and Gabard B. (2001) Photostabilization of butyl methoxydibenzoylmethane (Avobenzone) and methyl methoxycinnamate by bis-ethylhexyloxyphenol methoxyphenyl triazine (Tinosorb® S), a new UV broadband filter. *Photochem. Photobiol.* **74**: 401–406.
103. Pattanaargson S. and Limphong P. (2001) Stability of octyl methoxycinnamate and identification of its photodegradation product. *Int. J. Cosmet. Sci.* **23**: 153–160.
104. Pattanaargson S., Munhapol T., Hirunsupachot P. and Luangthongaram P. (2004) Photoisomerization of octyl methoxycinnamate. *J. Photochem. Photobiol., A* **161**: 269–274.
105. Cambon M., Issachar N., Castelli D. and Robert C. (2001) An *in vivo* method to assess the photostability of UV filters in a sunscreen. *J. Cosmet. Sci.* **52**: 1–11.
106. Moyal D., Refrégier J.-L. and Chardon A. (2002) In vivo measurement of the photostability of sunscreen products using diffuse reflectance spectroscopy. *Photodermatol., Photoimmunol. Photomed.* **18**: 14–22.
107. Pattanaargson S., Hongchinnagorn N., Hirunsupachot P. and Sritana-anant Y. (2003) UV Absorption and photoisomerization of *p*-methoxycinnamate grafted silicone. *Photochem. Photobiol.* **80**: 322–325.
108. Perugini P., Simeoni S., Scalia S., Genta I., Modena T., Conti B. and Pavanetto F. (2002) Effect of nanoparticles encapsulation on the photostability of the sunscreen agent 2-ethylhexyl *p*-methoxycinnamate. *Int. J. Pharm.* **246**: 37–45.
109. Carlotti M. E., Sapino S., Vione D., Pelizetti E., Ugazio E. and Morel S. (2005) Study on the photostability of octyl *p*-methoxycinnamate in SLN. *J. Dispersion Sci. Technol.* **26**: 209–226.
110. Hauri U., Lütolf B. and Hohl Ch. (2003) Determination of organic sunscreen filters in cosmetics with HPLC/DAD. *Mitt. Lebensmittelunters. Hyg.* **94**: 80–92.
111. Hauri U., Lütolf B., Schlegel U. and Hohl Ch. (2004) Determination of photodegradation of UV filters in sunscreens by HPLC/DAD and HPLC/MS. *Mitt. Lebensmittelunters. Hyg.* **95**: 80–92.
112. Gaspar L. R. and Maia Campos P. M. B. G. (2006) Evaluation of the photostability of different UV filter combinations in a sunscreen. *Int. J. Pharm.* **307**: 123–128.
113. Damiani E., Rosati L., Castagna R., Carloni P. and Greci L. (2006) Changes in ultraviolet absorbance and hence in protective efficacy against lipid peroxidation of organic sunscreens after UVA irradiation. *J. Photochem. Photobiol., B* **82**: 204–213.

114. Damiani E., Astolfi P., Cionna L., Ippoliti F. and Greci L. (2006) Synthesis and application of a novel sunscreen antioxidant. *Free Radical Res.* **40**: 485–494.
115. Venditti E., Spadoni T., Tiano L., Astolfi P., Greci L., Littaru G. P. and Damiani E. (2008) *In vitro* photostability and photoprotection studies of a novel 'multi-active' UV-absorber. *Free Radical Biol. Med.* **45**: 345–354.
116. Damiani E., Astolfi P., Giesinger J., Ehlis T., Herzog B., Greci L. and Baschong W. (2010) Assessment of the photodegradation of UV-filters and radical-induced peroxidation in cosmetic sunscreen formulations. *Free Radical Res.* **44**: 304–312.
117. Gonzales H., Tarras-Wahlberg N., Strömdahl B., Juzeniene A., Moan J., Larkö O., Rosén, A. and Wennberg A.-M. (2007) Photostability of commercial sunscreens upon sun exposure and irradiation by ultraviolet lamps. *BMC Dermatol.* **7**: 1–9.
118. Sayre R. M., Dowdy J. C., Gerwig, A. J., Shields, W. J., Lloyd, R. V. (2005) Unexpected photolysis of the sunscreen octinoxate in the presence of the sunscreen avobenzone. *Photochem. Photobiol.* **81**: 452–456.
119. Dondi D., Albini A. and Serpone N. (2006) Interactions between different solar UVB/UVA filters contained in commercial sunscreens and consequent loss of UV protection. *Photochem. Photobiol. Sci.* **5**: 835–843.
120. Charles A. K. and Darbre P. D. (2009) Oestrogenic activity of benzyl salicylate, benzyl benzoate and butylphenylmethylpropional (Lilial®) in MCF7 human breast cancer cells in vitro. *J. Appl. Toxicol.* **29**: 422–434.
121. Kammeyer A., Westerhof W., Bolhuis P. A., Ris A. J. and Hische E. A. (1987) The spectral stability of several sunscreening agents on stratum corneum sheets. *Int. J. Cosmet. Sci.* **9**: 125–136.
122. Fourtanier A., Labat-Robert J., Kern P., Berrebi C., Gracia A. M. and Boyer B. (1992) *In vivo* evaluation of photoprotection against chronic ultraviolet-A irradiation by a new sunscreen Mexoryl SX. *Photochem Photobiol.* **55**: 549–560.
123. Seite S., Moyal D., Richard S., de Rigal J., Leveque J. L. Hourseau C. and Fourtanier A. (1998) Mexoryl SX: a broad absorption UVA filter protects human skin from the effects of repeated suberythemal doses of UVA. *J. Photochem. Photobiol., B* **44**: 69–76.
124. Beck I., Deflandre A., Lang G., Arnaud R. and Lamaire J. (1981) Study of the photochemical behavior of sunscreens. Benzylidene camphor and derivatives. *Int. J. Cosmet. Sci.* **3**: 139–152.

125. Beck I., Deflandre A., Lang G., Arnaud R. and Lemaire J. (1985) Study of the photochemical behaviour of sunscreens. Benzylidene camphor and derivatives II: Photosensitized isomerization by aromatic ketones and deactivation of the 8-methoxypsoralen triplet state. *J. Photochem.* **30**: 215–227.
126. Benech-Kieffer F., Meuling W. J., Leclerc C., Roza L., Leclaire J. and Nohynek G. (2003) Percutaneous absorption of Mexoryl SX in human volunteers: comparison with in vitro data. *Skin Pharmacol. Appl. Skin Physiol.* **16**: 343–355.
127. Fourtanier A., Moyal D. and Seité S. (2008) Sunscreens containing the broad-spectrum UVA absorber, Mexoryl SX, prevent the cutaneous effects of UV exposure: a review of clinical study results. *Photodermatol., Photoimmunol. Photomed.* **24**: 164–174.
128. Gonzales H., Farbrot A., Larko O. and Wennberg A. M. (2006) Percutaneus absorption of the sunscreen benzophenone-3 after repeated whole-body applications, with and without ultraviolet irradiation. *Br. J. Dermatol.* **154**: 337–340.
129. Schallreuter K. U., Wood J. M., Farwell D. W., Moore J. and Edwards H. G. photoprotection versus antioxidant inactivation. *J. Invest. Dermatol.* **106**: 583–586.
130. Cantrell A., McGarvey D. J. and Truscott T. G. (2001) Photochemical and photophysical properties of sunscreens. In: *Sun protection in Man*, pp 495–519, Giacomoni, P. U. (ed.), Elsevier Science, Amsterdam.
131. Dubois M., Gilard P., Deflandre A. and Lefebvre M. A. (1998) *J. Chim. Phys.* **95**: 388–394.
132. Schwack W. and Rudolph T. (1995) Photochemistry of dibenzoylmethane UVA filters. Part I. *J. Photochem. Photobiol.* **28**: 229–2324.
133. Cantrell A. and McGarvey D. J. (2001) Photochemical studies of 4-*tert*-butyl-4'-methoxydibenzoylmethane (BM-DBM). *J. Photochem. Photobiol., B* **15**: 117–122.
134. Steenken S. (1989) One-electron redox reactions between radicals and molecules. Dominance of inner-sphere mechanisms. In: *Free Radicals in Synthesis and Biology*, pp 213–231, Minisci F. (ed.), Nato ASI Series, C260, Kluwer Academic Publishers, Dordrecht.
135. Fujita S. and Steenken S. (1981) Pattern of OH radical addition to uracil and methyl- and carboxyl-substituted uracils. Electron transfer of OH adducts with *N,N,N',N"*-tetramethyl-*p*-phenylenediamine and tetranitromethane. *J. Am. Chem. Soc.* **103**: 2540–2545.
136. Hazra D. K. and Steenken S. (1983) Pattern of OH radical addition to cytosine and 1-, 3-, 5-, and 6-substituted cytosines. Electron transfer

and dehydration reactions of the OH adducts. *J. Am. Chem. Soc.* **105**: 4380–4386.

137. Karlsson I., Hillerström, I., Stenfeldt A.-L., Mårtensson J. and Börje A. (2009) Photodegradation of dibenzoylmethanes: Potential Cause of photocontact allergy to sunscreens. *Chem. Res. Toxicol.* **22**: 1881–1892.
138. Herzog B., Hueglin D. and Osterwalder U. (2005) New sunscreen activities. In: *Sunscreens, Regulations and Commercial Development*, 3rd ed., pp 291–320, Shaath N. A. (ed.), Taylor & Francis, Boca Raton.
139. Inbaraj J. J., Bilski P. and Chignell C. F. (2002) Photophysical and photochemical studies of 2-phenylbenzimidazole and UVB sunscreen 2-phenylbenzimidazole-5-sulfonic acid. *Photochem. Photobiol.* **75**: 107–116.
140. Scalia S., Molinari A., Casolari A. and Maldotti A. (2004) Complexation of the sunscreen agent phenylbenzimidazolesulfonic acid with cyclodextrins: effect on stability and photoinduced free radical formation. *Eur. J. Pharm. Sci.* **22**: 241–249.
141. Bastien N., Millau J. F., Rouabhia M., Davies R. J. and Drouin R. (2010) The sunscreen agent 2-phenylbenzimidazole-5-sulfonic acid photosensitizes the formation of oxidized guanines in cellulo after UV-A or UV-B exposure. *J. Invest. Dermatol.* **130**: 2463–2471.
142. Stevenson C. and Davies R. J. (1999) Photosensitization of guanine-specific DNA damage by 2-phenylbenzimidazole and the sunscreen agent 2-phenylbenzimidazole-5-sulfonic acid. *Chem. Res. Toxicol.* **12**: 38–45.

G. Photochemistry of Inorganic Agents

The inorganic compounds titanium dioxide (TiO_2) and zinc oxide (ZnO) have been used together with organic sunscreens in commercial sunscreen products. Another inorganic compound, cerium dioxide (ceria, CeO_2) has been promulgated over the years; however, it seems that, to date, it has not been adopted for commercial sunscreens [1]. Nevertheless, it is included in some parts of the evaluations for comparison of its photophysical and photochemical properties with those of titanium and zinc oxides.

Titanium dioxide occurs in nature as the minerals rutile, anatase, brookite, ilmenite ($FeTiO_3$), and perovskite ($CaTiO_3$). The natural minerals are, of course, always contaminated with other elements. Pure titanium dioxide can be obtained from the minerals ilmenite and rutile, and from inorganic and organic titanium compounds and titanium metal by oxidations with molecular oxygen. Titanium dioxide is a very stable white solid with a melting point of about 1855 °C. It is of interest that titanium dioxide was detected on the planet Mars and in the atmosphere of the star Rho Cassiopeiae of our galaxy. Thus, the future traveler into outer space will conveniently find the reliable sunscreen for his or her protection from radiations. Titanium dioxide has been applied in a wide variety of commercial and industrial areas such as semiconductors; in welding, paints, enamels, lacquers, cements, white pigments, shoe whiteners, and in self-cleaning and anti-fogging agents; in skim milk, in toothpastes, in medicinal pills and tablets; as tattoo pigment; as coating of gem stones, e.g., mystic fire topaz; and alone or together with other catalysts in photocatalyzed oxidations and degradations.

Zinc oxide is found in nature as the mineral zincite. It can be prepared in pure form by reactions of zinc chloride with alkali and by the vaporization of zinc metal in an atmosphere of oxygen gas. Zinc oxide has been widely employed in various cosmetic and medicinal products, such as skin protectants, astringents, and antiseptics; in other areas as a white pigment, in the paper industry, glues, quick setting cements, inks, enamels, in car tires, fire retardants, and opaque and transparent glasses; and as a semiconductor in electronics.

Ceric oxide is found in nature as a mineral. It is practically insoluble in water and can be prepared in pure form by heating cerium salts at elevated temperatures. The element cerium is the most abundant element of the rare earth metals.

Inorganic sunscreens titanium and zinc oxides undergo photophysical and photochemical reactions on illumination with sunlight which contains the energies of the UVA and UVB radiations that are reflected, scattered, and mainly absorbed by the oxides. Titanium dioxide absorbs most effectively the energies of the UVB (280–320 nm) and UVA2 (320–340 nm) radiations, while zinc oxide absorbs the energies of the UVA (320–380 nm) and UVA1 (340–380 nm) radiations [1–10]. At present, the tendencies are to reduce the micronized forms of the oxides down to nano sizes below 100 nm in order to reduce the reflectance and scattering and increase the absorbance of the UV light. Furthermore, the absorptions will also undergo changes with changes of the nanosizes of particles [4, 8, 9].

The energies of the UV radiations absorbed by the oxides cause elevation of the electrons of valence bands of the oxides to the conductance bands resulting in pairs of electrons (e^-) and the positive, so-called e-holes that are denoted by $\overset{+}{h}$ [3, 4, 5, 8]. This stage is called the semiconductor photoexcited state **[Sch. 3G-1]**.

The energy difference between the valence and conduction bands is called the band gap. The gap energy for titanium dioxide is 3.0 eV, for zinc oxide 3.4 eV, and for cerium dioxide 3.1 eV, and the refractive indices for titanium dioxide are 2.5–2.7, for zinc oxide 2.0–2.1, and for cerium dioxide 2.1–2.2. Hence, on the basis of these values, it appears that the transparency of cerium dioxide is the same as that of zinc oxide and higher than the transparency of titanium dioxide. Furthermore, it was shown that the photochemistry of cerium dioxide is lower than those of zinc and titanium dioxides. Hence, it appears that cerium dioxide would be a suitable sunscreen agent [1]. Furthermore, it is important to bear in mind that the energies of UVB bands between 280 and 320 nm, with corresponding energies of 89 to 102 $kcal{\cdot}mol^{-1}$, and those in the UVA band between 75 to 89 $kcal{\cdot}mol^{-1}$ are of the same order of magnitude as those of the more common covalent bonds, such as, C–H ≈ 95–99 $kcal{\cdot}mol^{-1}$ at 300 nm, C–O ≈ 85–91 $kcal{\cdot}mol^{-1}$ at 325 nm, C–C ≈ 83–85 $kcal{\cdot}mol^{-1}$ at 345 nm and O–O = 52 $kcal{\cdot}mol^{-1}$.

Thus, the electron of the photoexcited semiconductor oxides can be transferred from the conduction band to the adsorbed molecular oxygen, which is a triplet in the ground state ($^3O_2$), with the formation of the superoxide radical anion($O_2{\cdot}^-$). This type of reduction process of molecular oxygen is known as the Type I sensitization [10, 11, 12, 13] **[Sch. 3G-1]**.

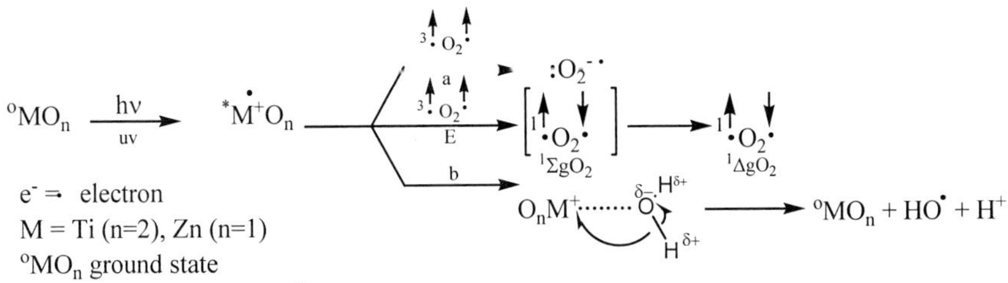

e^- = electron
M = Ti (n=2), Zn (n=1)
^oMO_n ground state
* MO_n excited state $e^- + h^+$
E = minimum energy required 22.7 kcal mol^{-1}
a = reactions at conduction band
b = reactions at valence band

Sch. 3G-1. UV radiation induced reactions of titanium dioxide and zinc oxide with (a) molecular oxygen and (b) water, and conversion of triplet oxygen to singlet oxygen. The transfer of the electron from the conduction band of the semiconductor to the adsorbed species is a reduction process. The transfer of the electron from the adsorbed species to the valence band of the semiconductor is an oxidation process of the adsorbed species.

The superoxide radical anion undergoes rapid protonation to the hydroperoxyl (HOO·) species, followed by a dismutation (disproportionation) reaction to produce hydrogen peroxide and molecular oxygen ($^3O_2$) and by a cascade of reactions producing various reactive oxygen species [**Sch. 3G-2** and **Sch. 3G-3**].

$$H_2O + O_2^{\bar{\bullet}} \longrightarrow HO_2^{\bullet} + HO^-$$
$$O_2^{\bar{\bullet}} + H^+ \rightleftharpoons HO_2^{\bullet}$$
$$2\,HO_2^{\bullet} \longrightarrow H_2O_2 + O_2$$
$$H_2O_2 + HO_2^{\bullet} \longrightarrow O_2 + HO^{\bullet} + H_2O$$
$$H_2O_2 + HO^{\bullet} \longrightarrow HO_2^{\bullet} + H_2O$$
$$H_2O_2 \rightleftharpoons HO_2^- + H^+$$
$$O_2^{\bullet} + 2H^+ \xrightarrow{e^-} H_2O_2$$
$$H_2O_2 \xrightarrow{e^-} HO^{\bullet} + HO^-$$
$$HO_2^{\bullet} \xrightarrow{e^-} HO_2^-$$

Sch. 3G-2. Propagation of reactive oxygen species derived from UV radiation induced reduction of molecular oxygen.

$$H_2O_2 + Fe^{2+}\,2X^- \longrightarrow HO\bullet + HO^- + Fe^{3+} + 2X^-$$

$$HO_2^- + Fe^{3+} \longrightarrow HO_2\bullet + Fe^{2+}$$

$$H_2O_2 + Cu^+X^- \longrightarrow HO\bullet + HO^- + Cu^{2+}X^-$$

$$X^- = \text{anion}$$

Sch. 3G-3. Fenton-type reactions that can occur at the human skin upon UV irradiations of titanium and zinc oxides.

Such reductions at the conduction band of the metal oxides can also occur with other molecular species in the cascade if absorbed at the semiconductor surface. Furthermore, the energies of the photoexcited metal oxide species are more than adequate to facilitate the conversion of molecular oxygen ($^3O_2$) to the singlet oxygen species $^1O_2$ [1, 2, 3, 5, 10–13, 16, 18, 20–22, 24]. The energy requirements for this conversion are only 22.7 kcal·mol^{-1} [5]. The first singlet oxygen species that is formed $^1\sum gO_2$ with paired electrons is very unstable and is rapidly converted to a more stable oxygen species, $^1\Delta gO_2$. This process is known as the Type II sensitization [10–13]. Such conversion of triplet oxygen $^3O_2$ to singlet species $^1O_2$ also readily occurs with many organic sunscreens, e.g., *p*-aminobenzoic acid (PABA) and 2-ethylhexyl 4-methoxycinnamate, since their excited triplet state species have energies of 57 kcal·mol^{-1} and 75 kcal·mol^{-1}, respectively [5]. Hence, it is not surprising that many organic filters readily undergo decompositions with generations of reactive oxygen species (ROS). The reactions of the energy rich species $\overset{+}{h}$ at the valence band can readily occur with adsorbed electron-rich molecules, such as water and hydrogen peroxide, whereby the electron donor undergoes an oxidation [3, 5]. The contact of the $\overset{+}{h}$ species with an electron donor could be facilitated by van der Waals forces. Thus, the reaction of $\overset{+}{h}$ at the valence band with water molecules produces hydroxyl radicals. The energy requirements are actually very high for homolysis of the HO–H bond, about 120 kcal·mol^{-1}.

Irradiation of titanium dioxide with UV light in the presence of hydrogen peroxide in aqueous media also produces hydroxyl radicals. This result is not surprising because of the weak oxygen–oxygen bond (52 kcal·mol^{-1}). Interestingly, this reaction can also produce the superoxide radical anion, probably in the protonated form as the hydroperoxyl radical

(HOO·). The requirements for this type of reaction to occur are about 90 kcal·mol^{-1} for the H–OOH bond [**Sch. 3G-4**].

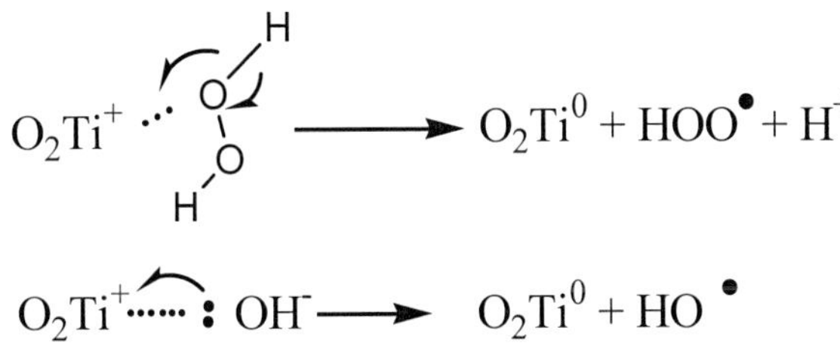

Sch. 3G-4. UV radiation induced reactions of $\overset{+}{h}$ species with hydrogen peroxide and hydroxide ion at the valence band.

When no mitigating conditions are in place, the decomposition of hydrogen peroxide to give hydroxyl radicals could also occur at the human skin by the well-known Fenton-type reaction, since the ubiquitous iron and copper salts are always present at the skin in ionized forms [**Sch. 3G-3**] [3, 9, 12, 17].

The generation of reactive oxygen species (ROS) by irradiation of titanium and zinc oxides can have either negative or positive effects on biological and other systems, and there exists a very large volume of literature attesting to these manifold photoinduced effects [25–40]. The following selected examples may adequately illustrate the photoinduced activities of inorganic sunscreens in the absence of mitigating conditions that would prevail in commercial products, such as encapsulations, doping, and other formulation practices. The prevalent ROS that are produced on UV irradiation of zinc oxide and titanium dioxide are the extremely reactive hydroxyl radicals (HO·) and the nonradical species singlet oxygen ($^1O_2$). The hydroxyl radicals very efficiently abstract hydrogen atoms from a variety of biological entities and other systems with formation of the "target" compound radicals, e.g., with the biologically important antioxidant vitamin E to give a resonance-stabilized vitamin E radical. The reactions of hydroxyl radicals with the heterobases of the DNA can cause severe damage. In addition, hydroxyl radicals can undergo addition reactions with heterobases of the DNA [1, 3, 12, 13, 23, 24, 25]. Singlet oxygen can also participate in reactions with the heterobases of the DNA, resulting in hydroperoxy derivatives followed by degradations. Singlet oxygen is involved with at least twenty other biological entities such as lipids and proteins, resulting in the formation of hydroperoxides, followed by their degradations to give ROS and other products [10, 12, 13].

Further examples of photoinduced activities of inorganic oxides exemplify the broad scope of biological effects that can be caused by these compounds, such as antibacterial effects, inactivation of *E. coli* by titanium dioxide [26, 27] and *Staphylococus aureus* by zinc oxide [28]; induction of cytotoxicity by zinc oxide, titanium dioxide, and other oxides [29, 30]; degradations down to mineralization of many organic compounds, including organic sunscreens [1, 3, 5, 6, 31–33]; anticancer properties of encapsulated titanium dioxide [34]; cell-specific antibodies–titanium dioxide conjugates for photodynamic therapy [35]; photokilling of malignant cells with ultrafine titanium dioxide [36]; nitration of proteins, such as tyrosine, by utilizing nitrates that are always present at the human skin [37, 38]; toxicity tests using ultrafine titanium dioxide in vitro and in vivo against mice, rabbits, and trout [39]; and photocatalytic treatment of water with titanium dioxide to remove natural and synthetic estrogens [40].

On the basis of these results, it is obvious that one would scarcely choose the inorganic oxides for the prevention of the harmful solar radiation at the human skin. Fortunately, these harmful effects caused by the photoexcited inorganic filters can be and should be reduced and even prevented by encapsulation, doping, and other formulation methods; and there exists ample information in the literature on this topic. A few examples may suffice to give a general idea about these methods. The metal oxide particles can be encapsulated using natural and synthetic polymers, such as liposomes multicomponent polymers, anionic polymers, waxes, dimethicon, a silicon polymer either alone or mixed with silicium dioxide, aluminum stearate, boric nitride, obtained by heating boric acid and urea, and doping with calcium oxide and silicium dioxide, and metal cations [1, 4, 5, 8, 9, 41–44].

The encapsulation methods either reduce or eliminate the oxygen and water content within the capsule and, thus, alleviate the photochemical reactions of metal oxides, resulting in the formation of ROS without interfering with absorption of the energy of UV radiations.

The inorganic sunscreens have a distinct advantage over the organic counterparts with respect to their permeation through the human skin and their chemical stability. Thus, the inorganic sunscreens, even in their fine micronized forms, are usually embedded in the outermost stratum corneum of the epidermis, and are not found in the deeper epidermis and dermal layers [6, 9, 44–55]. While the organic, mostly lipophilic, all aromatic [4, 8, 9] sunscreens—with molecular weights usually below 500, and seldom higher than 1000—can penetrate the deeper epidermis and even the dermal layers of the human skin, where the living cells can be encountered resulting in systemic absorptions with allergic, immunologic, and estrogenic responses. Furthermore, the organic sunscreens can facilitate the transport through the human skin of various xenobiotics that are prevalent in large cities. The extent of such penetrations may depend on the type of excipients in formulations and other conditions [4, 6, 9, 55–57].

The advent and rapid proliferations of nanosize materials in commerce and technologies have outpaced the thorough, impartial scrutinies and standardizations of these materials. The biological toxicities and health-related hazards of nanosize materials will, apparently, depend largely on the degree of micronization, the shape of the particles, and the type of materials. The risk factor will also depend on the mode of applications. In a series of recent investigations with carbon nanotubes, ranging in sizes between 1 and 20 nm, using either cell cultures in vitro or rodents, such as mice and rats in vivo, it was found that these materials have, with very few exceptions, a wide range of detrimental biological properties. Thus, these nanosize carbon tubes can cause antioxidant depletion and oxidative stress [58–63], induce pulmonary inflammations [62–66], retard bacterial clearance [62, 65], cause glaucoma formation and fibrogenesis [58], activate the tumor suppressor gene p53 and induce apoptosis [68], lead to mesothelioma, a cancer of the linings of the lungs [67, 69], induce cardiopulmonary diseases by pollutants [65], damage the mitochondrial DNA in aorta [65], induce atherosclerotic lesions in the brachiocephalic artery of the heart [65], cause respiratory functions impairments and stimulate mesenchymal cell growth [58, 64, 65], cause asthma on exposure to gas stoves [70], and can induce the release of proinflammatory cytokine interleukin 8 [71]. Nanotubes can be used for the delivery of anticancer drugs, such as a conjugate with paclitaxel for tumor suppression in mice [72]. The airborne carbon nanotubes, derived from combustions of fuels, may contribute to pollutions in urban habitats [65]. The inhalation of carbon nanoparticles of certain type and dimensions that resemble asbestos fibers cause inflammations of the linings of lungs, and, eventually, the mesothelioma cancer [67–70, 73].

These are, obviously, very alarming news if one recalls the problems that have been experienced over the years with the removal of asbestos from various installations, and the protracted litigations that are continuing to the present. Hence, it is of the foremost importance to avoid past mistakes, and to extend such investigations to other classes of nanosize materials in order to provide uniform safeguards and guidelines for the manufacture and applications of these materials.

On the basis of results that have been obtained, to date, with carbon nanotubes, there has been considerable concern over whether the inorganic sunscreens may have similar dangerous properties when used in nanosizes down to 1–20 nm. However, in recent investigations with titanium dioxide and zinc oxide using various micronized nanosize particles, it has been found that, apparently, neither the penetration through the human skin beyond the epidermic layers nor any other harmful properties could be detected with these oxides [9, 44, 55, 73–78, 79–88].

Hence, in conclusion, there is the notion that the inorganic sunscreens are superior to the organic sunscreens because of these and other favorable properties, such as lack of allergic reactions, safety, and stability, provided that the oxide particles are properly coated, and could be employed alone in commercial products in the absence of organic filters [10, 76, 77, 79, 88].

These products could be advantageously used for persons with sensitive skin, such as youngsters and persons who are sensitive to allergies and various dermatological conditions, e.g., chronic actinic dermatitis and psoriasis, just to mention a few.

At this stage, one should seriously consider abandoning altogether the organic filters and thereby simplify the manufacture, regulation, and application of sunscreen products.

References

1. Hidaka H., Kobayashi H., Koike T., Sato T. and Serpone N. (2006) DNA damage photoinduced by cosmetic pigments and sunscreen agents under solar exposure and artificial UV illumination. *J. Oleo Sci.* **55**: 249–261.
2. Serpone N., Dondi D. and Albini A. (2007) Inorganic and organic filters: their role and efficacy in sunscreens and suncare products. *Inorg. Chem. Acta* **360**: 794–802.
3. Banerjee S., Gopal J., Muraleedharan P., Tyagi A. K. and Raj B. (2006) Physics and chemistry of photocatalytic titanium dioxide: Visualization of bacterial activity using atomic force microscopy. *Curr. Sci.* **90**: 1378–1383.
4. Schlossman D. and Shao Y. (2005) Inorganic ultraviolet filters. In: *Sunscreens, Regulations and Commercial Development*, pp 137–161, Shaath N. A. (ed.), Taylor and Francis, Boca Raton.
5. Serpone N., Salinaro A., Emeline A. V., Horikoshi S., Hidaka H. and Zhao J. (2002) An in vitro systematic spectroscopic examination of the photostabilities of a random set of commercial sunscreen lotions and their chemical UVB/UVA active agents. *Photochem. Photobiol. Sci.* **1**: 970–981.

6. Dondi D., Albini A. and Serpone N. (2006) Interactions between different solar UVB/UVA filters contained in commercial sunscreens and consequent loss of UV protection. *Photochem. Photobiol. Sci.* **5**: 835–843.
7. Serpone N. and Emeline A. V. (2005) Modeling heterogeneous photocatalysis by metal-oxide nanostructured semiconductor and insulator materials: Factors that affect the activity and selectivity of photocatalysts. *Res. Chem. Intermed.* **31**: 391–432.
8. Anderson M. W., Hewitt Y. P. and Spruce S. R. (1997) Broad spectrum physical sunscreens: titanium dioxide and zinc oxide. In: *Sunscreens, Development, Evaluation and Regulatory Aspects*, pp 353–397, Lowe, N. J., Shaath N. A. and Pathak M. A. (eds.), Marcel Dekker, New York.
9. Bens, G. (2008) Sunscreens. In: *Sunlight, Vitamin D and Skin Cancer*, pp 137–161, Reichroth, J. (ed.), Springer Science and Business Media, New York.
10. Douki, T. (2007) UV-induced DNA damage. In: *Biological and Physiological Effects of Solar Radiation on Human Skin*, pp 227–269, Giacomoni P. V. (ed.), The Royal Society of Chemistry, Cambridge.
11. Foote C. S. (1991) Definition of Type I and Type II photosensitized oxidation. *Photochem. Photobiol.* **54**: 659.
12. Fuchs J. (1998) Potentials and limitations of the natural antioxidants *RRR*-α-tocopherol, L-ascorbic acid and β-carotene in cutaneous photoprotection. *Free Radical Biol. Med.* **25**: 848–873.
13. Girotti A. W. and Giacomoni P. U. (2007) Lipid and protein damage provoked by ultraviolet radiation: Mechanisms of indirect photooxidative damage. In: *Biophysical and Physiological Effects of Solar Radiation on Human Skin*, pp 271–292, The Royal Society of Chemistry, Cambridge.
14. Konaka R., Kasahara E., Dunlap W. C., Yamamoto Y., Chien K. C. and Inoue M. (1999) Irradiation of titanium dioxide generates both singlet oxygen and superoxide anion. *Free Radical Biol. Med.* **27**: 294–300.
15. Konaka R., Kashara E., Dunlap W. C., Yamamoto Y., Chien K. C. and Inoue M. (2001) Ultraviolet irradiation of titanium dioxide in aqueous dispersion generates singlet oxygen. *Redox Rep.* **6**: 319–325.
16. Harbour J. R., Tromp J. and Hair M. L. (1985) Photogeneration of hydrogen peroxide in aqueous TiO_2 dispersions. *Can. J. Chem.* **63**: 204–208.

17. Herrling Th., Groth N., Golz K., Zastrow L. (2000) The role of aggressive ·OH free radicals in skin – their generation, detection and prevention. *SÖFW–J.* **126**: 20–27.
18. Gogniat G. and Dukan S. (2007) TiO_2 photocatalysis causes DNA damage via Fenton reaction-generated hydroxyl radicals during the recovery period. *Appl. Environ. Microbiol.* **73**: 7740–7743.
19. Brezová V., Gabcová S., Dvoranová D. and Stasko A. (2005) Reactive oxygen species produced upon photoexcitation of sunscreens containing titanium dioxide (an EPR study). *J. Photochem. Photobiol., B* **79**: 121–134.
20. Lee M. C., Yoshino F., Shoji H., Takahashi S., Todoki K., Shimada S. and Kuse-Barouch K. (2005) Characterization by electron spin resonance spectroscopy of reactive oxygen species generated by titanium dioxide and hydrogen peroxide. *J. Dent. Res.* **84**: 178–182.
21. Yamamoto Y., Imai N., Mashima R., Konaka R., Inoue M. and Dunlap W. C. (1999) Singlet oxygen from irradiated titanium dioxide and zinc oxide. *Methods Enzymol.* **319**: 20–27.
22. Yamamoto Y., Imai N., Mashima R., Konaka R., Inoue M. and Dunlap W. C. (2000) Singlet oxygen from irradiated titanium dioxide and zinc oxide. *Methods Enzymol.* **319**: 29–37.
23. Dunford R., Salinaro A., Cai L., Serpone N., Horikoshi S., Hidaka H. and Knowland J. (1997) Chemical oxidation and DNA damage catalysed by inorganic ingredients. *FEBS Lett.* **418**: 87–90.
24. Wamer W. G., Yin J.-J. and Wei R. R. (1997) Oxidative damage to nucleic acids photosensitized by titanium dioxide. *Free Radical Biol. Med.* **27**: 851–858.
25. Wamer W. G., Yin J.-J. and Wei R. R. (1999) Oxidative damage to nucleic acids photosensitized by titanium dioxide generates both singlet oxygen and superoxide anion. *Free Radical Biol. Med.* **27**: 294–300.
26. Nagame S., Oku T., Kambara M. and Konishi K. (1989) Antibacterial effect of powdered semiconductor TiO_2 on the viability of oral micro-organisms. *J. Dent. Res.* **68**: 1696–1697.
27. Ireland J. C., Klosterman P., Rice E. W. and Clark R. M. (1993) Inactivation of E. coli by titanium dioxide photocatalytic oxidation. *Appl. Environ. Microbiol.* **59**: 1668–1670.
28. Jones N., Ray B., Ranjit K. T. and Manna A. C. (2008) Antibacterial activity of ZnO nanoparticle suspensions on a broad spectrum of microorganisms. *FEMS Microbiol. Lett.* **279**: 71–76.

29. Cai R., Kubota Y., Shuin T., Sakai H., Hashimoto K. and Fujishima A. (1992) Induction of cytotoxicity by photoexcited TiO_2 particles. *Cancer Res.* **52**: 2346–2348.
30. Soto K., Garza K. M. and Murr L. E. (2007) Cytotoxic effects of aggregated nanomaterials. *Acta Biomater.* **3**: 351–358.
31. Ricci A., Chretien M. N., Maretti L. and Scaiano J. C. (2003) TiO_2-promoted mineralization of organic sunscreens in water suspension and sodium dodecyl sulfate micelles. *Photochem. Photobiol. Sci.* **2**: 487–492.
32. Sayre R. M., Dowdy J. C., Ricci A., Chretien M. N. and Scaiano J. C. (2002) Mineralization of organic sunscreens: interesting, but relevant? Comment and response. *Photochem. Photobiol. Sci.* **2**: 1050–1051.
33. Hidaka H., Kubota H., Graetzel M., Pelizzetti E. and Serpone N. (1986) Photodegradation of surfactants II. Degradation of sodium dodecylbenzenesulfonate catalyzed by titanium dioxide particles. *J. Photochem.* **35**: 219–230.
34. Chihara Y., Fujimoto K., Kondo H., Moriwaka Y., Sasahira T., Hirao Y. and Kuniyasu H. (2007) Antitumor effects of liposome-encapsulated titanium dioxide in nude mice. *Pathobiology* **74**: 353–358.
35. Xu J., Sun Y., Huang J., Chen C., Liu G., Jiang Y., Zhao Y. and Jiang Z. (2007) Photokilling cancer cells using highly cell-specific antibody-TiO_2 bioconjugates and electroporation. *Bioelectrochemistry* **71**: 217–222.
36. Cai R., Hashimoto K., Itoh K., Kubota Y. and Fujishima A. (1991) Photokilling of malignant cells with ultrafine TiO_2 powder. *Bull Chem. Soc. Jpn.* **64**: 1268–1273.
37. Lu N., Zhu Z., Zhao X., Tao R., Yang X. and Gao Z. (2008) Nano-titanium dioxide photocatalytic protein tyrosine nitration: a potential hazard of TiO_2 on skin. *Biochem. Biophys. Res. Commun.* **370**: 675–680.
38. Nakagawa Y., Wakuri S., Sakamoto K. and Tanaka N. (1997) The photogenotoxicity of titanium dioxide particles. *Mutat. Res.* **394**: 125–132.
39. Warheit D. B., Hoke R. A., Finlay C., Donner E. M., Reed K. L. and Sayes C. M. (2007) Development of a base set of toxicity tests using ultrafine TiO_2 particles as a component of nanoparticle risk management. *Toxicol. Lett.* **171**: 99–110.
40. Ohko Y., Iuchi K., Niwa C., Tatsuma T., Nakashima T., Iguchi T., Kubota Y. and Fujishima A. (2002) 17beta-estradiol degradation by

TiO_2 photocatalysis as a means of reducing estrogenic activity. *Environ. Sci. Technol.* **36**: 4175–4181.
41. Cole C. A., Vollhardt J. and Mendrok C. (2009) Formulations and stability of sunscreen products. In: *Clinical guide to sunscreens and photoprotection*, pp 39–51, Lim H. W. and Draelos Z. D. (eds.), Informa Healthcare, New York.
42. Catlow B. (1993) Formulating of sunscreen with ultrafine titanium dioxide. *SÖFW-J.* **119**: 497–500.
43. Lee W. A., Pernodet N., Li B., Lin C. H., Hatchwell E. and Rafailovich M. H. (2007) Multicomponent polymer coating to block photocatalytic activity of TiO_2 nanoparticles. *Chem. Commun. (Camb.)* 4815–4817.
44. Couteau C., Alami S., Guitton M., Paparis E. and Coiffard L. J. (2008) Mineral filters in sunscreen products—comparison of the efficacy of zinc oxide and titanium dioxide by in vitro method. *Pharmazie* **63**: 58–60.
45. Pflücker F., Hohenberg H., Hölzle E., Will T., Pfeiffer S., Wepf R., Diembeck W., Wenck H. and Gers-Barlag H. (1999) The outermost stratum corneum layer is an effective barrier against dermal uptake of topically applied micronized titanium dioxide. *Int. J. Cosmet. Sci.* **21**: 399–405.
46. Lademann J., Weigmann H. J., Rickmeyer C., Barthelmes H., Schaefer H., Mueller G. and Sterry W. (1999) Penetration of titanium dioxide micro-particles in a sunscreen formulation into the horny layer and follicular orifice. *Skin Pharmacol. Appl. Skin Physiol.* **12**: 247–256.
47. Bennat C. and Müller-Goymann C. C. (2000) Skin penetration and stabilization of formulations containing microfine titanium dioxide as physical UV filter. *Int. J. Cosmet. Sci.* **22**: 271–283.
48. Brand R. M., Pike J., Wilson R. M. and Charron A. R. (2003) Sunscreen containing physical UV blockers can increase transdermal absorption of pesticides. *Toxicol. Ind. Health* **19**: 9–16.
49. Menzel T., Reinert T., Vogt J. and Butz T. (2004) Investigations of percutaneous uptake of ultrafine TiO_2 particles at the high energy ion nanoprobe LIPSION. *Nucl. Instrum. Methods Phys. Res., Sect. B*: **219–220**: 82–86.
50. Schulz J., Hohenberg H., Pflücker F., Gärtner E., Will T., Pfeiffer S., Wepf R., Wendel V., Gers-Barlag H. and Wittern K. P. (2002) Distribution of sunscreens on skin. *Adv. Drug Delivery Rev.* **54**: S157–63.

51. Mavon A., Miquel C., Lejeune O., Payre B. and Moretto P. (2007) In vitro percutaneous absorption and *in vivo* stratum corneum distribution of an organic and a mineral sunscreen. *Skin Pharmacol. Physiol.* **20**: 10–20.
52. Cross S. E., Innes B., Roberts M. S., Tsuzuki T., Robertson T. A. and McCormick P. (2007) Human skin penetration of sunscreen nanoparticles: in-vitro assessment of a novel micronized zinc oxide formulation. *Skin Pharmacol. Physiol.* **20**: 148–154.
53. Nohynek G. J., Ladermann J., Ribaud C. and Roberts M. S. (2007) Grey goo on the skin? Nanotechnology, cosmetic and sunscreen safety. *Crit. Rev. Toxicol.* **37**: 251–257.
54. Nohynek G. J., Dufour E. K. and Roberts M. S. (2008) Nanotechnology, cosmetics and the skin: is there a health risk? *Skin Pharmacol. Physiol.* **21**: 136–149.
55. Nash J. F. (2009) Systemic effects of topically applied sunscreen ingredients. In: *Clinical guide to sunscreens and photoprotection*, pp 139–154, Lim H. W. and Draelos Z. D. (eds.), Informa Healthcare, New York.
56. Chatelain E., Gabard B. and Surber C. (2003) Skin penetration and sun protection factor of five UV filters: effect of the vehicle. *Skin Pharmacol. Appl. Skin Physiol.* **16**: 28–35.
57. Klinubol P., Asawanonda P. and Wanichwecharungruang S. P. (2008) Transdermal penetration of UV filters. Skin penetration of UV filters. *Skin Pharmcol. Physiol.* **21**: 23–29.
58. Donaldson K., Aitken R., Tran L., Stone V., Duffin R., Forrest G. and Alexander A. (2006) Carbon nanotubes: a review of their properties in relation to pulmonary toxicology and workplace safety. *Toxicol. Sci.* **92**: 5–22.
59. Manna S. K., Sarkar S., Barr J., Wise K., Barrera E. V., Jejelowo O., Rice-Ficht A. C. and Ramesh G. T. (2005) Single-walled carbon nanotube induces oxidative stress and activates nuclear transcription factor-κB in human keratinocytes. *Nano Lett.* **5**: 1676–1684.
60. Fenoglio I., Tomatis M., Lison D., Muller J., Fonseca A., Nagy J. B. and Fubini B. (2006) Reactivity of carbon nanotubes: free radical generation of scavenging activity? *Free Radical Biol. Med.* **40**: 1227–1233.
61. Shvedova A. A., Castranova V., Kisin E. R., Schwegler-Berry D., Murray A. R., Gandelsman V. Z., Maynard A. and Baron P. (2003) Exposure to carbon nanotube material: assessment of nanotube cytotoxicity using human keratinocyte cells. *J. Toxicol. Environ. Health, Part A* **66**: 1909–1926.

62. Shedova A. A., Fabisiak J. P., Kisin E. R., Murray A. R., Roberts J. R., Tyurina Y. Y., Antonini J. M., Feng W. H., Kommineni C., Reynolds J., Barchowsky A., Castranova V. and Kagan V. E. (2008) Sequential exposure to carbon nanotubes and bacteria enhances pulmonary inflammation and infectivity. *Am. J. Respir. Cell Mol. Biol.* **38**: 579–590.
63. Duffin R., Mills N. L. and Donaldson K. (2007) Nanoparticles – a thoracic toxicology perspective. *Yonsei. Med. J.* **48**: 561–572.
64. Born P. J., Robbins D., Haubold S., Kuhlbusch T., Fissan H., Donaldson K., Schins R., Stone V., Kreyling W., Lademann J., Krutmann J., Warheit D. and Oberdorster. (2006) The potential risks of nanomaterials: a review carried out for ECETOC. *Part. Fibre Toxicol.* **3**: 11.
65. Lam C. W., James J. T., McCluskey R., Arepalli S. and Hunter R. L. (2006) A review of carbon nanotube toxicity and assessment of potential occupational and environmental health risks. *Crit. Rev. Toxicol.* **36**: 189–217.
66. Stern S. T. and McNeil S. E. (2008) Nanotechnology safety concerns revisited. *Toxicol Sci.* **101**: 4–21.
67. Poland C. A., Duffin R., Kinloch I., Maynard A., Wallace W. A., Seaton A., Stone V., Brown S., Macnee W. and Donaldson K. (2008) Carbon nanotubes introduced into the abdominal cavity of mice show asbestos-like pathogenicity in a pilot study. *Nat. Nanotechnol.* **3**: 423–428.
68. Zhu L., Chang D. W., Dai L. and Hong Y. (2007) DNA damage induced by multiwalled carbon nanotubes in mouse embryonic stem cells. *Nano Lett.* **7**: 3592–3597.
69. Takagi A., Hirose A., Nishimura T., Fukumori N., Ogata A., Ohashi N., Kitajima S. and Kanno J. (2008) Induction of mesothelioma in p53+/- mouse by interperitoneal application of multi-wall carbon nanotube. *J. Toxicol. Sci.* **33**: 105–116.
70. Murr L. E., Garza K. M., Soto K. F., Carrasco A., Powell T. G., Ramirez D. A., Guerrero P. A., Lopez D. A. and Venzor J. 3rd. (2005) Cytotoxicity assessment of some carbon nanotubes and related carbon nanoparticle aggregates and the implications for anthropogenic carbon nanotube aggregates in the environment. *Int. J. Environ. Res. Public Health* **2**: 31–42.
71. Monteiro-Riviere N. A., Nemanich R. J., Inman A. O., Wang Y. Y. and Riviere J. E. (2005) Multi-walled carbon nanotube interactions with human epidermal keratinocytes. *Toxicol. Lett.* **155**: 377–384.

72. Liu Z., Chen K., Davis C., Sherlock S., Cao Q., Chen X. and Dai H. (2008) Drug delivery with carbon nanotubes for *in vivo* cancer treatment. *Cancer Res.* **68**: 6652–6660.
73. Baan R. A. (2007) Carcinogenic hazards from inhaled carbon black, titanium dioxide, and talc not containing asbestos or asbestiform fibers: recent evaluations by an IARC Monographs Working Group. *Inhalation Toxicol.* **19**: 213–228.
74. Tsuji J. S., Maynard A. D., Howard P. C., James J. T., Lam C. W., Warheit D. B. and Santamaria A. B. (2006) Research strategies for safety evolution of nanomaterials, part IV: risk assessment of nanoparticles. *Toxicol. Sci.* **89**: 42–50.
75. Pinnell S. R., Fairhurst D., Gillies R., Mitchnick M. A. and Kollias N. (2000) Microfine zinc oxide is a superior sunscreen ingredient to microfine titanium dioxide. *Dermatol. Surg.* **26**: 309–314.
76. Ramanakumar A. V., Parent M. E., Latreille B. and Siemiatycki J. (2008) Risk of lung cancer following exposure to carbon black, titanium dioxide and talc: results from two case-control studies in Montreal. *Int. J. Cancer* **122**: 183–189.
77. Schauder S. (2001) Dermatologische Verträglichkeit von UV-Filtern, Duftstoffen and Konservierungsmitteln in Sonnenschutzpräparaten. *Bundesgesundheitsblatt-Gesundheits-forschung-Gesundheitsschutz* **44**: 471–479.
78. Wolf R., Matz H., Orion E. and Lipozencić J. (2003) Sunscreens—the ultimate cosmetic. *Acta Dermatovenerol. Croat.* **11**: 158–162.
79. Hayden C. G., Cross S. E., Anderson C., Saunders N. A. and Roberts M. S. (2005) Sunscreen penetration of human skin and related keratinocyte toxicity after topical application. *Skin Pharmacol. Physiol.* **18**: 170–174.
80. Cross S. E., Innes B., Roberts M. S., Tsuzuki T., Robertson T. A. and McCormic P. (2007) Human skin penetration of sunscreen nanoparticles: in-vitro assessment of a novel micronized zinc oxide formulation. *Skin Pharmacol. Physiol.* **20**: 148–154.
81. More B. D. (2007) Physical sunscreens: on the comeback trail. *Indian J. Dermatol. Venereol. Leprol.* **73**: 80–85.
82. Roberts M. S., Roberts M. J., Robertson T. A., Sanches W., Thörling C., Zou Y., Zhao X., Becker W. and Zvyagin A. V. (2008) In vitro and in vivo imaging of xenobiotic transport in human skin and in the rat liver. *J. Biophotonics* **1**: 478–493.
83. Wu J., Liu W., Xue C., Zhou S., Lan F., Bi L., Xu H., Yang X. and Zeng F. D. (2009) Toxicity and penetration of TiO_2 nanoparticles in

hairless mice and porcine skin after subchronic dermal exposure. *Toxicol. Lett.* **191**: 1–8.
84. Durand L., Habran N., Henschel V. and Amighi K. (2009) In vitro evaluation of the cutaneous penetration of sprayable sunscreen emulsions with high concentrations of UV filters. *Int. J. Cosmet. Sci.* **31**: 279–292.
85. Filipe P., Silva J. N., Silva R., Cirne de Castro J. L., Marques Gomes M., Alves L. C., Santus R. and Pinheiro T. (2009) Stratum corneum is an effective barrier to TiO_2 and ZnO nanoparticle percutaneous absorption. *Skin Pharmacol. Physiol.* **22**: 266–275.
86. Sadrieh N., Wokovich A. M., Gopee N. V., Zheng J., Haines D., Permiter D., Siltonen P. H., Cozart C. R., Patri A. K., McNeil S. E., Howard P. C., Doub W. H. and Buhse L. F. (2010) Lack of significant dermal penetration of titanium dioxide from sunscreen formulations containing nano- and submicron-size TiO_2 particles. *Toxicol. Sci.* **115**: 156–166.
87. Gulson B., McCall M., Korsch M., Gomez L., Casey P., Oytam Y., Taylor A., McCulloch M., Trotter J., Kinsley L. and Greenoak G. (2010) Small amounts of zinc from zinc oxide particles in sunscreens applied outdoors are absorbed through human skin. *Toxicol. Sci.* **118**: 140–149.
88. Schilling K., Bradford B., Castelli D., Dufour E., Nash J. F., Pape W., Schulte S., Tooley I., van den Bosch J. and Schellauf F. (2010) Human safety revive of "nano" titanium dioxide and zinc oxide. *Photochem Photobiol Sci.* **9**: 495–509.

CHAPTER FOUR

FORMATION AND REACTIONS OF REACTIVE OXYGEN SPECIES: OXIDATIVE STRESS

A. Radiation-Induced Formation of Reactive Oxygen Species (ROS)

Humans, other mammals, and plants have undergone the evolutionary process over millions of years in an atmosphere of oxygen, nitrogen, carbon dioxide, and argon gasses. Since the oxygen molecule was predestined during this evolutionary process to become a diradical, one would expect that the oxygen molecule would be readily involved in free radical reactions with various substances, resulting in oxygenated derivatives. Over the past decades, on the basis of extensive research efforts, molecular oxygen and reactive oxygen species (ROS) [1–28] have been implicated in various pathological and pathogenic conditions, such as, for example, the coronary heart and cardiovascular diseases, postichemic perfusion injuries, inflammations, xenobiotic toxicities, metabolism of chemotherapeutic agents, mutagenesis and carcinogenesis leading to cancer diseases, and radiation mediated, ROS inflicted injuries and damages to the vital DNA; to lipids, proteins, carbohydrates, and advanced glycation products derived from reactions of carbohydrates with amino acids; and to the skin and various cellular components [14, 16, 17, 23, 24, 27, 29–31]. Reactive oxygen species have also been detected and extensively investigated in plant materials [14, 24, 27]. The advanced glycation end-products (AGEs) have been found to be involved in aging processes and several grave diseases, such as Alzheimer's, Parkinson's, Creuzfeldt-Jakob, amyotrophic lateral sclerosis, diabetic complications, retinal aging, and macular degeneration [32–36]. AGEs are primarily formed by condensations of the amino groups of amino acids and peptides with the carbonyl groups of aldehydes, ketones, and large carbohydrates, resulting in the elimination of a water molecule to give a Schiff base, the so-called Maillard reaction. These intermediates undergo convoluted Amadori and Heyns rearrangements and other reactions to give AGEs and many byproducts. These types of reactions occur also in food processing. The UV light induced reactions of AGEs with molecular oxygen result in the damaging reactive oxygen species (ROS). (See **Sections 2 D** and **E**.)

The great variety of injuries to biological systems has been attributed to the so-called oxidative stress, i.e., a condition resulting from an imbalance of oxidants to antioxidants in favor of the former. This condition can develop in the human body endogenously, in various organs, and exogenously on the skin. Since the skin is one of the larger organs of the human body, the oxidative stress on the skin can lead to grave consequences and, ultimately, to cancers of the skin.

The oxidants involved in the oxidative stress can be various carbon-, sulfur-, nitrogen-, and oxygen-centered radicals. The carbon, alkoxy, and alkyl hydroperoxy-centered radicals are formed, e.g., during the peroxidation reactions of lipids. The all-important other oxygen-centered radical and other species derived from molecular oxygen can be formed endogenously in various organs of the human body. However, in connection with the topic on sunscreens, the generation of these species at the skin is of prime interest. Thus, many UV light energy absorbing substances, including sunscreen formulations, under solar UVA and UVB radiations can function as photosensitizers that can be quenched by molecular oxygen to generate the following species: hydroxyl radical ($HO\cdot$), hydroperoxy radical ($HOO\cdot$), superoxide anion radical ($O_2\cdot^-$), singlet oxygen ($^1O_2$), and hydrogen peroxide (H_2O_2), which is a source of further hydroxyl radicals.

The radiolysis reactions of oxygenated aqueous media yield the following species.

$$H_2O \longrightarrow H_2O_2 + H_2 + H_3O^+\cdot + HO\cdot + H\cdot + e^-_{aq}$$

e^-_{aq} = hydrated electron

The formation of the hydroxyl radical ($HO\cdot$) and hydrated electron occurs in 10^{-11} seconds, and molecular formations from recombinations and/or chemical reactions are complete in 10^{-8} seconds. The hydrated electron (e^-_{aq}) and $H\cdot$ react with oxygen at diffusion-controlled rates to give the superoxide anion radical ($O_2\cdot^-$) and hydroperoxy radical ($HOO\cdot$), respectively.

$$O_2 + e^-_{aq} \longrightarrow O_2\cdot^-$$

$$O_2 + H\cdot \longrightarrow HOO\cdot \rightleftharpoons H^+ + O_2\cdot^-$$

The superoxide anion radical species is a weak base and is rapidly protonated to give the hydroperoxy radical, $pK_a \cong 4.7$, whereby the equilibrium is shifted to the hydroperoxy radical. In aqueous media, the following dismutation reactions ensue to give hydrogen peroxide and molecular oxygen [2]. Thus, these species are precursors of hydrogen peroxide.

$$HOO\cdot + O_2\cdot^- + H^+ \rightarrow H_2O_2 + O_2 \qquad K = 1.0 \times 10^8\ M^{-1}s^{-1}$$
$$HOO\cdot + HOO\cdot \rightarrow H_2O_2 + O_2 \qquad K = 8.6 \times 10^5\ M^{-1}s^{-1}$$
$$O_2\cdot^- + O_2\cdot^- + 2\,H^+ \rightarrow H_2O_2 + O_2 \qquad K < 0.3\ M^{-1}s^{-1}$$

Similar results are obtained in aqueous media with non-ionizing ultraviolet A and B radiations. In the presence of substances that absorb the energy of the ultraviolet light, two primary reactions can occur, i.e., either the absorbed energy exceeds the bond energies and then the substance fragments, or the substance is excited to a singlet and triplet state species. These species can either return to the ground state with emissions of fluorescence and phosphorescence or they are quenched by various substances, but most efficiently by molecular oxygen to give reactive oxygen species (ROS). Molecular oxygen is in a triplet ground state and the best quencher of substances in the triplet state, but it can also quench very effectively species in the excited singlet state.

Two mechanisms have been proposed for the generation of ROS involving the quenching processes of excited states, i.e., Type I and Type II [**Sch. 4A-1**]. According to the Type I mechanism, an electron transfer occurs from the photosensitizer to oxygen to give the superoxide anion radical, and according to the Type II mechanism, the sensitizer in the singlet electronic state can undergo intersystem crossing to the triplet excited state and interact with oxygen to give the oxygen in the singlet state ($^1O_2$) [37–39], whereby a transfer of energy occurs from the triplet sensitizer to molecular oxygen in the ground state.

It has been found that many diverse classes of compounds can undergo these excitations resulting in ROS, e.g., aromatic ketones, quinones, phenols, naphthols, aromatic aldehydes, unsaturated aromatic hydroxy compounds such as salicylic acid and derivatives, aromatic sulfonic acids, flavins, porphyrins and related classes of compounds, amino acids and proteins containing aromatic components, condensation products of reducing carbohydrates and amino acids and peptides, many dyes with heterocyclic structures which may inadvertently be added to cosmetic formulations. Thus, melanins and various sunscreen components would be expected to undergo excitations to the singlet state on irradiation with ultraviolet light, followed by quenching processes of Type I and II.

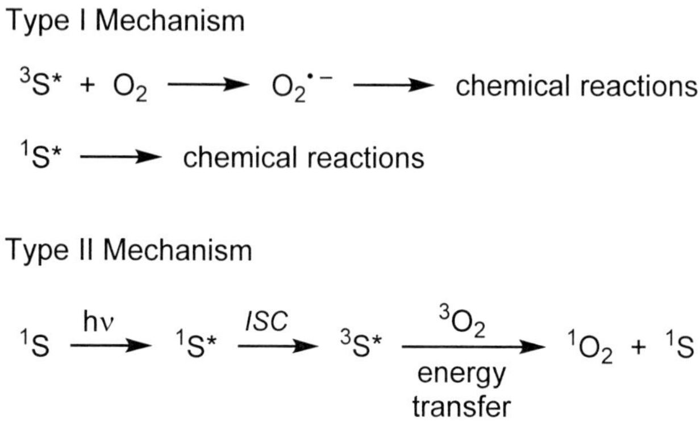

Sch. 4A-1. Proposed Mechanisms for the radiation-induced generation of ROS. ^1S = sensitizer in singlet electronic ground state; $^1S^*$ = sensitizer in singlet electronic excited state; $^3S^*$ = sensitizer in triplet electronic excited state; $^3O_2$ = oxygen in triplet electronic ground state; $^1O_2$ = oxygen in singlet electronic excited state; ISC = intersystem crossing.

B. Mechanisms of Hydrogen Peroxide Decomposition Reactions

Hydrogen peroxide can undergo homolytic decompositions in pure aqueous solutions, even in the absence of metal ion catalysts [**Sch. 4B-1**] [40–47].

$$H_2O \rightleftharpoons H^+ + HO^-$$
$$H_2O_2 + HO^- \rightleftharpoons HO_2^- + H_2O$$
$$HO_2^- + HO^- \rightleftharpoons O_2^{2-} + H_2O$$
$$O_2^{2-} + H_2O_2 \rightleftharpoons O_2^- + HO^- + HO\cdot$$
$$H_2O_2 + HO\cdot \rightleftharpoons H_2 + HO_2\cdot$$
$$O_2\cdot^- + H_2O \longrightarrow HO_2\cdot + HO^-$$
$$2HO_2\cdot \longrightarrow H_2O_2 + O_2$$

Sch. 4B-1. Homolytic decompositions of hydrogen peroxide in pure aqueous solutions.

The reactive oxygen species derived from the decomposition of hydrogen peroxide include the biologically important hydroxyl radicals ($HO\cdot$), the superoxide anion radical ($O_2\cdot^-$), and hydroperoxy radical ($HOO\cdot$). The analogous decomposition reactions of organic peroxide proceed by similar mechanisms. The chemistry of organic peroxide has been extensively studied over the years [40–47]. Acidic conditions have a stabilizing effect on aqueous hydrogen peroxide solutions, while alkaline conditions favor the decomposition reactions.

Transition-metal-cation catalyzed reactions of hydrogen peroxide are greatly important in industrial polymerizations, in synthesis, and in a biological environment. With respect to the present review, the more important cations are those of iron (Fe^{2+}/Fe^{3+}), copper (Cu^{1+}/Cu^{2+}), and titanium (Ti^{3+}/Ti^{4+}).

The iron-catalyzed Fenton Reaction was published in 1893 and the Ruff Degradation in 1898. However, the mechanistic interpretation was provided first by Haber and Weiss in 1934. The following mechanisms are based also on contributions by later investigators [**Sch. 4B-2**] [40–47].

$$H_2O_2 \rightleftharpoons H^+ + HO_2^-$$
$$H_2O_2 + Fe^{2+} \longrightarrow HO^- + HO\cdot + Fe^{3+}$$
$$HO_2^- + Fe^{3+} \rightleftharpoons HO_2\cdot + Fe^{2+}$$
$$H_2O_2 + HO\cdot \longrightarrow H_2O + HO_2\cdot$$
$$HO_2\cdot + H_2O_2 \longrightarrow O_2 + H_2O + HO\cdot$$

Further reactions occur with ferric cation:

$$H_2O_2 + Fe^{3+} \longrightarrow HO_2\cdot + H^+ + Fe^{2+}$$
$$HO\cdot + Fe^{2+} \longrightarrow Fe^{3+} + HO^-$$
$$HO_2^- + Fe^{3+} \longrightarrow Fe^{2+} + H^+ + O_2\cdot^-$$
$$H_2O_2 + O_2\cdot^- \longrightarrow O_2 + HO\cdot + HO^-$$

Sch. 4B-2. Proposed mechanism for the iron-catalyzed Fenton Reaction and Ruff Degradation.

Analogous mechanisms can be applied to other transition-metal cations and to organic peroxides [40–47]. It is evident that many of the ways of forming and transforming reactive oxygen species create an extremely complex, and not fully explored, redox environment in biological systems.

C. Properties of the Hydroxyl Radical

The highly electrophilic hydroxyl radical ($HO\cdot$) diffuses after its formation over a distance of about 5–10 molecule diameters with a half-life way of 1.8 mm and a half-life of only 0.3 ns. Hence, the reactions of the hydroxyl radical with the target are very site specific, and proceed with a second order rate constant of 10^{-9} to 10^{-10} M^{-1} s^{-1} [5, 48]. Thus, probably every molecule in a cell would be involved in reactions with hydroxyl radicals. It is estimated that the daily formation of oxidized species involving cellular components, the so-called hydroxyl adducts amount to about 10^4 – 10^8 molecules per cell. Clearly, the possible cellular damages involved in such processes can be severe unless mechanisms exist to either ameliorate or prevent such effects.

D. Identification of Reactive Oxygen Species

The reactive oxygen species, such as hydroxyl radical (HO·), hydroperoxy (HOO·) radical, and superoxide anion radical ($O_2\cdot^-$) can be detected, trapped, identified and quantified by electron paramagnetic resonance spectroscopy (EPR) using various nitrones, such as 5,5-dimethylpyrroline-1-oxide (DMPO, **1**, $R^1 = R^2 = H$, **Sch. 4D-1**), to produce stable nitroxyl (aminoxyl) radical derivatives **2**. More elaborate structures of nitrones have been designed over the years containing, e.g., fluorescent moieties, which allow fluorimetric analyses of the adducts in addition to the EPR analyses [9, 14, 16, 17, 23, 24, 27, 32, 49–52].

However, one has to be aware of possible interference reactions in cases where, in addition to oxygen-centered radicals, also singlet oxygen is formed, i.e., in reactions involving photosensitizers, such as various dyes, compounds used in photodynamic therapy and some sunscreen agents. In such cases, the reactions of singlet oxygen ($^1O_2$) with DMPO and other nitrones result in either the formation of hydroxyl radical adducts or oxidations to give acylnitroxyls (**3**) and degradation reactions of DMPO (**1**) yielding aliphatic nitroso and nitro derivatives [49, 50]. The reactions of DMPO and other nitrones and nitroso compounds with nitrogen dioxide also resulted in acylnitroxyls [**Sch. 4D-1**] [49, 50]. Nevertheless, the singlet-oxygen species can also be analyzed by EPR spectroscopy [14, 16, 23, 24, 32]. In this case, the reaction of singlet oxygen with sterically hindered alicyclic secondary amines (**4**) is utilized to produce nitroxyl (aminoxyl) radical derivatives (**5**) [**Sch. 4D-1**]. The secondary amines can be synthesized with various degrees of complexity to be used for specific purposes, including those containing a moiety that enables fluorimetric analysis.

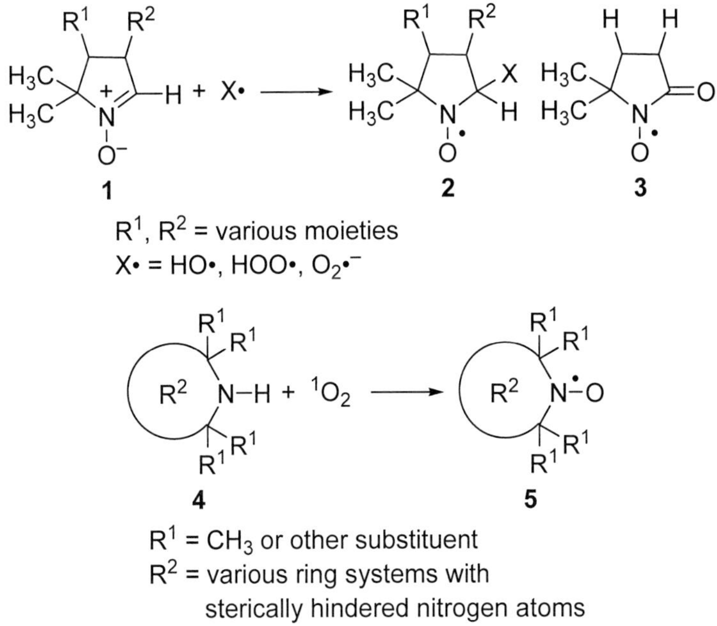

Sch. 4D-1. Identification of reactive oxygen species.

E. Nitroxyl (Aminoxyl) Radicals as Superoxide Dismutase Mimics

Considerable progress has been made in understanding the mechanisms involving the nitroxyl (aminoxyl) radicals as superoxide dismutase (SOD) mimics [18, 26, 53–59], and as inhibitors of the oxidative stress processes caused by peroxydations of lipids in biological systems. The mechanisms of the aminoxyl radical dismutase mimics and those of the natural SOD enzymes are analogous, i.e., in both cases redox processes are involved. The aminoxyl-catalyzed dismutation of superoxide anion radical in aqueous media can proceed by two mechanisms (A and B) depending on the redox potential of the aminoxyl mimic, whereby the protonated form of superoxide anion radical ($O_2\cdot^-$), the hydroperoxide radical (HOO·), is the dominant species [**Sch. 4E-1**].

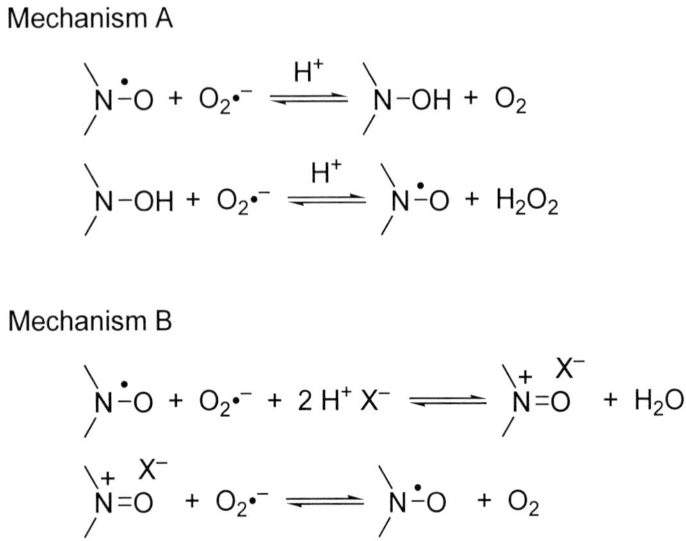

Sch. 4E-1. Mechanisms of the dismutation reactions of the superoxide anion radical and nitroxyl radicals. The open-ended nitroxyl is usually a part of various ring systems with sterically hindered nitrogen (X^- = a counterion).

F. Mechanisms of Autoxidations of Unsaturated Compounds and Reactions with Singlet Oxygen Species

The present discussion is restricted to the autoxidation of lipids, i.e., compounds containing unsaturated fatty acids, such as oleic, linoleic, linolenic, arachidonic, glycerides, fats, oils, waxes, cerebrosides, i.e., lipids of nerve tissues, and phosphatides.

The autoxidation reactions of these compounds commence with the abstraction of hydrogen atoms at allylic positions by molecular oxygen [60, 61]. The peroxidations of these radicals results in a mixture of isomeric hydroperoxides. The structures and number of isomers will depend on the initial number and positions of double bonds in the starting materials. Thus, the autoxidations of linoleic acid derivatives (**6**) containing two double bonds linked together with one methylene group proceed via the most favorable pentadienyl radical (**7**) to give, predictably, mainly, the two isomers 9- and 13-hydroperoxides (**9**, **10**) [**Sch. 4F-1**] [60, 61]. The oxidation of oleic acid derivatives containing only one double bond flanked by two methylene groups, $-CH_2-CH=CH-CH_2-$, will produce, predictably, mainly four isomers, namely the 8-, 9-, 10-, and 11-hydroperoxides [60, 61]. Hydroperoxides **9** and **10** can undergo thermal and transition-metal-cation catalyzed Fenton-type decomposition reactions to give allylic alkoxy radicals (**11**, **12**), which are converted either by reactions with hydrogen-atom donor compounds into the corresponding allylic alcohols (**13**, **14**), or by fragmentation into aldehydes (**15**, **18**) [**Sch. 4F-1**].

The reactions, in particular those involving thermal degradations, can be further complicated, e.g., by cis–trans isomerizations, additions of hydroxyl radicals to double bonds, abstraction of hydrogen atoms by hydroxyl radicals, and epoxidations.

Hydroperoxides **9** and **10** of methyl oleate can also be obtained by a non-radical reaction with singlet oxygen species [**Sch. 4F-2**]. This reaction is generally applicable to olefinic bonds [62, 63].

Furthermore, methyl oleate can be used as a specific reagent to prove that a given photooxidation reaction produces a singlet oxygen species. Thus, the ultraviolet light induced reaction of methyl oleate in the presence of the sunscreen agents titanium dioxide and zinc oxide produces only 9- and 10-hydroperoxides, as would be expected in the case of singlet oxygen formation, whereas an autoxidation reaction would yield four isomers [**Sch. 4F-1**] [62, 63].

The most reactive and damaging species in the human body is, without a doubt, the hydroxyl radical. Endogenously, hydroxyl radicals can be formed, e.g., during the respiratory process via the relatively nontoxic superoxide anion radical ($O_2{\cdot}^-$) and the degradations of hydroperoxides of lipids. The autoxidations of fatty acids in lipid membranes can be enhanced by UVA and UVB radiations, albeit with detrimental results, such as enhanced membrane leakages in human skin fibroblasts, changes of fluidity in human fibroblasts and keratinocytes, changes of permeability and transport properties in membranes, cytoskeletal damages and microtubule disassembly [64–72].

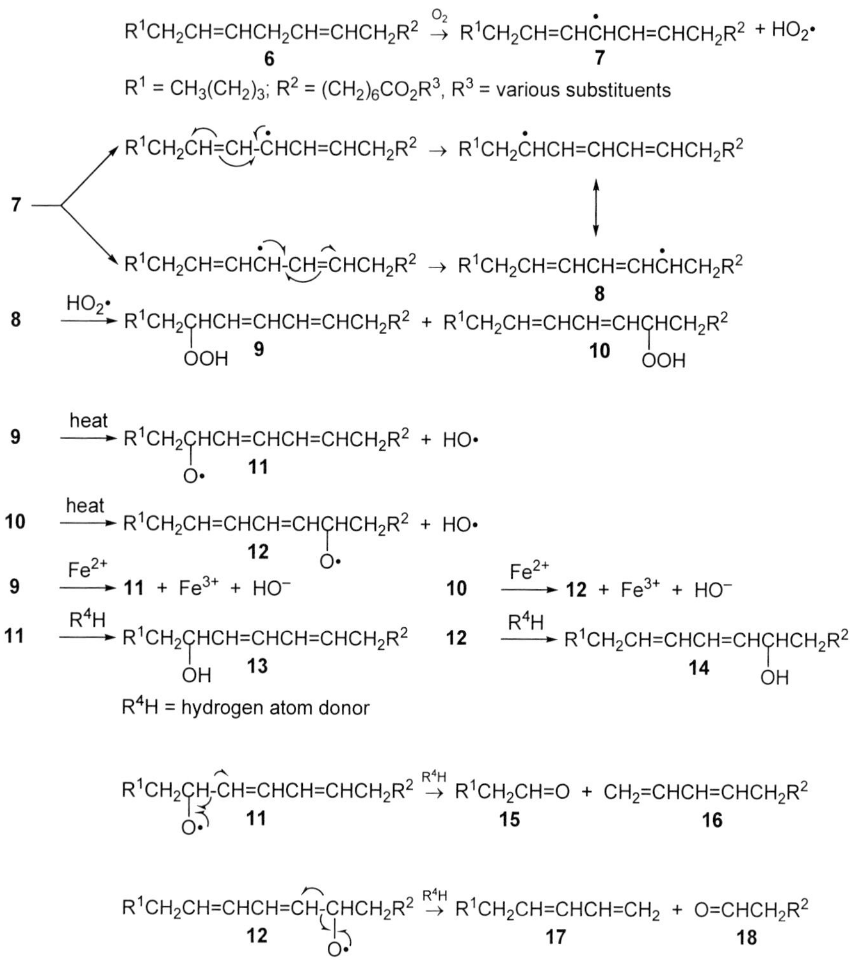

Sch. 4F-1. Mechanisms of autoxidation reactions of unsaturated compounds.

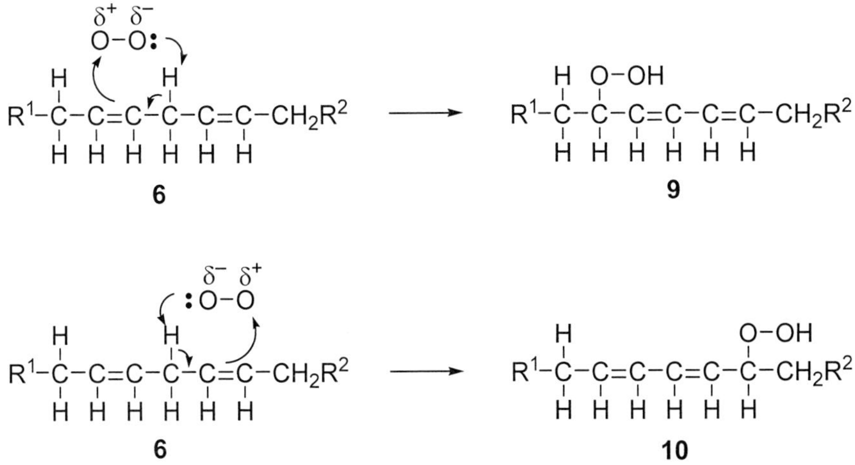

$R^1 = CH_3(CH_2)_3$, $R^2 = (CH_2)_6CO_2R^3$, R^3 = various substituents

Sch. 4F-2. Reactions of singlet oxygen with olefinic bonds.

References

1. Chance B., Sies H. and Boveris A. (1979) Hydrogen peroxide metabolism in mammalian organs. *Physiol. Rev.* **59**: 527–605.
2. Rodgers M. A. and Powers E. L. (eds.) (1981) *Oxygen and Oxyradicals in Chemistry and Biology*, Academic Press, New York.
3. McCord J. M. (1987) Oxygen-derived radicals: a link between reperfusion injury and inflammation. *Fed. Proc.* **46**: 2402–2406.
4. Fuchs J. and Packer L. (1991) Photooxidative stress in the skin. In: *Oxidative Stress: Oxidants and Antioxidants*, Sies H. (ed.), Academic Press, New York.
5. Fuchs J. (1992) *Oxidative Injury in Dermatopathology*, Springer Verlag, Berlin.
6. Fuchs J. and Parker L. (1993) *Oxidative Stress in Dermatology*, Marcel Dekker, New York.
7. Vessey D. A. (1993) Cutaneous antioxidant system. In: *Oxidative Stress in Dermatology*, pp 81–103, Fuchs J. and Packer L. (eds.), Marcel Dekker, New York.

8. Tyrrell R. M. (1984) The molecular and cellular pathology of solar ultraviolet radiation. *Mol. Aspects Med.* **15**: 1–77.
9. Chignell C. F., Bilski P., Krzysztof J., Reczka J., Motten A. G., Sik R. H. and Dahl T. A. (1994) Spectral and photochemical properties of curcumin. *Photochem. Photobiol.* **59**: 295–302.
10. McHugh P. and Knowland J. (1997) Characterization of DNA damage inflicted by free radicals from a mutagenic sunscreen ingredient and its location using an in vitro genetic reversion assay. *Photochem. Photobiol.* **66**: 276–281.
11. Scharffetter-Kochanek K., Weaschek M., Brenneisen P., Schauen M., Blaudschun R. and Wenk J. (1997) UV-induced reactive oxygen species in photocarcinogenesis and photoaging. *Biol. Chem.* **378**: 1247–1257.
12. Gabbianelli R. A., Falcioni G., Santroni A. M., Caulini G., Greci L. and Damiani E. (1997) Effect of aromatic nitroxides on homolysis of human erythrocytes entrapped with isolated hemoglobin chains. *Free Radical Biol. Med.* **23**: 278–284.
13. Antosiewicz J., Damiani E., Jassem W., Wozniak M., Orena M. and Greci L. (1997) Influence of structure of the antioxidant activity of indolinic nitroxide radicals. *Free Radical Biol. Med.* **22**: 249–255.
14. Hideg E., Kálai T., Hideg K. and Vass I. (1998) Photoinhibition of photosynthesis *in vivo* results in singlet oxygen production detection via nitroxide-induced fluorescence quenching in broad bean leaves. *Biochemistry* **37**:11405–11411.
15. Krishna M. C., DeGraff W., Hankovszky O. H., Sar C. P., Kálai T., Jekő J., Russo A., Mitchell J. B. and Hideg, K. (1998) Studies of structure–activity relationship of nitroxide free radicals and their precursors as modifiers against oxidative damage. *J. Med. Chem.* **41**: 3477–3492.
16. Kálai T., Hideg E., Vass I. and Hideg K. (1998) Double (fluorescent and spin) sensors for detection of reactive oxygen species in the thylakoid membrane. *Free Radical Biol. Med.* **24**: 649–652.
17. Hideg E., Takatsy A., Sar C., Vass I. and Hideg K. (1999) Utilizing new adamantyl spin traps in studying UV-B oxidative damage of photosystem II. *J. Photochem. Photobiol., B* **48**: 174–179.
18. Damiani R., Carloni P., Stipa P. and Greci L. (1999) Reactivity of an indolinonic aminoxyl with superoxide anion and hydroxy radicals. *Free Radical Res.* **31**: 113–121.
19. Damiani E., Greci L., Parson R. and Knowland J. (1999) Nitroxide radicals protect DNA from damage when illuminated in vitro in the

presence of dibenzoylmethane a common sunscreen ingredient. *Free Radical Biol. Med.* **26**: 809–816.

20. Damiani E., Carloni P., Biondi C. and Greci L. (2000) Increased oxidative modification of albumin when illuminated in vitro in the presence of a common sunscreen ingredient: protection by nitroxide radicals. *Free Radical Biol. Med.* **28**: 193–201.
21. Scharffetter-Kochanek K., Brenneisen P., Wenk J., Herrmann G., Ma W., Kuhr L., Meewes L. and Wlaschek M. (2000) Photoaging of the skin from phenotype to mechanisms. *Exp. Gerontol.* **35**: 307–316.
22. Li H., Xu K.Y., Zhou L., Kalai T., Zweier J. L., Hideg K. and Kuppusamy P. (2000) A pyrroline derivative of mexiletine offers marked protection against ischemia/reperfusion-induced myocardial contractile dysfunction. *J. Pharmacol. Exp. Ther.* **295**: 563–571.
23. Hideg E., Kálai T., Hideg K. and Vass I. (2000) Do oxidative stress conditions impairing photosynthesis in the light manifest as photoinhibition? *Philos. Trans. R. Soc., B* **355**: 1511–1516.
24. Hideg E., Vass I., Kálai T. and Hideg K. (2000) Singlet oxygen detection with sterically hindered amine derivatives in plants under light stress. *Methods Enzymol.* **319**: 77–85.
25. Damiani E., Kalinska B., Canapa A., Canestrari S., Wozniak M., Olmo E. and Greci L. (2000) The effects of nitroxide radicals on oxidative DNA damage. *Free Radical Biol. Med.* **28**: 1257–1265.
26. Raikov Z. D., Raikova E. T., Zheleva A. M. and Gradzheva V. (2000). In *Spin-labeled antitumor compounds,* Robev S. K. (ed.), ISBN 954-9736-02-5, Bulgaria.
27. Hideg E., Barta C., Kálai T., Vass I., Hideg K. and Asada K. (2002) Detection of singlet oxygen and superoxide with fluorescent sensors in leaves under stress by photoinhibition or UV radiation. *Plant Cell Physiol.* **43**: 1154–1164.
28. Pinnell S. R. (2003) Cutaneous photodamage, oxidative stress, and topical antioxidant protection. *J. Am. Acad. Dermatol.* **48**: 1–22.
29. Girotti A. W. (2001) Lipid photooxidative damage in biological membranes: reaction mechanisms, cytotoxic consequences, and defense strategies. In: *Sun Protection in Man*, pp 231–250, Giacomoni, P. U. (ed.), Elsevier, Amsterdam.
30. Davies M. J. and Truscott R. J. W. (2001) Photo-oxidation of proteins and its consequences. In: *Sun Protection in Man*, pp 251–275, Giacomoni, P. U. (ed.), Elsevier, Amsterdam.
31. Girotti A. W. and Giacomoni P. U. (2007) Lipid and protein damage provoked by ultraviolet radiation: mechanisms of indirect photooxidative damage. In: *Biophysical and Physiological Effects of Solar*

Radiation on Human Skin, pp 271–291, Giacomoni P. U. (ed.), The Royal Society of Chemistry, Cambridge.
32. Gottsch J. D., Pou S., Bynoe L. A. and Rosen G. M. (1990) Hematogenous Photosensitization. *Invest. Ophthalmol. Visual Sci.* **31**: 1674–1682.
33. Wondrak G. T., Roberts M. J., Jacobson M. K. and Jacobson E. L. (2002) Photosensitized growth inhibition of cultured human skin cells: mechanism and suppression of oxidative stress from solar irradiation of glycated protein. *J. Invest. Dermatol.* **119**: 489–498.
34. Howes K. A., Liu Y., Dunaief J. L., Milam A., Frederick J. M., Marks A. and Baehr W. (2004) Receptor for advanced glycation and products and age-related macular degeneration. *Invest. Ophthalmol. Visual Sci.* **45**: 3713–3720.
35. Takeuchi M., Kikuchi S., Sasaki N., Suzuki T., Watai T., Iwaki M., Bucala R. and Yamagishi S. (2004) Involvement of advanced glycation end-products (AGEs) in Alzheimer's disease. *Curr. Alzheimer Res.* **1**: 39–46.
36. Glenn J. V. and Stitt A. W. (2009) The role of advanced glycation end products in retinal ageing and disease. *Biochim. Biophys. Acta, Gen. Subj.* **1790**: 1109–1116.
37. Foote C. S. (1991) Definition of Type I and Type II photosensitized oxidation. *Photochem. Photobiol.* **54**: 659.
38. Fuchs J. (1998) Potentials and limitations of the natural antioxidants *R,R,R*-α-tocopherol, L-ascorbic acid and β-carotene in cutaneous photoprotection. *Free Radical Biol. Med.* **25**: 848–873.
39. Gnewuch C. T. and Sosnovsky G. (2002) Critical appraisals of approaches for predictive designs in anticancer drugs. *Cell. Mol. Life Sci.* **59**: 859–1023.
40. Nagiev T. M. (2001) *Interaction of synchronized reactions in chemistry and biology* (Russian), Baku, Azerbaijan, ISBN 5-8066-1329-1, and references therein.
41. Sosnovsky G. and Zaret E. H. (1970) Base catalyzed autoxidation. In: *Organic Peroxides*, Vol. I, pp 517–560, Swern D. (ed.), John Wiley & Sons, New York.
42. Sosnovsky G. and Rawlison D. J. (1970) Metal ion-catalyzed reactions of symmetric peroxides. In: *Organic Peroxides*, Vol. I, pp 561–584, Swern D. (ed.), John Wiley & Sons, New York.
43. Sosnovsky G. and Rawlison D. J. (1970) Metal ion-catalyzed reactions of peroxyesters. In: *Organic Peroxides*, Vol. I, pp 585–608, Swern D. (ed.), John Wiley & Sons, New York.

44. Hiatt R. (1971) Hydroperoxides. In: *Organic Peroxides*, Vol. II, pp 1–151, Swern D. (ed.), John Wiley & Sons, New York.
45. Sosnovsky G. and Rawlison D. J. (1971) Chemistry of hydroperoxides in the presence of metal ions. In: *Organic Peroxides*, Vol. II, pp 153–268, Swern D. (ed.), John Wiley & Sons, New York.
46. Sosnovsky G. (1971) Metal ion-catalyzed reactions of hydrogen peroxide and peroxydisulfate. In: *Organic Peroxides*, Vol. II, pp 269–336, Swern D. (ed.), John Wiley & Sons, New York.
47. Davies A. G. (1971) Formation of organometallic peroxides by autoxidation. In: *Organic Peroxides*, Vol. II, pp 337–354, Swern D. (ed.), John Wiley & Sons, New York.
48. Herrling T., Groth K., Golz K. and Zastrow L. (2000) The role of aggressive ·OH free radicals in skin – their generation, detection and prevention. *SÖFW–J.* **126**: 20–27.
49. Bilski P., Reszka K., Bilska M. and Chignell C. F. (1996) Oxidation of the spin trap 5,5-dimethyl-1-pyrroline *N*-oxide by singlet oxygen in aqueous solution. *J. Am. Chem. Soc.* **118**: 1330–1338.
50. Astolfi P., Greci L. and Panagiotaki M. (2005) Spin trapping of nitrogen dioxide and of radicals generated from nitrous acid. *Free Radical Res.* **39**: 137–144.
51. Sar C. P., Hideg E., Vass I. and Hideg K. (1998) Synthesis of α-aryl-*N*-adamant-1-nitrones and using them for spin trapping of hydroxyl radicals. *Bioorg. Med. Chem. Lett.* **8**: 379–384, and references therein.
52. Kálai T., Hideg E., Jekö J. and Hideg K. (2003) Synthesis of paramagnetic BODIPY dyes as new double (spin and fluorescence) sensors. *Tetrahedron Lett.* **44**: 8497–8499.
53. Finkelstein E., Rosen G. M. and Rauckmann E. J. (1984) Superoxide–dependent reduction of nitroxides by thiols. *Biochem. Biophys. Acta* **802**: 90–98.
54. Mitchell J. B., Biaglow Y. E. and Russo A. (1988) A role of glutathione and endogeneous thiols in radiation protection. *Pharmacol. Ther.* **39**: 274.
55. Samuni A., Krishna M. C., Riesz P., Finkelstein E. and Russo A. (1998) A novel metal-free low molecular weight superoxide dismutase mimic. *J. Biol. Chem.* **263**: 1792.
56. Mitchell J. B., Samuni A., Krishna M. C., DeGraff W. G., Ahn M. S., Samuni V. and Russo A. (1990) Biologically active metal-independent superoxide dismutase mimic. *Biochemistry* **29**: 2802–2807.

57. Krishna M. C., Grahame D. A., Samuni A., Mitchell J. B. and Russo A. (1992) Oxoammonium cation intermediate in the nitroxide-catalyzed dismutation of superoxide. *Proc. Natl. Acad. Sci. U. S. A.* **89**: 5537–5541.
58. Sledzinski A., Wozniak M., Antosiewicz J., Lezoche E., Familiari M., Bertoli E., Greci L., Bonelli A., Mazera N. and Wajda Z. (1995) Protective effect of 4-hydroxy-TEMPO, a low molecular weight superoxide dismutase mimic on free radical toxicity in experimental pancreatitis. *Int. J. Pancreatol.* **18**: 153–160.
59. Greci L., Damiani E., Carloni P. and Stipa P. (1997) Indolinic and quinolinic aminoxyls as biological antioxidants. In: *Free Radical in Biological Environment*, pp 223–232, Minisci, F. (ed.), Kluwer Academic Publisher, The Netherlands.
60. Frankel E. N., Neff W. E., Rohwedder W. K., Khambay B. P. S., Garwood R. F. and Weedon B. C. L. (1977) Analysis of autoxidized fats by gas chromatography–mass spectrometry. I. Methyl oleate. *Lipids* **12**: 901–907.
61. Frankel E. N., Neff W. E., Rohwedder W. K., Khambay B. P. S., Garwood R. F. and Weedon B. C. L. (1977) Analysis of autoxidized fats by gas chromatography–mass spectrometry. II. Methyl oleate. *Lipids* **12**: 908–913.
62. Yamamoto Y., Imai N., Mashima R., Konaka R., Inoue M. and Dunlap W. C. (2000) Singlet oxygen from irradiated titanium dioxide and zinc oxide. *Methods Enzymol.* **319**: 29–37.
63. Zhang W., Sun M. and Salomon R. G. (2006) Preparative singlet oxygenation of linoleate provides doubly allylic dihydroperoxides: putative intermediates in the generation of biologically active aldehydes *in vivo*. *J. Org. Chem.* **71**: 5607–5615.
64. Desai I. D., Sawant P. L. and Tappel A. L. (1964) Peroxidative and radiation damage to isolated lysosomes. *Biochim. Biophys. Acta* **86**: 227–285.
65. Roshchupkin D. I., Pelenitsyn A. B., Potapenko A. Y., Talitsky V. V. and Vladimirov Y. A. (1975) Study of the effects of ultraviolet light on biomembranes–IV. The effect of oxygen on UV-induced hemolysis and lipid photoperoxidation in rat erythrocytes and liposomes. *Photochem. Photobiol.* **21**: 63–69.
66. Putvinsky A. V., Sokolov A. I., Roshchupkin D. I. and Vladimirov Y. A. (1979) Electric breakdown of bilayer phospholipid membranes under ultraviolet irradiation induced lipid peroxidation. *FEBS Lett.* **106**: 53–55.

67. Azizova A. O., Islomov A. I., Roshchupkin D. J., Predvoditelev D. A., Remizov A. N. and Vladimir Y. A. (1980) Free radicals formed on ultraviolet irradiation of the lipids of biological membrane. *Biophysics* **24**: 407–414.
68. Mandal T. K. and Chatterjee S. N. (1980) Ultraviolet- and sunlight-induced lipid peroxidation in liposomal membrane. *Radiat. Res.* **83**: 290–302.
69. Bose B., Agarwal S. and Chatterjee S. N. (1989) UV-A induced lipid peroxidation in liposomal membrane. *Radiat. Environ. Biophys.* **28**: 59–65.
70. Punnonen K., Puniela A. and Ahotupa M. (1991) Effects of ultraviolet A and B irradiation and activity of the antioxidant enzymes in keratinocytes in culture. *Photodermatol., Photoimmunol. Photomed.* **8**: 3–6.
71. Gaboriau F., Morliere P., Marquis I., Moysan A., Goegze M. and Dubertret L. (1993) Membrane damage induced in cultured human skin fibroblasts by UVA irradiation. *Photochem. Photobiol.* **58**: 515–520.
72. Morliere P., Moysan A., Santus R., Huppe G., Maziere J. P. and Dubertret L. (1991) UVA-induced lipid peroxidation in cultured human fibroblasts. *Biochem. Biophys. Acta* **1084**: 248–261.

CHAPTER FIVE

ENDOGENOUS ANTIOXIDANTS AGAINST ROS IN HUMAN SKIN

A. Enzymes

i. Superoxide Dismutase and Nitroxyl (Aminoxyl) Radicals as SOD Mimics

Superoxide dismutases can be formed in various tissues and organs of the human body, such as muscles, liver, kidney, and lung, and in the epidermis, dermis, and subcutis of the skin [1–25]. The superoxide dismutases (SODs) are involved in the detoxification processes of superoxide anion radical species ($O_2\cdot^-$) [8–10]. This species is formed by one-electron reduction processes of molecular oxygen in aerobic cellular metabolisms and photochemical reactions [1]. Excessive quantities of the superoxide anion radical in cells can damage various cellular components, in particular by the transformation of the $O_2\cdot^-$ species into hydroxyl radical (HO·). Superoxide anion radical also interacts with transition metal cations by reducing the metal cations, which can then participate in reactions for the generation of hydroxyl radicals [11].

Two SOD enzymes are involved in the reaction with superoxide anion radical, the Cu^{+2}/Zn^{+2} and the Mn^{+2} SODs. In this reaction, hydrogen peroxide is formed as a byproduct.

$$O_2\cdot^- + O_2\cdot^- \xrightarrow[SOD]{2H^+} H_2O_2 + O_2$$

Since hydrogen peroxide is toxic to the biological environment, it must be reduced to water. Therefore, the action of SOD is accompanied by the action of hydrogen peroxide metabolizing enzymes, such as catalase and glutathione peroxidase [12, 25]. The SOD activity can be detected in the skin of humans and other mammals, although, in the skin, the levels of

SOD are lower than in other tissues [13]. The levels of SOD tend to increase in the epidermis and dermis with an increase in the oxidative stress, i.e., with the formation of reactive oxygen species. However, reduced levels of SOD activity were found in cases of non-cutaneous cancers and in skin cancers, squamous cell carcinoma, and basal cell epitheliomas [14]. There were also observed oxidative processes mediated by SOD and resulting in peroxidations of lipids and increased formation of hydrogen peroxide.

In the past decade, extensive investigations have been conducted on various aspects of the nonenzymatic nitroxyl (aminoxyl) radicals that can mimic the reactions of superoxide dismutases [15–21, 25]. (See also **Section 4E**.)

ii. Catalase

The catalase enzyme activity is mainly displayed in the peroxysomes. However, the enzyme is present in all aerobic cells of mammals, including humans, e.g., in brain, liver, and skin cells. The catalase presence in the skin is of importance in the case of photosensitized oxidations involving reactive oxygen species [1–3, 12, 13, 25].

The catalase enzyme mediates several reactions. Probably the most important reaction involves the metabolism of hydrogen peroxide to water and molecular oxygen.

$$2\,H_2O_2 \xrightarrow{\text{cat}} 2\,H_2O + O_2$$

The enzyme can further catalyze the peroxidation reactions of type a and b of various substrates.

a. $RCH_2OH + H_2O_2 \rightarrow RCHO + 2\,H_2O$
b. $RH + RO\text{–}OH \rightarrow 2\,ROH + H_2O$
R = various organic groups

iii. Selenium-Dependent Glutathione Peroxidases

These enzymes metabolize hydrogen peroxide and various organic hydroperoxides, including lipid hydroperoxides [1–7, 12, 13, 25]. Hydrogen peroxide and hydroperoxides are formed by autoxidations of various compounds and in the photosensitized formation of ROS. The toxicity of these compounds increases in the presence of transition metal cations, such as those of iron and copper, which catalyze the decompositions of these compounds into very reactive and toxic hydroxyl radical (HO·) species. The reductions of hydrogen peroxide and hydroperoxides by glutathione peroxidases are mediated by glutathione (GSH) [22–26].

$$H_2O_2 + 2\,GSH \rightarrow 2\,H_2O + GSSG$$
$$ROOH + 2\,GSH \rightarrow ROH + GSSG + H_2O$$
R = various organic groups

The glutathione peroxidase activity can be detected in many human organs, such as the brain, heart, lung, and skin. In the epidermis, the activity is higher than in the dermis. The activity can appreciably vary in response to oxidative stress, cancer-promoting chemicals, anticancer drugs, and UV radiation. Thus, glutathione reductase is deactivated by the alkylating anticancer drug *N,N*-bis(2-chloroethyl)-*N*-nitrosourea (BCNU).

iv. NADPH quinone reductase (NQR)

The ubiquitous enzyme NQR, found in biological systems, is readily reduced to semiquinone radicals by one-electron reductions mediated by flavoproteins [1, 12, 24]. The semiquinone radicals can react with oxygen to give the superoxide anion radical which undergoes oxidative reactions with the thiol groups of proteins and other biomolecules. In particular, the formation of semiquinone radicals from xenobiotic quinones is undesirable, and biologically it is more favorable to convert the semiquinone groups either into hydroxyl groups or, by two-electron reductions, into quinols. The enzyme NADPH quinone reductase catalyzes this type of reaction. The activity of this enzyme is particularly high in the epidermis of the skin. The activity of NQR in the skin can by induced by various compounds, e.g., polycyclic hydrocarbons and 2,6-di-*tert*-butyl-4-methylphenol (BHT) [25, 26, 28, 29].

v. Thioprotein Reductase (Thioredoxin Reductase)

The thioprotein reductase system can be found in many mammalian tissues and organs [1, 13, 27]. Thioredoxin is a thiol-dependent, electron-transport system. The reduced form of the enzyme, containing two thiol groups, is produced by the flavin-containing redox enzyme thioredoxin reductase and NADPH. In the oxidized form, the thiol groups are converted into the redox active disulfide groups. The reduced thioredoxin functions as a hydrogen donor for other enzymes, and as a reductant of disulfide bonds in such molecules as insulin. In the epidermis, thioredoxin is an inhibitor of free radicals which are derived from oxidative stress processes, and is thus contributing to the defense against damage to epidermis tissues by free radicals. Studies in this connection have been conducted on the reduction of nitroxyl (aminoxyl) radicals, since these radicals can function as nonenzymatic singlet oxygen dismutase (SOD) mimics. (See **Section 4E**.) However, the thioredoxin enzyme has little SOD-like activity.

B. Nonenzymatic Hydrophilic Antioxidants

i. Vitamin C

Ascorbic acid (vitamin C, **1**) is the main water-soluble vitamin in nature, and is found in all parts of the skin and in many human organs [1, 25, 26, 29–34]. It has been widely used as an antioxidant in the food industry, which unwittingly played a decisive part in the past during the scurvy epidemics. It is believed that additions of **1** to sunscreen formulations could have a beneficial effect on the elimination of ROS that are formed by the UV radiation. Since vitamin C can participate in the important regeneration of vitamin E, which is present in some sunscreen formulations, the idea seems to be not too farfetched. It is also believed that **1** may be involved in cancer prevention processes. The stratum corneum, i.e., the outer part of human skin, contains only little vitamin C, and, hence, the epidermal vitamin C probably offers little protection against the UV radiation of the sun, although it was reported that ascorbic acid prevents injuries to the eye lens.

Vitamin C can be used both in one-electron and two-electron reductions, whereby ascorbic acid is converted via the ascorbyl anion radical (**2**) into dehydroascorbate (**3**), and then into 2,3-diketo-L-gulonic acid (**4**) [**Sch. 5B.i-1**] [35, 36]. Ascorbic acid can undergo reactions with a variety of oxidants, such as peroxy radicals, superoxide anion radical ($O_2\cdot^-$), hydroxyl radical (HO·), thiyl radicals, hydrogen peroxide, and singlet oxygen. The reaction of ascorbic acid with α-tocopheryl radical will restore α-tocopherol (**5**) [13, 37]. Dehydroascorbate (**3**) can be reduced to ascorbic acid (**1**) enzymatically by NADPH and glutathione, mediated by dehydroascorbate reductase.

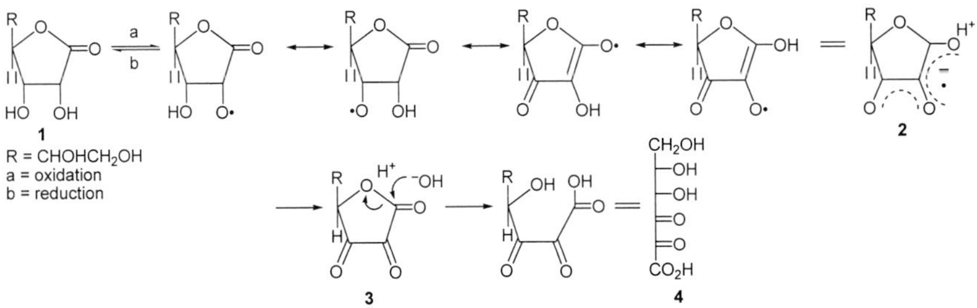

Sch. 5B.i-1. Redox reactions of vitamin C.

However, there are a number of less known reactions of **1** that could play a role, for example, in diminishing the effectiveness of **1** as an antioxidant in sunscreens. Ascorbate has the potential to generate prooxidant effects in cells and cell free systems [38, 39]. Thus, it has been known that ene diols, such as vitamin C, are readily autoxidized to diketones (**6**) and hydrogen peroxide [**Sch. 5B.i-2**].

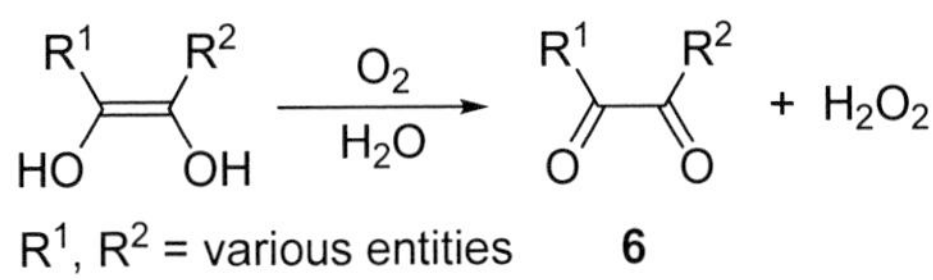

Sch. 5B.i-2. Oxidation of ene diols to diketones (**6**)

This reaction is greatly accelerated by catalytic amounts of transition-metal cations, such as the biologically ubiquitous copper and iron cations. It was shown that cupric cations are initially the actual oxidant of ascorbic acid, and that the oxygen species serve to continuously regenerate the cupric ions from the cuprous ions [37]. Molecular oxygen is converted in this process into superoxide anion radical or its protonated form (HOO·) that is more stable. At the final stage, a Fenton-type reaction of hydrogen peroxide results in the formation of hydroxyl radicals [35, 36]. Hence, vitamin C mediated reactions result in the formation of toxic reactive oxygen species that were presupposed to be scavenged by vitamin C [**Sch. 5B.i-3**].

$$\begin{array}{lllll}
\mathbf{1} & + & Cu^{++} & \longrightarrow & \mathbf{2} + Cu^{+} + H^{+} \\
Cu^{+} & + & O_2 & \longrightarrow & Cu^{++} + O_2\cdot^{-} \text{ or } HOO\cdot \\
\mathbf{2} & + & Cu^{++} & \longrightarrow & \mathbf{3} + Cu^{+} + H^{+} \\
O_2\cdot^{-} & + & Cu^{+} + 2\,H^{+} & \longrightarrow & H_2O_2 + Cu^{++} \\
2\,O_2\cdot^{-} & + & 2\,H^{+} & \longrightarrow & H_2O_2 + O_2 \\
H_2O_2 & + & Cu^{+} & \longrightarrow & HO^{-} + HO\cdot + Cu^{++}
\end{array}$$

Sch. 5B.i-3. Autoxidation of vitamin C and the catalytic, acid-mediated formation of ROS.

Another aerobic oxidation of vitamin C can be mediated by the enzyme ascorbic acid oxidase, a copper-containing protein of about 140,000 molecular weight, which can be found in various vegetables, including the cucumber [41].

In high concentrations, in the presence of transition metal cations, ascorbic acid can also function as an oxidizing agent in lipid peroxidations and degradation reactions. It was found that vitamin C can cause the degradation of lipid hydroperoxides to give genotoxic products [42]. Lipid hydroperoxides are readily formed from fatty acids by reactions of oxygen and other reactive oxygen species, and also by enzyme-mediated processes. The lipid hydroperoxides can undergo a transition-metal-ion-catalyzed decomposition reaction resulting, in part, in the formation of genotoxic α,β-unsaturated aldehydes, i.e., 4-oxononetal, 4-hydroxynonetal, and 4,5-epoxy-2-decenal from the chosen fatty acid. Lipid hydroperoxides can undergo this decomposition, even in the absence of metal cations at 37 °C, to give unsaturated aldehydes [42]. One of these aldehydes is a precursor of etheno-2-deoxyadenosine found in the human DNA as a highly mutagenic lesion product. The cytotoxic and mutagenic effects of ascorbate on isolated cells probably involve transition-metal ions [43].

In addition to the aforementioned properties, vitamin C (**1**) at the cellular level inhibits UVR-induced p53 activation [44], inhibits JNK/AP-1 pathway, modulates the expression of AP-1 regulated genes [45], prevents UVR-induced induction of contact hypersensitivity, prevents induction of tolerance [46], and decreases sunburn cell formation [47]. Ascorbic acid also is an excellent reagent for the reduction of various nitroxyls (aminoxyls) which could be used to mimic superoxide dismutase [48–51]. (See **Section 4E**.) Nevertheless, the nitroxyls are more efficient inhibitors of the UVA radiation induced damages of the calf skin collagen than the natural inhibitors antioxidant vitamins C and E [51].

The molecular pathways leading to UVR-induced inflammation are presumably different from the biochemical cascade causing immunosuppression, aging, and cancer [52]. Thus, the UVR-induced erythema may not be a valid indicator for assessing the protective effect of antioxidants in the prevention of photoimmunosuppression [53, 54], photoaging, and photocarcinogenesis [55].

It must be emphasized that although ascorbate has the potential to cause prooxidant effects in vitro, it was not firmly established whether this property is relevant in vivo [35, 38, 39].

ii. Glutathione

Glutathione (GSH, **7**) is a tripeptide composed of γ-glu-cys-gly amino acids. Glutathione is a cofactor for the glutathione peroxidase enzyme, but it can also function independently as an antioxidant, whereby the thiol group (SH) of cysteine is the active antioxidant moiety. GSH can inactivate a variety of radical and non-radical reactive oxygen species, such as hydrogen peroxide, alkoxy radicals, superoxide anion radical ($O_2\cdot^-$), and singlet oxygen ($^1O_2$), and it can quench the excited triplets of carbonyl groups including those of sunscreens [1, 12, 25, 26, 56–59]. The reactions with radical species (R·) may proceed as follows, although more complex reaction paths can be envisaged.

$$2\,GSH + 2\,R\cdot \rightarrow 2\,RH + GSSG$$

Another type of reaction involves the regeneration of sulfhydryl groups of proteins (R^1SH and R^2SH) that had become oxidized.

$$R^1S{-}SR^2 + GSH \rightarrow R^1S{-}SG + R^2SH$$
$$R^1S{-}SG + GSH \rightarrow R^1SH + GS{-}SG$$

Glutathione disulfide (GS–SG), which is formed in these reactions, is then reduced by the enzyme GSH reductase to give glutathione [30].

Glutathione is present in various organs of the human body, including the skin. The concentration of GSH in the epidermis is higher than in the dermis [13]. Processes that drastically increase the oxidative stress, such as the UV light of solar radiation, cause a decrease of the levels of GSH and GSSG in the skin [13, 59]. Thus, the UVA irradiation of human keratinocytes in vitro produced significant cell mortality, release of lactate dehydrogenase, oxidative stress caused by reactive oxygen species (ROS), lipid peroxidation, and apoptosis. In the presence of the UVA irradiation absorbing sunscreen 4-*tert*-butyl-4'-methoxydibenzoylmethane, these effects were significantly enhanced because of additional formation of ROS derived from the sunscreen agent. In the presence of glutathione (GSH), but in the absence of the sunscreen agent, the formation of ROS was decreased, whereas in the presence of the sunscreen agent the protective effect of GSH was diminished [59].

Under certain conditions, glutathione can react as a nucleophile, i.e., as a thiolate anion (GS^-), e.g., with electrophilic quinones to give hydroquinone derivatives (7) [**Sch. 5B.ii-1**] [13].

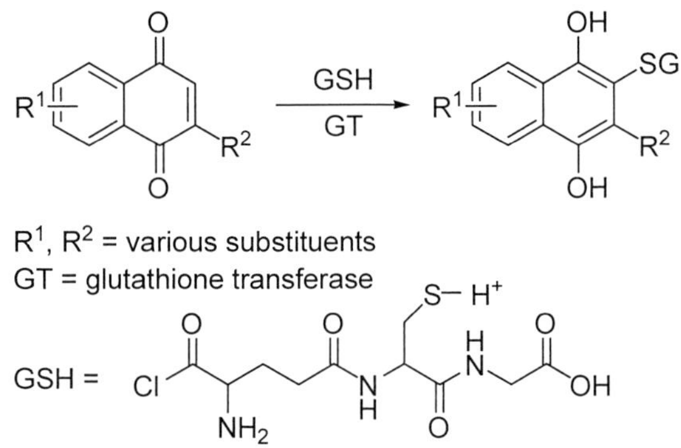

Sch. 5B.ii-1. Reactions of quinones with glutathione as the GS^- thiolate anion.

iii. Uric Acid

Uric acid (2,6,8-trioxypurine, **8**) is formed in the human body as an end product of the degradations of purines. Uric acid is considered to be the major antioxidant in the human body [1, 12]. It is a particularly effective antioxidant in human blood. Reactions of compound **8** proceed readily with radicals, such as peroxy radicals, alkoxy radicals, hydroxyl radicals, and the non-radical species singlet oxygen. Furthermore, uric acid absorbs and tightly binds transition-metal cations, such as those of copper and iron, and, thus, helps to prevent the participation of these cations in radical initiation reactions. Uric acid is considered to be a more efficient antioxidant than vitamin C. Uric acid is also present in the human skin. The oxidations of uric acid by reactive oxygen species results in the formation of allantoin (**9**) [**Sch. 5B.iii-1**].

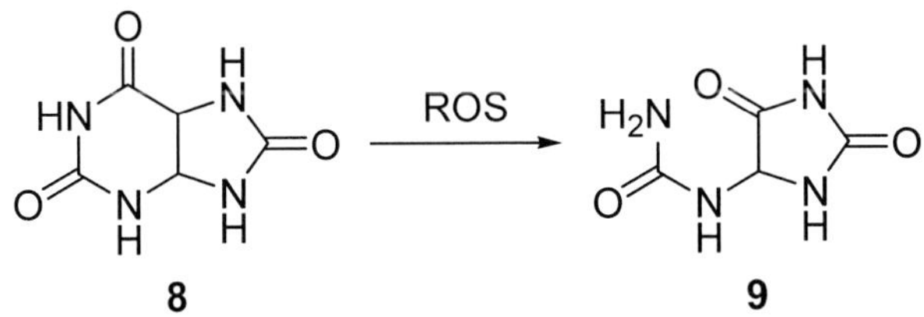

ROS = reactive oxygen species

Sch. 5B.iii-1. Oxidations of uric acid by reactive oxygen species.

C. Nonenzymatic Lipid-Soluble Antioxidants

i. Vitamin E and Congeners

The name vitamin E encompasses eight naturally occurring isomers with the same type but different degrees of biological activity [1, 25, 26, 29–34]. The isomer d-α-tocopherol (*R,R,R*-α-tocopherol, **5**) has the highest potency. Synthetic vitamin E is usually a racemic mixture of all isomers with a potency of about 60%, comparable to that of the α-isomer. In the present review, the terms vitamin E and α-tocopherol are used interchangeably to represent the d-α-isomer. Vitamin E is a powerful lipid-soluble antioxidant in humans and other mammals. Vitamin E readily interacts with various radicals, including xenobiotic radicals and photogenerated reactive oxygen species (ROS). Thus, vitamin E inhibits the lipid peroxidation processes in membranes, and is oxidized by superoxide anion radical and by singlet oxygen. Vitamin E is also a quencher of photoexcited triplet state species derived from compounds containing carbonyl groups and other chromophores, including those of some sunscreens.

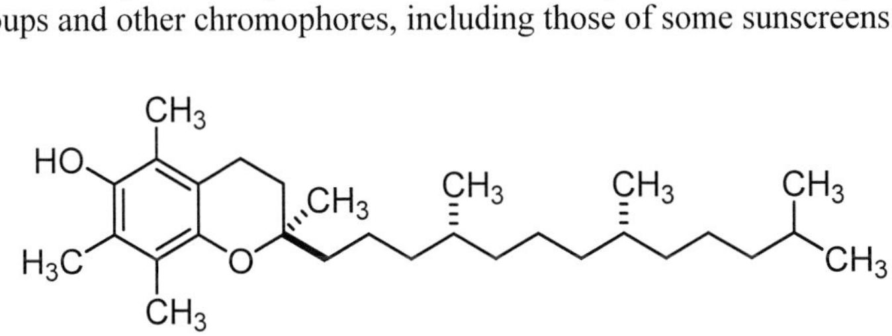

Structure of d-α-tocopherol (**5**)

The oxidation of **5** results in the formation of the oxygen-centered, resonance-stabilized phenoxyl radical (**5a**) [**Sch. 5C.i-1**].

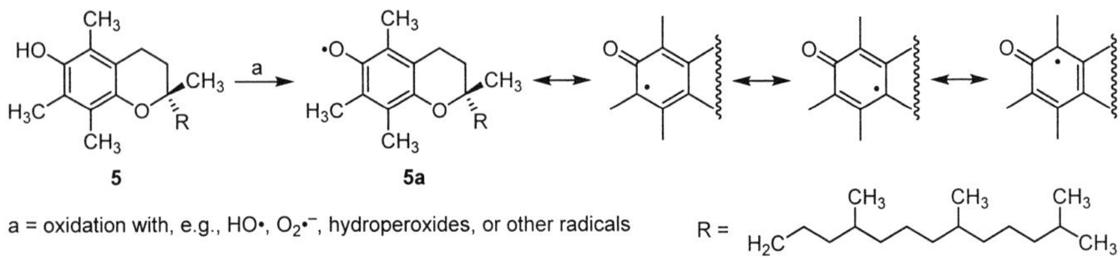

Sch. 5C.i-1. Reactions of vitamin E with free radical species.

This radical, **5a**, can be oxidized to the quinone (**5b**), which can be further degraded [**Sch. 5C.i-2**].

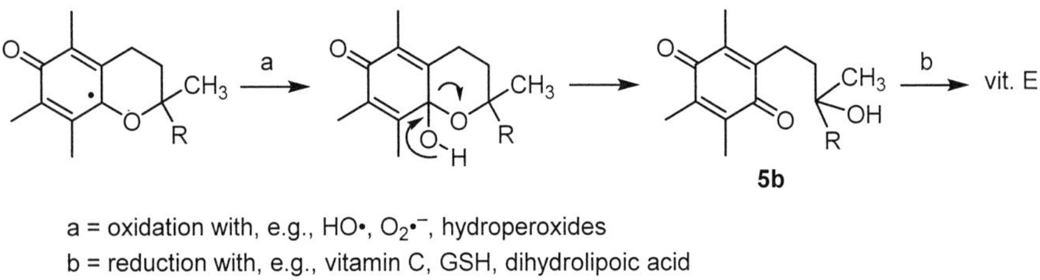

Sch. 5C.i-2. Oxidative degradation of vitamin E.

The regeneration of **5** from the tocopheryl radical (**5a**) is readily accomplished by glutathione (**7**), ubiquinol (**10a**), dihydrolipoic acid (**14a**) and, in particular, by ascorbic acid (**1**). However, the recycling of α-tocopherol (**5**) causes a depletion of other antioxidants, such as ascorbate, thiols, and ubiquinols [60–64]. High concentrations of **5** have a prooxidant effect in vitro in autoxidation reactions of unsaturated compounds, such as lipids. The binding of transition-metal cations by vitamin E (**5**) causes a reduction of biologically active cations in biomembranes [13].

Vitamin E can be formed in various human tissues and organs, such as the adrenal gland, heart, skeletal muscle, lung, brain, kidney, fat, and skin, to mention a few [13, 30]. The concentrations of vitamin E in the human body vary considerably. The highest levels are in the lipid-rich cell fractions. The concentrations of vitamin E in various human tissue are as follows: erythrocytes 2.3, kidney 7.0, uterus 9.0, plasma 9.5, ovary 11.0, liver 13.0, muscle 19.0, heart 20.0, platelets 30.0, testis 40.0, pituary 40.0, adrenal 132.0, and adipose 150 [63]. In spite of low concentrations of vitamin E in human tissue, it is the most effective lipid-soluble antioxidant [64, 65]. Orally administered high doses of vitamins E and C can render some protection against erythema in humans [66]. Similar results were reported for topically applied mixtures of vitamins E and C. Vitamin E absorbs UV light at 290 nm and, as a result, some photoprotective effect can be anticipated. However, vitamin E could also function as a photosensitizer and interact with molecular oxygen to produce ROS.

It has been shown that, at cellular levels, α-tocopherol can affect various cell functions in the following ways: decrease the cell cycling and Nf-κB activation [67], protect against UVR-mediated cell death and growth arrest [68], reduce UVA-induced ROS and inhibit transcription factor STATl [69], protect against UVR-induced immunosuppression and lipid peroxidation [70, 71], inhibit UVR-induced p53 [72], inhibit the formation of thymidine dimers [73–75], inhibit the formation of cyclobutane pyrimidine dimers in the p53 gene [76], decrease the UVR-induced erythema, and decrease the proteases MMP-1 and MMP-9 [77]. However, the blocked vitamin E and methyl ether derivatives are either marginally active or ineffective [73–75]. It should be emphasized that the clinical efficacy of α-tocopherol **(5)** in the prevention of solar radiation induced reactions of skin is largely unproven [77–80].

The effectiveness of vitamin E as an inhibitor of oxidative processes that occur in the presence of sunscreen agents has been investigated in vitro [81–86], since many commercial sunscreen products contain vitamin E, and compared to nitroxyl radical inhibitors. Thus, irradiation with UVA light of DNA plasmids [81], BSA protein [82], and lipids [83, 84] in the presence of sunscreen agent 4-*tert*-butyl-4-methoxydibenzoylmethane either alone [81–83] or together with 2-ethylhexyl 4-methoxycinnamate and 2-ethylhexyl 2-cyano-3,3,-diphenylacrylate [84] resulted in severe oxidative degradations of DNA, proteins, and lipids caused by reactive oxygen species (ROS) that were generated by the UVA-induced degradation of sunscreens. In the presence of either vitamin E or nitroxyls, considerable reductions of the oxidative damage resulted only in the presence of nitroxyl radicals, whereas with vitamin E there was either no inhibitory effect [81, 83] or a lesser effect [84] than that found with a nitroxyl radical inhibitor. Hence, it appears that the nitroxyl radical inhibitors would be a better choice for topical sunscreen formulations than vitamin E [83]. Applications of nitroxyl (aminoxyl) radicals as antioxidants in sunscreen formulations should not cause any problems to the human skin, since it was shown [87–89] on many occasions that these stable free radicals are neither cytotoxic nor mutagenic. They have been successfully used in contrast agents in magnetic resonance imaging (MRI), in anticancer drugs, and in many biological studies. Recently, novel nitroxyl-labeled sunscreen agents were prepared containing the nitroxyl label as part of the 2-ethylhexyl cinnamate structure, i.e., the molecules contain a sun protection component and an antioxidant component in the same molecule [90]. The compound 2,2,6,6-tetramethyl-piperidin-4-yl-*p*-methoxycinnamyloxy-1-oxyl was patented [90]. The antioxidant component 4-hydroxy-2,2,6,6-tetramethylpiperidine-1-oxyl (TEMPOL) of the patented sunscreen agent [90] has not only a very low toxicity [87–89] but also a high thermal stability [91]. Thus, in a boiling *n*-octane solution at 128 ± 2 ºC, there was no sign of decomposition during a period of 44 hours when the test was terminated [91]. The photostabilities of five frequently used commercial sunscreen filters were investigated using UVA and UVB radiations and various combinations of stable and unstable filters and the antioxidant esters of vitamins A, C, and E. Unfortunately, under the UV radiations, the mixture composed of the vitamin esters turned out to be the most unstable combination [92].

Similar to vitamin E, the congeners containing phenolic structures would be expected to undergo analogous reactions with various reactive oxygen species and other oxidants to give the corresponding phenoxy radicals which are resonance-stabilized, and, hence, can neither initiate nor propagate chain reactions. Compounds with alkene moieties attached to the aromatic ring could have additional resonance-stabilized structures. Therefore, all compounds with phenolic moieties can basically be involved in analogous reactions as vitamin E, including photosensitized reactions leading to ROS. (See **Section 6**.)

ii. Ubiquinone/Ubiquinols

The ubiquinone/ubiquinol redox complexes (**10a**, **10b**) range in molecular weight from n = 1 to n = 12 [**Fig. 5C.ii-1**]. The compound with n = 10 is found in various biological tissues of humans, including the skin. The compounds function in the transport of protons and electrons across membranes and as antioxidants. Thus, ubiquinol (**10b**) helps to protect membranes against lipid peroxidations, and ubiquinone (**10a**) interacts with singlet oxygen and may inhibit lipid peroxidations [93]. α-Tocopherol (**5**) is regenerated from α-tocopheryl radical (**5a**) by ubiquinol and by ascorbic acid, whereby ubiquinol is converted into ubiquinone and ascorbic acid (**1**) into dehydroascorbic acid (**3**). The redox properties of **10a** and **10b** were thoroughly studied [94].

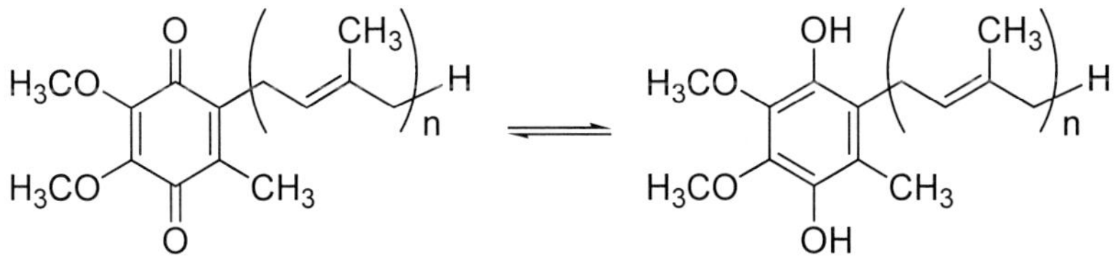

10a n = 1–12 **10b**

Fig. 5C.ii-1. The ubiquinone/ubiquinol redox complexes.

iii. β-Carotene and Congeners

The carotenoid pigments are widely distributed in plants and mammals [1, 13, 25, 26, 29, 31, 95, 96]. They play a protective role in plants, and it was logical to determine if they would act as photoprotective agents in the treatment of human photosensitivity [34]. The main carotenoids include the red pigment lycopene (**11**) and the yellow pigment β-carotene (**12**) [**Fig. 5C.iii-1**]. β-Carotene (**12**) is a precursor of vitamin A, and both compounds can be found in the epidermis, dermis, and subcutis of human skin. Furthermore, skin surface lipids contain **12** and vitamin A.

In human skin, carotenoids were shown [97] to scavenge peroxy radicals and inhibit lipid peroxidations. Compounds **11** and **12** were also shown [98] to be efficient scavengers of molecular oxygen and peroxy radicals generated during photooxidations. Carotenoids readily react with peroxy radicals of the fatty acids of lipids and undergo reactions with other ROS to give various products [99–101]. In general, it appears that the reactions with singlet oxygen are more efficient than those of vitamin E. β-Carotene readily undergoes autooxidative processes to give β-carotene peroxy radicals. (See **Section F** for reactions of singlet oxygen with alkenes.)

Carotenoids might enhance free radical reactions under special conditions [99, 100]. UVB radiation induces the formation of excited states of β-carotene, which may participate in free radical pathways. Compound **12** is a good radical-trapping antioxidant at low partial pressures of oxygen, which are found in most tissues under physiological conditions. However, at higher oxygen partial pressures, **12** was shown to have a prooxidant effect in vitro [13, 101, 102].

At the cellular level, β-carotene quenches singlet oxygen [103], inhibits UVR-induced erythema [104], enhances UVA induction of heme oxygenase-1 (HO-1) and IL-6 [105], inhibits the UVB radiation induced lipid peroxidation [106], causes growth arrest in transformed cells by stimulating gap junction communication [107], and inhibits UVR-induced carcinogenesis [108]. A retardation was observed [78] in the development of the UVB-induced erythema by oral administration to volunteers for 112 days of a food supplement consisting of low doses of vitamin E acetate (10 mg), β-carotene (2.4 mg), ascorbic acid (60 mg), and selenium (60 mg).

Dietary **12** was found to protect against UVR-induced carcinogenesis in mice [106], and this effect was independent of the conversion of **12** to vitamin A [107]. However, in another study, it was found that a diet rich in vitamin A caused increased UV carcinogenesis in hairless mice [108]

β-Carotene was found [104] to protect from erythema formation in humans. However, in human skin, the carotenoids are not particularly effective as protecting agents against the UV radiation of the sun, and orally administered **12** was shown to be ineffective [109, 110].

In a clinical study, it was demonstrated that neither UVA and UVB radiation induced erythema, nor UVB radiation mediated DNA damage in humans was significantly influenced by oral β-carotene [111]. In a double-blind, placebo-controlled study, the effect of **12** supplementation on the human sunburn response and on the induction of sunburn cells was examined, and it was concluded that the use of **12** provided no significant photoprotection [112]. However, in another investigation, it was shown that using an oral presupplementation prior to the topical sunscreen application was more effective than the application of sunscreen agent alone [113].

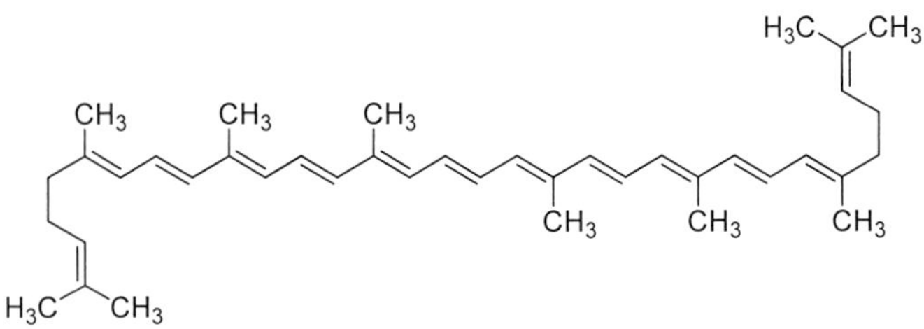

Lycopene (**11**)

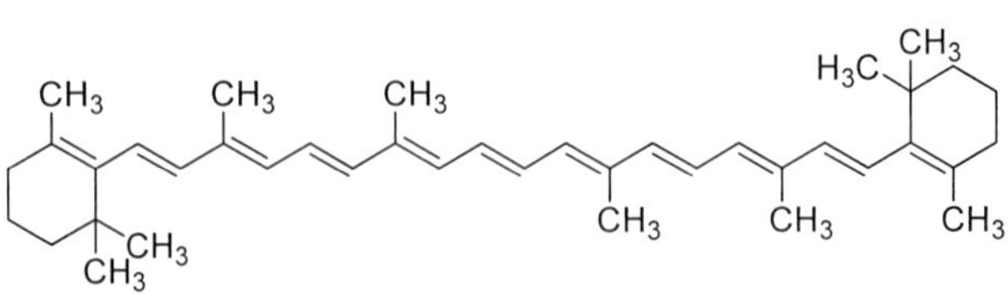

β-Carotene (**12**)

Fig. 5C.iii-1. Structures of lycopene (**11**) and β-carotene (**12**).

iv. Bilirubin

Bilirubin (**13**) [**Fig. 5C.iv-1**] is produced during the metabolism of heme in mammals. The reactions of the methylene group (CH_2) in **13** with lipid peroxy radicals produce resonance-stabilized bilirubin radicals, which can react with peroxy radicals to form adducts [13]. At low oxygen concentrations, bilirubin is considered to be a more efficient antioxidant than vitamin E. It is uncertain whether bilirubin is involved in the human skin as an antioxidant. However, one would expect that bilirubin, containing the same building elements as the heme and hemoglobin, would be an excellent photosensitizer on irradiation with UV light, i.e., would be excited to the singlet and triplet states, and would be efficiently quenched by molecular oxygen to give ROS.

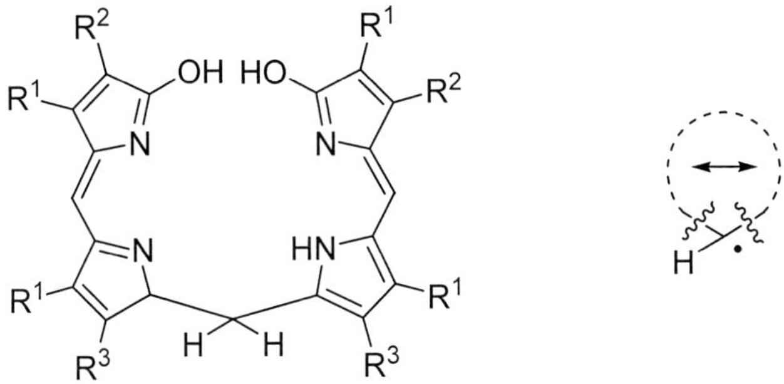

a **b**

13a (bilirubin); $R^1 = CH_3$, $R^2 = H_2C{=}CH$, $R^3 = CH_2CH_2CO_2H$
13b; partial structure of the resonance-stabilized radical of **13a**

Fig. 5C.iv-1. Structure of bilirubin.

v. Lipoic and Dihydrolipoic Acids

The lipoic acid (**14**)/dihydrolipoic (**14a**) couple has various redox functions in mammals, including human tissues [**Fig. 5C.v-1**]. Thus, **14** is readily oxidized by hydroxyl radicals and can convert glutathione disulfide (GS–SG) into glutathione (**7**), and the dehydroascorbyl anion radical (**2**) and dehydroascorbate (**3**) into ascorbic acid (**1**) [13]. Similarly, **14a** probably can participate in the regeneration of α-tocopherol (**5**) from α-tocopheryl radical (**5a**). Dihydrolipoic acid (**14a**) cannot react with singlet oxygen, while lipoic acid can scavenge singlet oxygen and inhibit the photochemical peroxidation reactions of unsaturated compounds. Dihydrolipoic acid was reported to alleviate the UV light induced erythema in human skin. However, the autoxidations of dihydrolipoic acid in the presence of transition-metal cations, such as ferric and cupric ions, result in the generation of ROS and reduced cations, i.e., ferrous and cuprous cations, which can participate in the further generation of ROS.

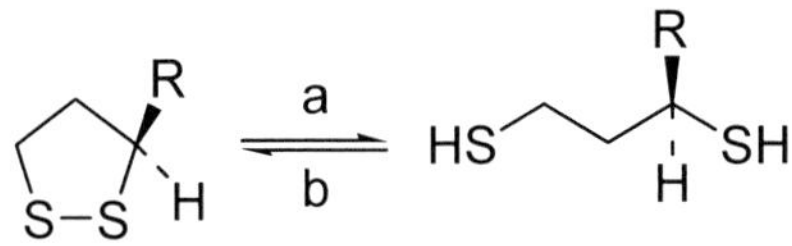

14 **14a**

R = $(CH_2)_4CO_2H$
a = reduction
b = oxidation

Fig. 5C.v-1. The lipoic acid (**14**)/dihydrolipoic (**14a**) couple.

In the end, it is important to reiterate and emphasize the fact that a number of antioxidants in this section are composed of conjugated chromophores [**Fig. 5C.v-2**, Structures **a**, **b**, and **c**]. These chromophores, on irradiation with UV light, absorb the energies of the radiations to undergo n,π^* and π,π^* transitions to excited singlet-state species. The singlet-state species then undergo intersystem crossing (ISC) to the lower-energy triplet state.

In the presence of air, the triplet species is readily quenched by molecular oxygen ($^3O_2$). Molecular oxygen is the best quencher of the triplet-state species, resulting in a cascade of reactive oxygen species (ROS). Thus, the antioxidants can become producers of oxidative stress.

O=C–C=C–C=O	–C=C–C=C–C=C–	–N=C–C=C–C=N–
a	**b**	**c**

Fig. 5C.v-2. Structures of conjugated chromophores.

References

1. Vessey D. A. (1993) The cutaneous antioxidant systems. In: *Oxidative Stress in Dermatology*, pp 81–103, Fuchs J. and Packer L. (eds.), Marcel Dekker, New York.

2. Pigeolet E., Corleisier P., Houbion A., Lambert D., Michiels C., Raes M., Zachary M. and Remacle J. (1990) Glutathione peroxidase, superoxide dismutase, and catalase inactivation by peroxides and oxygen derived free radicals. *Mech. Ageing Dev.* **31**: 283–297.
3. Halliwell B. (1993) Reactive oxygen species in pathology with special reference to the skin. In: *Oxidative Stress in Dermatology*, pp 3–11, Fuchs J. and Packer L. (eds.), Marcel Dekker, New York.
4. Carraro C. and Pathak M. A. (1988) Characterization of superoxide dismutase from mammalian skin epidermis. *J. Invest. Dermatol.* **90**: 31–36.
5. Ohkuma N., Matsuo S., Iizuka H. and Ohkawara A. (1987) Superoxide dismutase in epidermis. *J. Dermatol.* (Tokyo) **14**: 218–223.
6. Ueda H. and Sugiura K. (1988) Lipid peroxide and superoxide dismutase in human skin. In: *Cutaneous Aging*, pp 449–457, Klingman A. M. and Takase Y. (eds.), University of Tokyo Press, Tokyo.
7. Oguia R., Ueta H., Sugiyama M. and Hidaka T. (1990) Distribution of superoxide dismutase activity in the epidermis: measurement with electron spin resonance trapping. *J. Invest. Dermatol.* **94**: 227–229.
8. Fridovich I. (1981) The biology of superoxide and of superoxide dismutases – in brief. In: *Oxy-radicals in Chemistry and Biochemistry*, pp 197–204, Rodgers M. A. J. and Powers E. L. (eds.), Academic Press, New York.
9. Nanni E. J., Stallings M. D. and Sawyer D. T. (1980) Does superoxide ion oxidize catechol, α-tocopherol and ascorbic acid by direct electron transfer? *J. Am. Chem. Soc.* **102**: 4481–4485.
10. Omar B. A., Flores S. C. and McCord J. M. (1992) Superoxide dismutases: pharmacological developments and applications. *Adv. Pharmacol.* **23**: 109–161.
11. Gutteridge J. M. C. (1977) The protective action of superoxide dismutase on metal-ion catalyzed peroxidation of phospholipids. *Biochem. Biophys. Res. Commun.* **77**: 379–386.
12. Katiyar S. K., Afaq F. and Mukhtar H. (2001) Effects of solar radiation on detoxification mechanisms in the skin. In: *Sun Protection in Man*, pp 419–436, Giacomoni, P. U. (ed.), Elsevier, Amsterdam.
13. Fuchs J. (1992) The skin and oxidative stress. In: *Oxidative Injury in Dermatopathology*, pp 5–85, Springer Verlag, New York.
14. Oberly L. W. and Buettner G. R. (1979) The role of superoxide dismutase in cancer: a review. *Cancer Res.* **39**: 1141–1149.
15. Raikov Z. D., Raikova E. T., Zheleva A. M. and Gadzheva V. G. (2000). In: *Spin-labeled Antitumour Compounds*, Robev S. K. (ed.), ISBN 954-9736-02-5, Bulgaria.

16. Gadzheva V., Ichimori K., Nakazawa H. and Raikov Z. D. (1994) Superoxide scavenging activity of spin labeled nitrosourea and triazine derivatives. *Free Radical Res.* **21**: 177–186.
17. Fuchs J., Groth N. and Herrling T. (1998) Cutaneous tolerance of nitroxide free radicals in human skin. *Free Radical Biol. Med.* **24**: 643–648.
18. Antosiewicz Y., Damiani E., Jassem W., Wozniak M., Orena M. and Greci L. (1997) Influence of structure on the antioxidant activity of indolinic nitroxide radicals. *Free Radical Biol. Med.* **22**: 249–255.
19. Mitchell J. B., Samuni A., Krishna M. C., DeGraff W. G., Ahn M. S., Samuni V. and Russo A. (1990) Biologically active metal-independent superoxide dismutase mimics. *Biochemistry* **29**: 2802–2807.
20. Samuni A., Krishna M. C., Riesz P., Finkelstein F. and Russo A. (1988) A novel metal free low molecular weight superoxide dismutase mimic. *J. Biol. Chem.* **263**: 17921–17924.
21. Finkelstein E., Rosen G. M. and Rauckman E. J. (1984) Superoxide-dependent reduction of nitroxides by thiols. *Biochem. Biophys. Acta* **802**: 90–98.
22. Wendel A. (1980) Glutathione peroxidase. In: *Enzymatic Basis of Detoxification*, Vol. 1, pp 333–353, Jakoby W. B. (ed.), Academic Press, New York.
23. Blum J. and Fridovich I. (1985) Inactivation of glutathione peroxidase by superoxide radical. *Arch. Biochem. Biophys.* **240**: 500–508.
24. Flohe L., Gunzies W. and Ladenstein R. (1976) Glutathione peroxidase. In: *Glutathione, Metabolism and Function*, Arias I. and Jacoby W. (eds.), Raven Press, New York.
25. Sorg O., Antille C. and Saurat J.-H. (2004) Retinoids, other topical vitamins, and antioxidants. In: *Photoaging*, pp 89–115, Rigel D. S., Weiss R. A., Lim H. W. and Dover J. S. (eds.), Marcel Dekker, New York and Basel.
26. Chaudhuri R. K. (2005) Role of antioxidants in suncare products. In: *Sunscreens, Regulations, Commercial Development*, 3rd ed., pp 603–638, Taylor and Francis, Boca Raton.
27. Merk H., Jugert F., Bonnekoh B. and Mahrle O. (1991) Induction and inhibition of NADPH quinone reductase in murine and human skin. *Skin Pharmacol.* **4**: 183–190.
28. Koone M. D. and Black H. S. (1986) A mode of action for butylated hydroxytoluene-mediated photoprotection. *J. Invest. Dermatol.* **87**: 343–347.

29. Black H. S. and Rhodes L. E. (2001) Systemic photoprotection, dietary intervention and therapy. In: *Sun Protection in Man*, pp 573–591, Giacomoni, P. U. (ed.), Elsevier, Amsterdam.
30. Pinnell S. R. (2003) Cutaneous photodamage, oxidative stress, and topical antioxidant protection. *J. Am. Acad. Dermatol.* **48**: 1–22.
31. Strickland F. M. (2001) Boosting the immune system. In: *Sun Protection in Man*, pp 613–636, Giacomoni, P. U. (ed.), Elsevier, Amsterdam.
32. Stahl W. and Sies H. (2001) Protection Against Solar Radiation – Protective properties of antioxidants. In: *Sun Protection in Man*, pp 561–572, Giacomoni, P. U. (ed.), Elsevier, Amsterdam
33. González S. and Gilaberte-Calzada Y. (2009) Oral and other non-sunscreen photoprotective agents. In: *Clinical Guide to Sunscreen and Photoprotection*, pp 207–222, Lim H. W. and Draelos Z. D. (eds.), Informa Healthcare, New York.
34. F'guyer S., Afaq F. and Mukhtar J. (2003) Photochemoprevention of skin cancer by botanical agents. *Photodermatol., Photoimmunol. Photomed.* **19**: 56–72.
35. Halliwell B. and Whiteman M. (1997) Antioxidant and prooxidant properties of vitamin C. In: *Vitamin C in Health and Disease*, pp 59–73, Parker L. and Fuchs J. (eds.), Marcel Dekker, New York.
36. Swartz H. M. and Dodd N. J. F. (1981) The role of ascorbic acid on radical reactions *in vivo*. In: *Oxygen and Oxy-radicals in Chemistry and Biology*, pp 161–168, Rodgers M. A. I. and Powers E. L. (eds.), Academic Press, New York.
37. Nishikimi M. and Jagi K. (1977) Oxidations of ascorbic acid and α-tocopherol by superoxide. In: *Biochemical and Medical Aspects of Active Oxygen*, p 79, Hayaishi O. and Asada K. (eds.), University Park Press, New York.
38. Trommer H., Bottcher R., Poppl A., Hoentsch J., Wartewig S. and Neubert R. H. (2002) Role of ascorbic acid in stratum corneum lipid models exposed to UV irradiation. *Pharm. Res.* **19**: 982–990.
39. Jenkins G. J., Stephens L. A., Masnavi N. and Parry J. M. (2002) Molecular analysis of the chemoprotective effect of topical sunscreen and vitamin C in preventing UV-induced and reactive oxygen species-induced DNA damage, respectively, using the PCR inhibition methodology. *Anticancer Res.* **22**: 3873–3877.
40. Walling C. (1957) *Free Radicals in Solution*, pp 457–462, John Wiley & Sons, New York.

41. Dawson C. R. (1966) Ascorbate oxidase. In: *The Biochemistry of Copper*, p 305, Peisach J., Aisen P. and Blumberg W. E. (eds.), Academic Press, New York.
42. Lee S. H., Oe T. and Blair I. A. (2001) Vitamin C-induced decomposition of lipid hydroperoxides to endogeneous genotoxins. *Science* **292**: 2083–2086.
43. Shamberger R. J. (1984) Genetic toxicology of ascorbic acid. *Mutat. Res.* **133**: 135–159.
44. Vile G. F. (1997) Active oxygen species mediate the solar ultraviolet radiation-dependent increase in the tumour suppressor protein p53 in human skin fibroblasts. *FEBS Lett.* **412**: 70–74.
45. Catani M. V., Rossi A., Costanzo A., Sabatini S., Levrero M., Melino G. and Avigliano L. (2001) Induction of gene expression via activator protein-1 in the ascorbate protection against UV-induced damage. *Biochem. J.* **356**: 77–85.
46. Nakamura T., Pinnell S. R., Darr D., Kurimoto I., Itami S., Yoshikawa K. and Streilein J. W. (1997) Vitamin C abrogates the deleterious effects of UVB radiation on cutaneous immunity by a mechanism that does not depend on TNF-alpha. *J. Invest. Dermatol.* **109**: 20–24.
47. Darr D., Dunston S., Faust H. and Pinnell S. (1996) Effectiveness of antioxidants (vitamins C and E) with and without sunscreens as topical photoprotectants. *Acta Derm.-Venereol.* **76**: 264–268.
48. Paleos C. M. and Dais P. (1977) Ready reduction of some nitroxide free radicals with ascorbic acid. *J. Chem. Soc., Chem. Commun.* 345–346.
49. Gutierrez P. L. (1988) The influence of ascorbic acid on the free-radical metabolism of xenobiotics: the example of diaziquone. *Drug Metab. Rev.* **19**: 319–343.
50. Sosnovsky G. and Konieczny M. (1977) Preparation of four phosphorylated 1,4-dihydroxy-2,2,6,6-tetramethylpiperidines by reduction of nitroxyls with ascorbic acid. *Synthesis* 619–622.
51. Venditti E., Scire A., Tanfani F., Greci L. and Damiani E. (2008) Nitroxides are more efficient inhibitors of oxidative damage to calf skin collagen than antioxidant vitamins. *Biochim. Biophys. Acta* **1780**: 58–68.
52. Wolf P., Donawho C. K. and Kripke M. L. (1994) Analysis of the protective effect of different sunscreens on ultraviolet radiation-induced local and systemic suppression of contact hypersensitivity and inflammatory responses in mice. *J. Invest. Dermatol.* **100**: 254–259.

53. Moyal D. D. and Fourtanier A. M. (2008) Broad-spectrum sunscreens provide better protection from solar ultraviolet-simulated radiation and natural sunlight-induced immunosuppression in human beings. *J. Am. Acad. Dermatol.* **58** (S Suppl. 2): 149–154.
54. Halliday G. M. and Hönigsmann H. (2009) Sunscreens, photoimmunosuppression, and photoaging. In: *Clinical Guide to Sunscreens and Photoprotection*, pp 101–116, Lim H. W. and Draelos Z. D. (eds.), Informa Healthcare, New York.
55. Healy E., Reynolds N. J., Smith M. D., Campbell C., Farr P. M. and Rees J. L. (1994) Dissociation of erythema and p53 protein suppression in human skin following UVB irradiation and induction of p53 protein and RNA following application of skin irritants. *J. Invest. Dermatol.* **103**: 493–499.
56. Connor M. J. and Wheeler L. A. (1987) Depletion of cutaneous glutathione by ultraviolet light radiation. *Photochem. Photobiol.* **46**: 239–245.
57. Reed D. J. (1986) Regulation of reduction processes by glutathione. *Biochem. Pharmacol.* **35**: 7–13.
58. Mitchell J. B., Biaglow J. E. and Russo Y. E. (1988) Role of glutathione and endogeneous thiols in radiation protection. *Pharmacol. Ther.* **39**: 269–274.
59. Armeni T., Damiani E., Battino M., Greci L. and Principato M. (2004) Lack of in vitro protection by a common sunscreen ingredient of UVA-induced cytotoxicity in keratinocytes. *Toxicology* **203**: 165–178.
60. Krol E. S., Kramer-Stickland K. A. and Liebler D. C. (2000) Photoprotective actions of topically applied vitamin E. *Drug Metab. Rev.* **32**: 413–420.
61. Packer J. E., Slater T. F. and Willson R. L. (1979) Direct observation of a free radical interaction between vitamin E and vitamin C. *Nature* **278**: 737–738.
62. Packer L., Maguire J. J., Mehlhorn R. J., Serbinova E. and Kagan V. E. (1989) Mitochondrial and microsomal membranes have a free radical reductase activity that prevents chromanoxyl radical accumulation. *Biochem. Biophys. Res. Commun.* **159**: 229–235.
63. Machlin L. J. (1984) Vitamin E. In: *Handbook of Vitamins: Nutritional, Biochemical and Clinical Aspects*, pp 99–145, Machlin L. J. (ed.), Marcel Dekker, New York and Basel.
64. Burton G. W., Joyce A. and Ingold K. U. (1982) First proof that vitamin E is major lipid soluble, chain-breaking antioxidant in human blood plasma. *Lancet* **2**: 327.

65. Ingold K. U., Webb A. C., Witter D., Burton G. W., Metcalfe T. A. and Muller D. P. R. (1987) Vitamin E remains the major lipid soluble, chain-breaking antioxidant in human plasma even in individuals suffering severe vitamin E deficiency. *Arch. Biochem. Biophys.* **259**: 224–225.
66. Cecarini J. P., Michel L., Marette J. M., Adhoute H. and Bejot M. (2003) Immediate effects of UV radiation on the skin: modification by antioxidant complex containing carotenoids. *Photodermatol., Photoimmunol. Photomed.* **19**: 182–189.
67. Maalouf S., El-Sabban M., Darwiche N. and Gali-Muhtasib H. (2002) Protective effect of vitamin E on ultraviolet B light-induced damage in keratinocytes. *Mol. Carcinog.* **34**: 121–130.
68. Werninghaus K., Handjani R. M. and Gilchrest B. A. (1991) Protective effect of alpha-tocopherol in carrier liposomes on ultraviolet-mediated human epidermal cell damage in vitro. *Photodermatol., Photoimmunol. Photomed.* **8**: 236–242.
69. Mazière C., Dantin F., Dubois F., Santus R. and Mazière J. (2000) Biphasic effect of UVA radiation on STATl activity and tyrosine phosphorylation in cultured human keratinocytes. *Free Radical Biol. Med.* **28**: 1430–1437.
70. Djavaheri-Mergny M. and Dubertret L. (2001) UV-A induced Ap-1 activation requires the Raf/ERK pathway in human NCTC 2544 keratinocytes. *Exp. Dermatol.* **10**: 204–210.
71. Yuen K. S. and Halliday G. M. (1997) Alpha-tocopherol, an inhibitor of epidermal lipid peroxidation, prevents ultraviolet radiation from suppressing the skin immune system. *Photochem. Photobiol.* **65**: 587–592.
72. Vile G. F. (1997) Active oxygen species mediate the solar ultraviolet radiation-dependent increase in the tumour suppressor protein p53 in human skin fibroblasts. *FEBS Lett.* **412**: 70–74.
73. McVean M. and Liebler D. C. (1997) Inhibition of UVB induced DNA photodamage in mouse epidermis by topically applied alpha-tocopherol. *Carcinogenesis* **18**: 1617–1622.
74. McVean M. and Lieber D. C. (1999) Prevention of DNA photodamage by vitamin E compounds and sunscreens: roles of ultraviolet absorbance and cellular uptake. *Mol. Carcinog.* **24**: 169–176.
75. Berton T. R., Conti C. J., Mitchell D. L., Aldaz C. M., Lubet R. A. and Fischer S. M. (1998) The effect of vitamin E acetate on ultraviolet-induced mouse skin carcinogenesis. *Mol. Carcinog.* **23**: 175–184.
76. Chen W., Barthelman M., Martinez J., Alberts D. and Gensler H. L. (1997) Inhibition of cyclobutane pyrimidine dimer formation in epi-

dermal p53 gene of UV-irradiated mice by alpha-tocopherol. *Nutr. Cancer* **29**: 205–211.
77. Fuchs J. and Kern H. (1998) Modulation of UV-light-induced skin inflammation by D-alpha-tocopherol and L-ascorbic acid: a clinical study using solar simulated radiation. *Free Radical Biol. Med.* **25**: 1006–1012.
78. Greul A.-K., Grundmann J.-U., Heinrich F., Pfitzner I., Bernhardt J., Ambach A., Biesalski H.-K. and Gollnick H. (2002) Photoprotection of UV-irradiated human skin: an antioxidative combination of vitamins E and C, carotenoids, selenium and proanthocyanidins. *Skin Pharmacol. Appl. Skin Physiol.* **15**: 307–315.
79. Eberlein-König B., Placzek M. and Przybilla B. (1998) Protective effect against sunburn of combined systemic ascorbic acid (vitamin C) and d-α-tocopherol (vitamin E). *J. Am. Acad. Dermatol.* **38**: 45–48.
80. Fuchs J. (1998) Potentials and limitations of the natural antioxidants RRR-alpha-tocopherol, L-ascorbic acid and β-carotene in cutaneous photoprotection. *Free Radical Biol. Med.* **25**: 848–873.
81. Damiani E., Greci L., Parsons R. and Knowland J. (1999) Nitroxide radicals protect DNA from damage when illuminated in vitro in the presence of dibenzoylmethane and a common sunscreen ingredient. *Free Radical Biol. Med.* **26**: 809–816.
82. Damiani E., Carloni P., Biondi C. and Greci L. (2000) Increased oxidative modification of albumin when illuminated in vitro in the presence of a common sunscreen ingredient: protection by nitroxide radicals. *Free Radical Biol. Med.* **28**: 193–201.
83. Damiani E., Castagna R. and Greci L. (2002) The effects of derivatives of the nitroxide Tempol on UVA-mediated in vitro lipid and protein oxidation. *Free Radical Biol. Med.* **33**: 128–136.
84. Damiani E., Rosati L., Castagna R., Carloni P. and Greci L. (2006) Changes in ultraviolet absorbance and hence in protective efficacy against lipid peroxidation of organic sunscreens after UVA irradiation. *J. Photochem. Photobiol.* **82**: 204–213.
85. Damiani E., Astolfi P., Cionna L., Ippoliti F. and Greci L. (2006) Synthesis and application of a novel sunscreen-antioxidant. *Free Radical Res.* **40**: 485–494.
86. Venditti E., Spadoni T., Tiano T., Astolfi P., Greci L., Littarru G. P. and Damiani E. (2008) In vitro photostability and photoprotection studies of a novel "multiactive" UV-absorber. *Free Radical Biol. Med.* **45**: 345–354.

87. Sosnovsky G. (1992) A critical evaluation of the present status of toxicity of aminoxyl radicals. *J. Pharm. Sci.* **81**: 496–499.
88. Zhdanov R. I. (1992) The toxicity of aminoxyl radicals. In: *Bioactive Spin Labels*, pp 429–438, Zhdanov R. I. (ed.), Springer-Verlag, Berlin.
89. Gadjeva V., Lazarova G. and Zheleva A. (2003) Spin labeled antioxidants protect bacteria against the toxicity of alkylating antitumor drug CCNU. *Toxicol. Lett.* **144**: 289–294.
90. Damiani E., Astolfi P. and Greci L. (2007) Synthesis of a nitroxide antioxidant and methods of use in cosmetic and dermatological compositions. *U.S. Pat. Appl.* 20070140996A.
91. Sosnovsky G., Jawdosiuk M. and Clumpner J. M. (2000) Di-*tert*-alkyl nitroxyl radicals. Synthesis, physical properties and applications as inhibitors of vinyl polymerization at elevated temperatures. *Z. Naturforsch.* **55b**: 109–126.
92. Gaspar L. R. and Campos P. M. (2007) Photostability and efficacy of topical formulations containing UV-filters combination and vitamins A, C and E. *Int J. Pharm.* **343**: 181-191.
93. Battino M., Ferri E., Gattavecchia E., Sassi S. and Lenaz G. (1991) Coenzyme Q10 as possible membrane protecting agent against irradiation damages. In: *Biomedical and Clinical Aspects of Coenzyme Q10*, Vol. 6, pp 181–190, Folkers K., Yamagami T. and Littaru G. P. (eds.), Elsevier, The Netherlands.
94. Giorgini E., Tommasi G., Stipa P., Tosi G., Littarru G. and Greci L. (2001) Reactivity of ubiquinones and ubiquinols with free radicals. *Free Radical Res.* **35**: 63–72.
95. Petrucci R., Giorgini E., Damiani E., Carloni P., Marrosu G., Trazza A., Littaru G. P. and Greci L. (2000) A study on the interactions between coenzyme Q_0 and superoxide anion. Could ubiquinones mimic superoxide dismutase (SOD)? *Res. Chem. Intermed.* **26**: 269–282.
96. Britton G., Liaaen-Jensen S. and Pfander H. (eds.) (2004) *Carotenoids: Handbook*, Birkhauser, Boston.
97. Mortensen A. (2002) Scavenging of benzylperoxyl radicals by carotenoids. *Free Radical Res.* **36**: 211–216.
98. Eichler O., Sies H. and Stahl W. (2002) Divergent optimum levels of lycopene, beta-carotene and lutein protecting against UVB irradiation in human fibroblasts. *Photochem. Photobiol.* **75**: 503–506.
99. Terao J., Yamauchi R., Murakami H. and Matsusnita S. (1980) Inhibitory effects of tocopherols and β-carotene on singlet oxygen initiated photooxidation of methyl linoleate and soybean oil. *J. Food Process. Preserv.* **4**: 79–93.

100. Faria J. A. F. and Mukai M. K. (1983) Use of a gas chromatographic reactor to study lipid photooxidation. *J. Am. Oil Chem. Soc.* **60**: 77–81.
101. Burton G. W. and Ingold K. U. (1984) β-Carotene: an unusual type of lipid antioxidant. *Science* **224**: 569–573.
102. Palozza P., Luberto C., Calviello G., Ricci P. and Bartoli G. M. (1997) Antioxidant and prooxidant role of β-carotene in murine normal and tumor thymocytes: effects of oxygen partial pressure. *Free Radical Biol. Med.* **22**: 1065–1073.
103. Stratton S. P. and Liebler D. C. (1997) Determination of singlet oxygen-specific versus radical-mediated lipid peroxidation in photosensitized oxidation of lipid bilayers: effect of beta-carotene and alpha-tocopherol. *Biochemistry* **36**: 12911–12920.
104. Stahl W., Heinrich U., Jungmann H., Sies H. and Tronnier H. (2000) Carotenoids and carotenoids plus vitamin E protect against ultraviolet light-induced erythema in humans. *Am. J. Clin. Nutr.* **71**: 795–798.
105. Obermüller-Jevic U. C., Schlegel B., Flaccus A. and Biesalski H. K. (2001) The effect of beta-carotene on the expression of interleukin-6 and heme oxygenase-1 in UV-irradiated human skin fibroblasts in vitro. *FEBS Lett.* **509**: 186–190.
106. Epstein J. H. (1977) Effects of beta-carotene on ultraviolet induced cancer formation in the hairless mouse skin. *Photochem. Photobiol.* **25**: 211–213.
107. Mathews-Roth M. M. and Krinsky N. I. (1985) Carotenoid dose level and protection against UV-B induced skin tumors. *Photochem. Photobiol.* **42**: 35–38.
108. Mikkelsen S., Berne B., Staberg B. and Vahlquist A. (1998) Potentiating effect of dietary vitamin A on photocarcinogenesis in hairless mice. *Carcinogenesis* **19**: 663–666.
109. Mathews-Roth M. M., Pathak M. A., Parrish J., Fitzpatrick T. B., Kass E. H., Toda K. and Clemens W. (1972) A clinical trial of the effects of oral beta-carotene on the responses of human skin to solar radiation. *J. Invest. Dermatol.* **59**: 349–353.
110. Greenberg E. R., Baron J. A., Stukel T. A., Stevens M. M., Mandel J. S., Spencer S. K., et al. (1990) The alpha-tocopherol, beta-carotene cancer prevention study group. A clinical trial of beta-carotene to prevent basal-cell and squamous-cell cancer on the skin. *N. Engl. J. Med.* **323**: 789–795.
111. Wolf C., Steiner A. and Hönigsmann H. (1988) Do oral carotenoids protect human skin against ultraviolet erythema, psoralen phototoxi-

city and ultraviolet-induced DNA damage? *J. Invest. Dermatol.* **90**: 55–57.

112. Garmyn M., Ribaya-Mercado J. D., Russel R. M., Bhawan J. and Gilchrest B. A. (1995) Effect of beta-carotene supplementation on the human sunburn reaction. *Dermatology* **4**: 104–111.
113. Grundmann J.-U. and Gollnick H. (1999) Prevention of ultraviolet ray damage: external and internal sunscreens. *Ther. Umsch.* **56**: 225–232.

CHAPTER SIX

EXOGENOUS ANTIOXIDANTS TOPICALLY APPLIED TO HUMAN SKIN: PLANT ANTIOXIDANTS FOR PHOTOCHEMOPREVENTION OF SKIN CANCER

The incidence of non-melanoma skin cancer, consisting of basal- and squamous-cell carcinomas, continues to increase in the world. Ultraviolet B radiation (UVBR) has been implicated as its main cause although UVA radiation, which penetrates deeper through the skin, is definitely contributing to the initiation of skin cancers. UV radiation is known to cause excessive generation of reaction oxygen species (ROS), leading to cancer initiation and promotion [1–4]. Antioxidants can quench these ROS and some of them can inhibit many UVR-induced signal transduction pathways [3–7]. One approach to reducing the occurrence of skin cancer is by photochemoprotection, which is defined as the use of agents capable of ameliorating the adverse effects of UVBR on the skin [3–14]. An emerging important class of chemoprotective agents is naturally occurring plant antioxidants [3–14]. These compounds may play a role in protecting the skin's antioxidant system resulting in an inhibition of carcinogenesis in mouse "models" in vitro as well as in vivo.

Some common ring structures can be discerned among these natural plant products **[Fig. 6-1**]. Apigenin (**15a**), kaempferol (**15b**), luteolin (**15c**), quercitin (**15d**), rutin (**15e**), and silymarin (**15f**) contain a 2-phenyl flavone ring system [15, 16]. The flavonoid apigenin (**15a**), present in the leaves and stems of vascular plants, fruits, and vegetables is a 5,7,4'-trihydroxyflavone, i.e., a polyphenol ring system. Topical application of **15a** prior to UV exposures was shown [17] to decrease the UV-induced mouse skin tumorigenesis, as manifested by a reduction in cancer incidence and an increase in cancer-free survivals. Apigenin was found to inhibit the UV-mediated induction of ornithine decarboxylase (ODC) activity [17], to cause G1 cell-cycle arrest [19], and to inhibit cdk2 activity [17–19].

Silymarin, a polyphenolic flavonoid from milk thistle plant (*Silybum marianum*, L. Gaertn) is a mixture of several flavonolignans, which include silybin, silibinin, silidianin, silychristin, and isosilybin [20]. Silybin (silymarin, **15f**) has been shown to be the main compound responsible for the antioxidant and anticarcinogenic effects [20–22]. It also contains a polyphenol ring structure, which can absorb UVR, resulting in the formation of reactive oxygen species. A number of these flavonoids can be found in Ginkgo biloba extract, prepared from the leaves of the ginkgo biloba tree, including apigenin (**15a**), luteolin (**15c**), quercetin (**15d**), rutin (**15e**), catechin (**16a**), and epicatechin (**16b**) [23]. These compounds are also polyphenols containing the flavone ring system. Ginkgo biloba acts as an antioxidant and anti-inflammatory agent in the prevention of carcinogenesis [22, 23]. Ginkgo biloba extract reduces inflammation [14], decreases SOD activity [23, 24], reduces the number of sunburn cells [25], and reduces catalase activity [26].

Closely related to these compounds are the 3-phenyl isoflavones, such as daidzein (**17a**), genistein (**17b**), and formonetin (**17c**). Genistein, a 4',5,7-trihydroxyisoflavone, is found in soy, ginkgo biloba extract, and Greek oregano and sage. It has been shown [26, 27] to possess antioxidant and anticarcinogenic effects in the skin, to reduce the inflammatory edema reaction, and to suppress the contact hypersensitivity induced by moderate doses of solar-simulated UV radiation [28]. It was assumed that **17b** causes the inhibition of photocarcinogenesis through the inhibition of DNA adduct formation and reduction of oxidative stress and inflammation [5].

A close structural relationship exists between the above compounds and analogs of the chroman ring system. These compounds include the 3-phenyl chromans, catechin (**16a**) and its isomer epicatechin (**16b**), found in green tea and other sources. The green tea polyphenols (GTPs) are 3,3',4',5,7-flavanpentol derivatives, which absorb UVB radiation and can scavenge ROS, such as lipid free radicals, superoxide radical, hydroxyl radical, hydrogen peroxide and singlet oxygen [5]. GTPs have antimutagenic and anticarcinogenic properties in vitro [29]. Topical application of GTPs 30 minutes prior to UVB irradiation resulted in a reduced production of cyclobutane pyrimidine dimers (CPDs) in the epidermis and dermis of human volunteers [31, 32].

The chroman system is also contained in α-tocopherol **(5)**, the chief lipid-soluble vitamin. (See discussion in Section 5.) A number of in vitro tests have been conducted on the photoprotective effect of **5** on cultured animal and human cells [5]. α-Tocopherol was found to prevent UVB-induced formation of mutagenic thymidine dimers [32] and cyclobutane pyrimidine dimers in the epidermal p53 gene of mice [33]. Since cyclobutane dimers are formed directly by photoexcitation, it was suggested that **5** acts directly as a sunscreen [33]. In other experiments, the application of **5** to mice prevented UVB-induced local immunosuppression by inhibiting lipid peroxidation without affecting post irradiation inflammatory edema [34, 35]. The photoprotection afforded by **5** is probably the result of the quenching of UVR-generated lipid peroxides and ROS. In a clinical study, it was found that the topical application of a combination of **5** with other antioxidants, such as ascorbic acid, provided effective skin photoprotection [36].

The compound curcumin (diferuloylmethane, **18**), a natural yellow-orange dye obtained from the root of the tumeric plant (*Curcuma longa*, Linn), contains a phenol structure as well as a cinnamoyl side chain. Curcumin has been found [37–44] to possess a variety of properties. Thus, curcumin is an anti-inflammatory agent, an oral and topical antioxidant, a scavenger of reactive oxygen species, a potential inhibitor of skin carcinogenesis in humans, a potential chemoprotective agent of premalignant lesions, and an inhibitory agent of various cancers. Various in vitro and in vivo studies of curcumin and tumor growth inhibition have been reported [37–44]. Curcumin binds irreversibly to CD13/aminopeptidase N (APN), a membrane-bound metalloproteinase that plays a key role in cancer invasion and angiogenesis [45]. This observation may explain curcumin's property of slowing tumor cell growth by inhibition of angiogenesis [45]. A p53-dependent apoptosis is caused by curcumin in human basal cell carcinoma [46], while in human melanoma cells apoptosis is induced by a p53-independent pathway [47]. The inhibition of the glutathione S-transferase activity in human melanoma cells is caused by a number of unrelated carbonyl compounds, including curcumin [48].

Curcumin has also been considered as a possible adjunct agent in sunscreen formulations [48]. However, it was shown that irradiation of curcumin with a light source of <400 nm results in phototoxicity through the production of excited species which emit fluorescence and phosphorescence, and in the formation of singlet oxygen ($^1O_2$), superoxide anion radical ($O_2{\cdot}^-$), and degradation products [49]. Although these results were obtained [49] mainly in non-aqueous systems, it is believed [4] that, under biological conditions, singlet oxygen and superoxide anion radical could also be produced, resulting in phototoxicity. Hence, these results cast some doubt on the suitability of curcumin as a sunscreen agent or as an adjunct agent. Furthermore, the use of curcumin as an anticancer drug is not likely to materialize because of its low activity and poor intestinal absorption properties [50]. Instead, a structurally related compound, the diphenyl difluoroketone, was proposed for gastrointestinal cancers [50]. However, new curcumin analogs, 3,5-bis(arylidene)-4-piperidones, containing various aminoxyl labels and fluorine, were found to have low toxicities and high antioxidant and anti-inflammatory properties. These compounds could have potential applications as safe and effective anticancer agents [51–53].

Sunscreen agents with analogous 1,3-dione structures, such as dibenzoylmethane derivatives, could be expected to undergo analogous photosensitized reactions, and, thus, exhibit toxicity on the skin with solar radiation. Hence, while protecting the skin from erythema, this type of sunscreen agent would also contribute to the damaging effects on the skin. This photosensitivity of the dibenzoylmethanes has been confirmed [54, 55]. Thus, irradiation with UVA light of either 4-isopropyldibenzoylmethane or the sunscreen agent 4-*tert*-butyl-4'-methoxydibenzoylmethane resulted in a mixture of various degradation products [54].

Resveratrol (*trans*-3,4',5-trihydroxystilbene, **19**) is similar in structure to curcumin, and contains both a phenolic and a conjugated double bond system. Found in grape nuts, fruits, and red wine, it is a potent antioxidant with strong anti-inflammatory and antiproliferative properties [56]. Application of resveratrol to the skin of mice resulted in a significant decrease in UVB-induced generation of hydrogen peroxide and infiltration of leucocytes [57]. In addition, resveratrol was found to inhibit UVB-mediated increased level of lipid peroxidation [57], inhibit UVB-induced skin thickening, skin inflammation and edema, hydrogen peroxide generation, leucocyte infiltration, lipid peroxidation, cyclooxygenase (COX) and ornithine decarboxylase (ODC) enzyme activities [57, 58], the UVBR-induced activation of nuclear transcription factors NF-κB, Ikkα, and phosphorylation and degradation of IκBα [60]. Paramagnetic aminoxyl spin labeled resveratrol analogs were found to have potent ROS scavenging antioxidant and anti-inflammatory properties [61]. Furthermore, some plants, herbs, and lichens, many belonging to the rutaceae family, such as lime, lemon, bergamot, and to the family of umbelliferae like fennel, dill, carrot, fig, and members of other botanical families can cause sun sensitivity in some persons [62].

Aspirin™ (acetylsalicylic acid, 2-acetoxybenzoic acid, **20**), the well-known analgesic, antipyretic, and anti-inflammatory drug is derived from naturally occurring salicylic acid. Salicylic acid (**21**) is an endogenous growth regulator, and a regulator of resistance to pathogens in plants. It has also other functions, and is widely distributed including in the bark of the willow tree. Aspirin™, in comparison to other nonsteroidal anti-inflammatory drugs (NSAIDs) has a low toxicity, with LD_{50} values for mice and rats of 1.1 and 1.5 g/kg [63].

The drug was prepared originally by the French chemist Charles Frederic Gerhardt in 1853 from acetyl chloride and sodium salicylate [64]. Aspirin™ and all other NSAIDs are highly selective inhibitors of lipooxygenase (LOX) and cyclooxygenase (COX-2) enzymes [65]. The biodegradation of Aspirin™ by Aspirin™ esterases initially produces salicylic (**21**) and 2,5-dihydroxybenzoic (gentisic, **22**) acids. The liberated acetoxy group undergoes, in part, decarboxylation to give carbon dioxide, and, in part, becomes attached by acetylation to various biomolecules, such as proteins, glycoproteins, lipids, and other entities. Salicylic acid and gentisic acid undergo conjugation reactions with glycine, forming amide bonds and leading to salicyluric and gentisuric acids. Salicylic acid also undergoes condensation with glucoronic acid to give two salicyl glucuronides. These conjugations occur primarily in the liver, kidney, and the intestinal tract. Excretion of Aspirin™ and salicylic acid occurs primarily though the urine [63].

The antioxidative properties of all compounds containing phenolic moieties can be attributed to the facile reduction of various reactive oxygen species and other oxidation products whereby the phenol group is converted into oxygen-centered phenoxyl radicals, as shown in the case of α-tocopherol resulting in the α-tocopheroxyl radical. The original phenol moieties can be restored by various reducing agents, in particular, by the ubiquitous ascorbic acid. The oxygen-centered radicals of all these compounds are resonance-stabilized and can neither initiate nor propagate chain reactions. Analogous reactions can occur with salicylic acid (**21**). The photochemistry of plant antioxidants can be attributed to certain distinctive structural features in their molecules, i.e., the chromophores and abundance of hydroxyl auxochromes, such as, **a** in silymarin and related compounds, **b** in salicylic acid, daidzein, and analogs, **c** in curcumin, and **d** in resveratrol [**Fig. 6-2**]. In these chromophores, the interactions of the bonding electrons of the double bonds of C=C and C=O groups with solar UVA and UVB radiations result in π,π^* and n,π^* transitions, respectively, i.e., in excited singlet and triplet states. These species are readily quenched by molecular oxygen to give reactive oxygen species. Hence, many plant antioxidants can become, under UV radiations, inadvertently, also sources of oxidative stress.

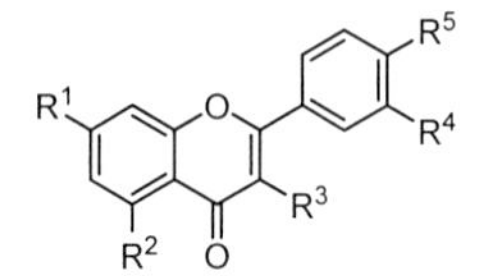

Apigenin (**15a**); $R^1 = R^2 = R^5 = OH$, $R^3 = R^4 = H$
Kaempferol (**15b**); $R^1 = R^2 = R^3 = R^5 = OH$, $R^4 = H$
Luteolin (**15c**); $R^1 = R^2 = R^4 = R^5 = OH$, $R^3 = H$
Quercitin (**15d**); $R^1 = R^2 = R^3 = R^4 = R^5 = OH$
Rutin (**15e**); $R^1 = R^2 = R^4 = R^5 = OH$, R^3 = *O*-rutinuside

Silymarin (**15f**); $R^1 = R^2 = R^3 = OH$, R^4,R^5 =

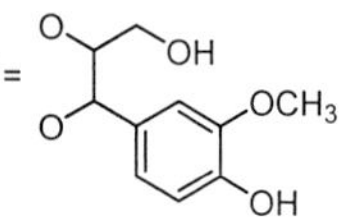

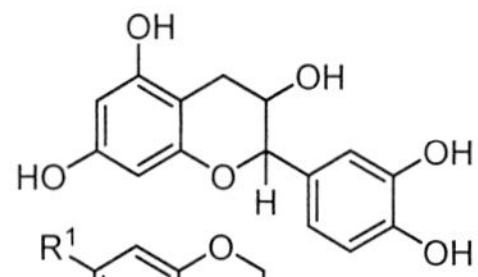

(+) Catechin (*trans*) (**16a**)
(–) Epicatechin (*cis*) (**16b**)

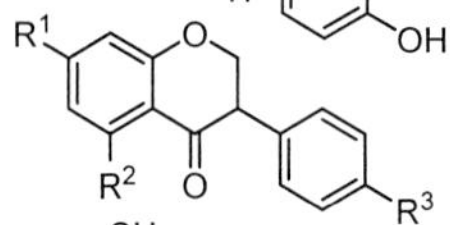

Daidzein (**17a**); $R^1 = R^3 = OH$, $R^2 = H$
Genistein and Biochanin (A and B) (**17b**); $R^1 = R^2 = R^3 = OH$
Formonetin (**17c**); $R^1 = OH$, $R^2 = H$, $R^3 = OCH_3$

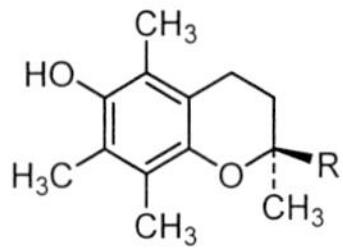

R,R,R-α-Tocopherol, Vitamin E (**5**)

R =

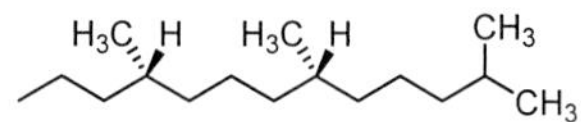

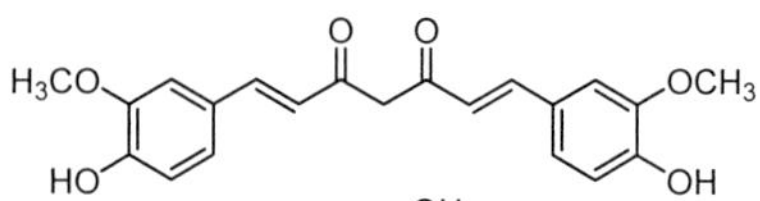

Curcumin (**18**)

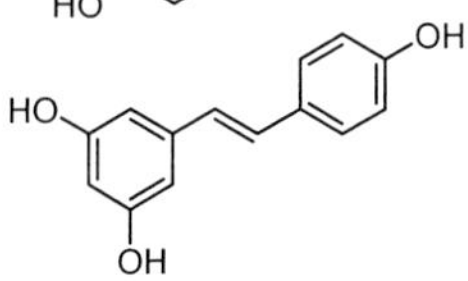

Resveratrol (**19**)

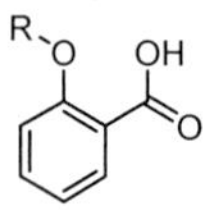

Aspirin™, R = $COCH_3$ (**20**)
Salicylic acid, R = H (**21**)

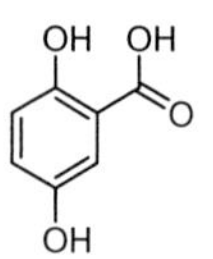

2,5-Dihydroxybenzoic acid (gentisic acid, **22**)

Fig. 6-1. Structures of antioxidants derived from plant sources.

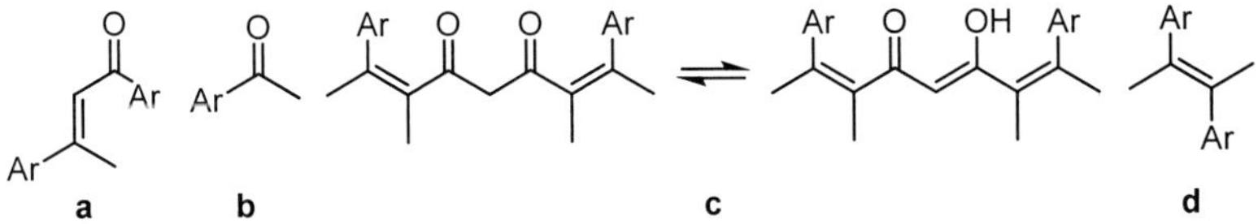

Fig. 6-2. Structures of chromophores of plant antioxidants. Ar = aromatic groups; **a** = silymarin and analogues; **b** = salicylic acid, daidzein, and analogues; **c** = curcumin tautomers; **d** = resveratrol.

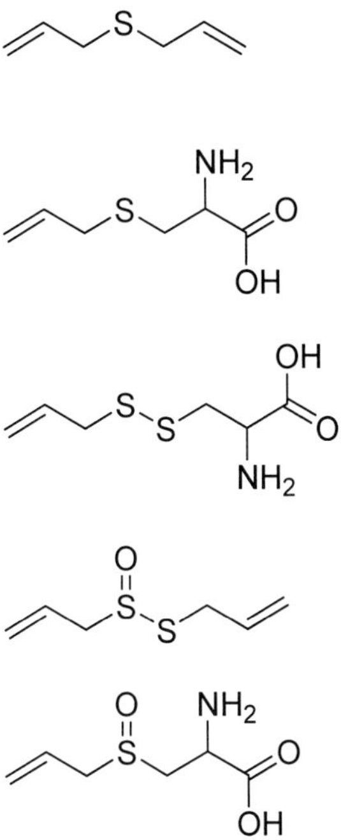

Diallyl sulfide (**23**)

S-Allylcysteine (SAC, **24**)

S-Allylmercaptocysteine (SAMC, **25**)

Diallyldisulfide oxide (Allicin, **26**)

S-Allyl-l-cysteine sulfoxide (Alliin, **27**)

Fig. 6-3. Structures of several compounds found in garlic and onions.

$$\underset{\mathbf{28}}{CH_2{=}CH{-}CH_2{-}S{-}OH} \xrightarrow{R\cdot} \underset{\mathbf{29}}{CH_2{=}CH{-}CH_2{-}S{-}O\cdot} + RH$$

Sch. 6-1. ROS oxidation of allicin.

Garlic, the European bulbous herb *Allium sativum*, and onion, the Asiatic herb *Allium cepa*, both of the lily family of *L. Lilliaceae* contain a number of unique organosulfur compounds, including diallyl sulfide (**23**), a powerful antioxidant with photochemopreventive properties [66–77]. Aged garlic extract contains two major water-soluble organosulfur compounds, *S*-allylcysteine (**24**), *S*-allylmercaptocysteine (**25**), or diallyldisulfide oxide (allicin, **26**), and *S*-allyl-L-cysteine sulfoxide (alliin, **27**), which have antioxidant activity [**Fig. 6-3**]. Mice fed a diet containing 4% aged garlic extract and exposed to moderate doses of UVBR had a large decrease in the suppression of the systemic contact hypersensitivity induced by UVBR [69]. The mechanism of this protection probably involves an antagonism of the *cis*-urocanic acid induced immunosuppression [5].

The garlic and onion compounds have very strong antioxidant scavenging properties. Thus, it was found that, in the presence of reactive oxygen species (ROS), the decomposition of allicin (**26**) produces propenyl sulfenic acid (**28**), which rapidly interacts with ROS (R·), similar to the hydroxyl groups, e.g. in vitamin E, to give a neutral radical (**29**) [**Sch. 6-1**] [78].

Garlic and onion compounds have not only antioxidation properties but also antibiotic, antithrombotic, anti-inflammatory, and antibacterial properties. Hence, they might be of potential medicinal value in causing a reduction of risk in such diseases as cardiovascular, diabetic, bowel, and neurodegenerative diseases, and, in general, as LOX and COX inhibitors [65, 70, 75–77]. A large number of studies have been conducted in recent years using endogenous and exogenous naturally occurring antioxidants in vitro and in vivo with animals and humans to establish the efficiencies of protection against UV radiation induced damages. The topical applications of antioxidants are somewhat limited by poor diffusion properties into the epidermis and their instabilities requiring reapplications to the skin. Studies with humans have provided some evidence that carotenoids and, to a lesser extent, α-tocopherol and ascorbate can be used to moderately protect against the UV radiation induced formation of erythema, although in most studies only a modest protection was obtained. Similarly, studies with large numbers of botanicals have rendered, in general, only modest efficiencies in protection. The oral photoprotection with supplements of naturally occurring antioxidants is easier than the topical applications. The oral supplementations with β-carotene and to a lesser extent with α-tocopherol, combined with ascorbate, were found to have a modest protection against photoinduced erythema, while the separate use of the antioxidants was ineffective, probably because of the essential restoration of the α-tocopherol by ascorbate. In any case, orally administered antioxidants cannot replace the regular topical sunscreen agents, but only serve as supplements. In conclusion, the results of many investigations could not provide unambiguous information on the efficiencies of prevention by topically and orally administered natural antioxidants against the photoinduced damages [2, 11, 14, 79].

References

1. Pinnell S. R. (2003) Cutaneous photodamage, oxidative stress, and topical antioxidant protection. *J. Am. Acad. Dermatol.* **48**: 1–22.
2. Cecarini J. P., Michel L., Marette J. M., Adhoute H. and Bejot M. (2003) Immediate effects of UV radiation on the skin: modification by antioxidant complex containing carotenoids. *Photodermatol., Photoimmunol. Photomed.* **19**: 182–189.
3. Afaq F. and Mukhtar H. (2002) Photochemoprevention by botanical antioxidants. *Skin Pharmacol. Appl. Skin Physiol.* **15**: 297–306.
4. Afaq F., Adhami V. M., Ahmad N. and Mukhtar H. (2002) Botanical antioxidants for chemoprevention of photocarcinogenesis. *Front. Biosci.* **7**: d784–792.
5. F'guyer S., Afaq F. and Mukhtar J. (2003) Photochemoprevention of skin cancer by botanical agents. *Photodermatol., Photoimmunol. Photomed.* **19**: 56–72.
6. Uliasz A. and Spencer J. M. (2004) Chemoprevention of skin cancer and photoaging. *Clin. Dermatol.* **22**: 178–182.
7. Spencer J. M. (2006) The exciting field of chemoprevention. *Skin Cancer Found. J.* **24**: 45–47.
8. Stratton S. P., Dorr R. T. and Alberts D. S. (2000) The state-of-the-art in chemoprevention of skin cancer. *Eur. J. Cancer* **36**: 1292–1297.
9. Koo S. W., Hirakawa S., Fujii S., Kawasumi M. and Nghiem P. (2007) Protection from photodamage by topical application of caffeine after ultraviolet irradiation. *Br. J. Dermatol.* **156**: 957–964.
10. Strickland F. M. (2001) Boosting the immune system. In: *Sun Protection in Man*, pp 613–636, Giacomoni, P. U. (ed.), Elsevier, Amsterdam.
11. Black H. S. and Rhodes L. E. (2001) Systemic photoprotection, dietary intervention and therapy. In: *Sun Protection in Man*, pp 573–591, Giacomoni, P. U. (ed.), Elsevier, Amsterdam.
12. Sorg O., Antille C. and Saurat J.-H. (2004) Retinoids, other topical vitamins, and antioxidants. In: *Photoaging*, pp 89–115, Rigel D. S., Weiss R. A., Lim H. W. and Dover J. S. (eds.), Marcel Dekker, New York and Basel.

13. Chaudhuri R. K. (2005) Role of antioxidants in sun care products. In: *Sunscreens. Regulations and Commercial Development*, 3rd ed., pp 603–638, Shaath N. A (ed.), Taylor and Francis, Boca Raton.
14. González S. and Gilaberte-Calzada Y. (2009) Oral and other non-sunscreen photoprotective agents. In: *Clinical Guide to Sunscreens and Photoprotection*, pp 207–222, Lim H. W. and Draelos Z. D. (eds.), Informa Healthcare, New York.
15. Nijveldt R. J., van Nood E., van Hoom D. E., Boelens P. G., van Norren K. and van Leeuwen P. A. M. (2001) Flavonoids: a review of probable mechanisms of action and potential applications. *Am. J. Clin. Nutr.* **74**: 418–425.
16. Balentine D. A., Wiseman S. A. and Bouwens L. C. (1997) The chemistry of tea flavonoids. *Crit. Rev. Food Sci. Nutr.* **37**: 693–704.
17. Birt D. F., Mitchell D., Gold B., Pour P. and Pinch H. C. (1997) Inhibition of ultraviolet light induced skin carcinogenesis in SKH-1 mice by apigenin, a plant flavonoid. *Anticancer Res.* **17**: 85–91.
18. McVean M., Weinberg W. C. and Pelling J. C. (2002) A p21(waf1)-independent pathway for inhibitory phosphorylation of cyclin-dependent kinase p34(cdc2) and concomitant G(2)/M arrest by the chemopreventive flavonoid apigenin. *Mol. Carcinog.* **33**: 36–43.
19. Lepley D. M. and Pelling J. C. (1997) Induction of p21/WAF1 and G1 cell-cycle arrest by the chemopreventive agent apigenin. *Mol. Carcinog.* **19**: 74–82.
20. Wagner J., Diesel P. and Seitz M. (1974) The chemistry and analysis of silymarin from Silybum marianum Gaertn. *Arzneimittelforschung* **24**: 466–471.
21. Comoglio A., Leonarduzzi G., Carini R., Busolin D., Basaga H., Albano E, Tomasi A., Poli G., Morazzoni P. and Magistretti M. J. (1990) Studies on the antioxidant and free radical scavenging properties of IdB 1016 a new flavanolignan complex. *Free Radical Res. Commun.* **11**: 109–115.
22. Katiyar S. K., Korman N. J., Mukhtar H. and Agarwal R. (1997) Protective effects of silymarin against photocarcinogenesis in a mouse skin model. *JNCI, J. Natl. Cancer Inst.* **89**: 556–566.
23. Shi H. and Niki E. (1998) Stoichiometric and kinetic studies on Ginkgo biloba extract and related antioxidants. *Lipids* **33**: 365–370.
24. Ozkur M. K., Bozkurt M. S., Balabanli B., Aricioglu A., Ilter N., Gurer M. A. and Inaloz H. S. (2002) The effects of Egb 761 on lipid peroxide levels and superoxide dismutase activity in sunburn. *Photodermatol., Photoimmunol. Photomed.* **18**: 117–120.

25. Lin S. Y. and Chang, H. P. (1997) Induction of superoxide dismutase and catalase activity in different rat tissues and protection from UVB irradiation after topical application of Ginkgo biloba extracts. *Methods Find. Exp. Clin. Pharmacol.* **19**: 367–371.
26. Wei H., Wei L., Frenkel K., Bowen R. and Barnes S. (1993) Inhibition of tumor promoter-induced hydrogen peroxide formation in vitro and in vivo by genistein. *Nutr. Cancer* **20**: 1–12.
27. Wei H., Bowen R., Zhang X. and Lebwohl M. (1998) Isoflavone genistein inhibits the initiation and promotion of two-stage skin carcinogenesis in mice. *Carcinogenesis* **19**: 1509–1514.
28. Widyarini S., Spinks N., Husband A. J. and Reeve V. E. (2001) Isoflavonoid compounds from red clover (*Trifolium pratense*) protect from inflammation and immune suppression induced by UV radiation. *Photochem. Photobiol.* **74**: 465–470.
29. Mukhtar H., Wang Z. Y., Katiyar S. K. and Agarwal R. (1992) Tea components: antimutagenic and anticarcinogenic effects. *Prev. Med.* **21**: 351–360.
30. Elmets C. A., Singh D., Tubesing K., Matsui M., Katiyar S. and Mukhtar H. (2001) Cutaneous photoprotection from ultraviolet injury by green tea polyphenols. *J. Am. Acad. Dermatol.* **44**: 425–432.
31. Katiyar S. K., Perez A. and Mukhtar H. (2000) Green tea polyphenol treatment to human skin prevents formation of ultraviolet light B-induced pyrimidine dimers in DNA. *Clin. Cancer Res.* **6**: 3864–3869.
32. McVean M. and Liebler D. C. (1997) Inhibition of UVB induced DNA photodamage in mouse epidermis by topically applied alpha-tocopherol. *Carcinogenesis* **18**: 1617–1622.
33. Chen W., Barthelman M., Martinez J., Alberts D. and Gensler H. L. (1997) Inhibition of cyclobutane pyrimidine dimer formation in epidermal p53 gene of UV-irradiated mice by alpha-tocopherol. *Nutr. Cancer* **29**: 205–211.
34. Yuen K. S. and Halliday G. M. (1997) Alpha-tocopherol, an inhibitor of epidermal lipid peroxidation, prevents ultraviolet radiation from suppressing the skin immune system. *Photochem. Photobiol.* **65**: 587–592.
35. Sorg O., Tran C., Carraux P., Didierjean L., Falson F. and Saurat J. H. (2002) Oxidative stress-independent depletion of epidermal vitamin A by UVA. *J. Invest. Dermatol.* **118**: 513–518.
36. Mireles-Rocha H., Galindo I., Huerta M., Trujillo-Hernandez B., Elizalde A. and Cortes-Franco R. (2002) UVB photoprotection with antioxidants: effects of oral therapy with d-alpha-tocopherol and

ascorbic acid on the minimal erythema dose. *Acta Derm.-Venereol.* **82**: 21–24.
37. Conney A. H., Lysz T., Ferraro T., Abidi T. F., Manchand P. S., Laskin J. D. and Huang M. T. (1991) Inhibitory effect of curcumin and some related dietary components on tumor promotion and arachidonic acid metabolism in mouse skin. *Adv. Enzyme Regul.* **31**: 385 –396.
38. Huang M. T., Lou Y. R., Newmark H. L., Reuhl K. R. and Conney A. H. (1994) Inhibitory effects of dietary curcumin on forestomach, duodenal, and colon carcinogenesis in mice. *Cancer Res.* **54**: 5841–5847.
39. Huang M. T., Newmark H. L. and Frenkel K. (1997) Inhibitory effects of curcumin on tumorigenesis in mice. *J. Cell Biochem.* **27** (Suppl.): 26–34.
40. Huang M. T., Smart R. C., Wong C. Q. and Conney A. H. (1988) Inhibitory effect of curcumin, chlorogenic acid, caffeic acid, and ferulic acid on tumor promotion in mouse skin by 12-O-tetradecanoylphorbol-13-acetate. *Cancer Res.* **48**: 5941–5946.
41. Sharma R. A., McLelland H. R., Hill K. A., Ireson C. R., Euden S. A., Manson M. M., Pirmohamed M., Marnett L. J., Gescher A. J. and Steward W. P. (2001) Pharmacodynamic and pharmacokinetic study of oral curcumin extract in patients with colorectal cancer. *Cancer Clin. Cancer Res.* **7**: 1894–1900.
42. Cheng A. L., Hsu C. H., Lin J. K., Hsu M. M., Ho Y. F., Shen T. S., et al. (2001) Phase I clinical trial of curcumin, a chemopreventive agent, in patients with high-risk or pre-malignant lesions. *Anticancer Res.* **21**: 2895–2900.
43. Aggarwal B. B., Kumar A. and Bhart A. C. (2003) Anticancer potential of curcumin: preclinical and clinical studies. *Anticancer Res.* **23**: 363–398.
44. Nakamura Y., Ohto Y., Murakami A., Osawa T. and Ohigashi H. (1998) Inhibitory effects of curcumin and tetrahydrocurcuminoids on the tumor promoter-induced reactive oxygen species generation in leukocytes in vitro and in vivo. *Jpn. J. Cancer Res.* **89**: 361–370.
45. Shim J. S., Kim J. H., Cho H. Y., Yum Y. N., Kim S. H., Park H. J., Shim B. S, Choi S. H, Kwon H. J. (2003) Irreversible inhibition of CD13/amino-peptidase N by the antiangiogenic agent curcumin. *Chem. Biol.* **10**: 695–704.
46. Jee S. H., Shen. S. C., Tseng C. R., Chiu H. C. and Kuo M. L. (1998) Curcumin induces a p53-dependent apoptosis in human basal cell carcinoma cells. *J. Invest. Dermatol.* **111**: 656–661.

47. Bush J. A., Cheung K. J. Jr. and Li G. (2001) Curcumin induces apoptosis in human melanoma cells through a Fas receptor/caspase-8 pathway independent of p53. *Exp. Cell Res.* **271**: 305–314.
48. Iersel M. L., Ploemen J. P., Struik I., van Amersfoort C., Keyzer A. E., Schefferlie J. G. and van Bladeren P. J. (1996) Inhibition of glutathione S-transferase activity in human melanoma cells by alpha,beta-unsaturated carbonyl derivatives. Effects of acrolein, cinnamaldehyde, citral, crotonaldehyde, curcumin, ethacrynic acid, and *trans*-2-hexenal. *Chem.-Biol. Interact.* **102**: 117–132.
49. Chignell C. F., Bilski P., Reszka K. J., Motten A. G., Sik R. H. and Dahl T. A. (1994) Spectral and photochemical properties of curcumin. *Photochem. Photobiol.* **59**: 295–302.
50. Subramaniam D., May R., Sureban S. M., Lee K. B., George R., Kuppusamy P., Ramanujam R. P., Hideg K., Dieckgraefe B. K., Houchen C. W. and Anant S. (2008) Diphenyl difluoroketone: a curcumin derivative with potent *in vivo* anticancer activity. *Cancer Res.* **66**: 1962–1969.
51. Kálai T., Kuppusamy M. L., Balog M., Selvendiran K., Rivera B. K., Kuppusamy P. and Higed K. (2011) Synthesis of N-substituted 3,5-bis(arylidene)-4-piperidones with high antitumor and antioxidant activity. *J. Med. Chem.* **54**: 5414–5421.
52. Selvendiran K., Ahmed S., Dayton A., Kappusamy M. L., Rivera B. K., Kálai T., Hideg K. and Kappusamy P. (2011) HO-3867, a curcumin analog, sensitizes cisplatin-resistant ovarian carcinoma, leading to therapeutic synergy through STAT3 inhibition. *Cancer Biol. Ther.* **12**: 837–845.
53. Dayton A., Selvendiran K., Kappusamy M. L., Rivera B. K., Meduru S., Kálai T., Hideg K. and Kappusamy P. (2011) Cellular uptake, retention and bioabsorption of HO-3867, a fluorinated curcumin analog with potential antitumor properties. *Cancer Biol. Ther.* **12**: 1027–1032.
54. Schwack W. and Rudolph T. (1995) Photochemistry of dibenzoylmethane UVA filters. Part 1. *J. Photochem. Photobiol., B* **28**: 229–234.
55. Damiani E., Greci L., Parsons R. and Knowland J. (1999) Nitroxide radicals protect DNA from damage when illuminated in vitro in the presence of dibenzoylmethane and a common sunscreen ingredient. *Free Radical Biol. Med.* **26**: 809–816.
56. Jang M., Cai L., Udeani G. O., Slowing K. V., Thomas C. F., Beecher C. W., Fong H. H., Farnsworth N. R., Kinghorn A. D., Mehta R. G., Moon R. C. and Pezzuto J. M. (1997) Cancer chemopreventive

activity of resveratrol, a natural product derived from grapes. *Science* **275**: 218–220.
57. Afaq F., Adhami V. M. and Ahmad N. (2003) Prevention of short-term ultraviolet B radiation-mediated damages by resveratrol. *Toxicol. Appl. Pharmacol.* **186**: 28–37.
58. Subbaramaiah K., Chung W. J., Michaluart P., Telang N., Tanabe T., Inoue H., Jang M., Pezzuto J. M. and Dannenberg A. J. (1998) Resveratrol inhibits cyclooxygenase-2 transcription and activity in phorbol ester-treated human mammary epithelial cells. *J. Biol. Chem.* **273**: 21875–21882.
59. Subbaramaiah K., Michaluart P., Chung W. J., Tanabe T., Telang N. and Dannenberg A. J. (1999) Resveratrol inhibits cyclooxygenase-2 transcription in human mammary epithelial cells. *Ann. N. Y. Acad. Sci.* **889**: 214–223.
60. Adhami V. M., Afaq F. and Ahmad N. (2003) Prevention of skin neoplasia by resveratrol: involvement of nuclear transcription factor NF-κB. *Neoplasia* **5**: 74–82.
61. Kálai T., Borza E., Antus C., Radnai B., Gulyás-Fekete G., Fehér A., Sümegi B. and Hideg K. (2011) Synthesis and study of new para-magnetic resveratrol analogues. *Bioorg. Med. Chem.* **19**: 7311–7317.
62. Orentreich D., Leone A.-S., Arpino G. and Burack H. (2001) Sun-screens: practical application. In: *Sun Protection in Man*, pp 535–559, Giacomoni P. U. (ed.), Elsevier Science, Amsterdam.
63. Rainsford K. D. (1985) Salicylates. In: *Anti-Inflammatory and Anti-Rheumatic Drugs*, pp 109–148, Rainsford K. D. and Path M. R. S. (eds.), CRC Press, Boca Raton.
64. Gerhardt C. (1853) Untersuchungen über die wasserfreien organ-ischen Säuren. *Ann. Chem. Pharm.* **87**: 149–179.
65. Méric J.-B., Rottey S., Olaussen K., Soria J.-C., Khayat D., Rixe O. and Spano J. P. (2006) Cyclooxygenase-2 as a target for anticancer drug development. *Crit. Rev. Oncol./Hematol.* **59**: 51–64.
66. Amagase H., Petesch B. L., Matsuura H., Kasuga S. and Itakura Y. (2001) Intake of garlic and its bioactive components. *J. Nutr.* **131**: 955S–962S.
67. Block E. (1985) The chemistry of garlic and onions. *Sci. Am.* **252**: 114–119.
68. Rouvray D. (2004) Benefiting from bad breath. *Chem. World* **1**: 36–40.
69. Moriguchi T., Saito H. and Nishiyama N. (1997) Anti-ageing effect of aged garlic extract in the inbred brain atrophy mouse model. *Clin. Exp. Pharmacol. Physiol.* **24**: 235–242.

70. Takasu J., Uykimpang R., Sunga M., Amagase H. and Niihara Y. (2006) Aged garlic extract is a potential therapy for sickle-cell anemia. *J. Nutr.* **136**: 803S–805S.
71. Amagase H., Schaffer E. M. and Milner J. A. (1996) Dietary components modify the ability of garlic to suppress 7,12-dimethylbenz[*a*]-anthracene-induced mammary DNA adducts. *J. Nutr.* **126**: 817–824.
72. Ide N. and Lau B. H. (1997) Garlic compounds protect vascular endothelial cells from oxidized low-density lipoprotein-induced injury. *J. Pharm. Pharmacol.* **49**: 908–911.
73. Imai J., Ide N., Nagae S., Moriguchi T., Matsuura H. and Itakura Y. (1994) Antioxidant and radical scavenging effects of aged garlic extract and its constituents. *Planta Med.* **60**: 417–420.
74. Reeve V. E., Bosnic M., Rozinova E. and Boehm-Wilcox C. (1993) A garlic extract protects from ultraviolet B (280–320) radiation-induced suppression of contact hypersensitivity. *Photochem. Photobiol.* **58**: 813–817.
75. Chung L. Y. (2006) The antioxidant properties of garlic compounds: allyl cysteine, alliin, allicin, and allyl disulfide. *J. Med. Food* **9**: 205–213.
76. Wilson E. A. and Demmig-Adams B. (2007) Antioxidant, anti-inflamatory, and antimicrobial properties of garlic and onion. *Nutr. Food Sci.* **37**: 178–183.
77. Block E. (2009) *Garlic and other alliums. The lore and the science*, RSC Publishing, Cambridge.
78. Vaidya V., Ingold K. U. and Pratt D. A. (2009) Garlic: source of the ultimate antioxidants – sulfenic acids. *Angew. Chem., Int. Ed.* **48**: 157–160.
79. Blade H. S. and Rodes L. E. (2001) Systemic photoprotection. Dietary intervention and therapy. In: *Sun Protection in Man*, pp 575–591, Giacomoni P. U. (ed.), Elsevier Science, Amsterdam.

CHAPTER SEVEN

CRITICAL APPRAISALS OF ORAL SUPPLEMENTATIONS OF ENDOGENOUS AND EXOGENOUS ANTIOXIDANTS IN MEDICINAL EVALUATIONS

A. Evaluations of Vitamin E and Other Endogenous Antioxidants as Drugs against Various Diseases Including Cancers

It is believed that exogenous and hereditary factors are involved in the initiation and development of various diseases including cancers, and it has been estimated that 75–80% of all human maladies are environmentally induced and perhaps 30–40% of them by diet. On the basis of very extensive research over the years, it is now believed that free radicals, in particular reactive oxygen species (ROS), have an important role in the initiation and promotions of various diseases, including cancers. Hence, it is not unreasonable to conclude that various endogenous and exogenous antioxidants, such as vitamin E, vitamin C, alpha-lipoic acid, carotenoids, and nonsteroidal anti-inflamatory drugs, when orally administered could be used to alter the incidences of various diseases, including cancers, and function either as preventive agents or drugs for cure.

A very large number of investigations have been conducted in the past fifty years, such as case-control studies, cohort studies and meta-analysis trials in order to establish the usefulness of antioxidants, such as vitamin E, vitamin C, α-lipoic acid, β-carotene, other carotenoids, and occasionally other antioxidative species like selenium as possible drugs either for prevention or cure for various diseases, including various cancers.

At the onset, it is apparent that the use of test substances for oral supplementations at the dietary endogenous level like those found in the human body, and various exogenous substances found in various plants, herbs and extracts, such as green tea would not produce the desired effects in a foreseeable timespan. Hence, the question arises as to what dosage levels of various antioxidants would be required to achieve the desired results. By inspecting a large number of various studies, one has the impression that the dosage levels have been chosen at random. Nevertheless, the dosages for vitamin E ranging between 16.5–3200 IU were covered, although it was stated in many cases that 400–600 IU (267–400 mg) are high doses and could produce ill health effects. This kind of cautious attitude is not warranted [1], since, on a conversion of IU to milligram, it is evident that these doses are equivalent to about one Aspirin™ tablet or a half tablet of Tylenol®, which are real drugs consumed by large numbers of people without any dangerous consequences.

In various medicinal trials, it is often not clear what type of vitamin E is used for oral supplementation. It has been known for many years [2] that vitamin E exists as eight different stereoisomers [**Table 7A-1**].

Table 7A-1. The biologically important vitamin E is the stereoisomer 2*R*,4*R*,8*R* = RRR-d-α-tocopherol. Synthetic vitamin E is a mixture of eight stereoisomers, including d-α-tocopherol. This mixture is called all-racemic-dl-tocopherol. Isolating the individual stereoisomers is a difficult task. In this table, all stereoisomers are shown as well as their activities in percent compared to RRR-α-tocopherol. In addition, interconversions from IU to milligram are shown for d-α-tocopherol. The 667 mg dose of d-α-tocopherol equals in size but not in activity two 325 mg Aspirin™ tablets, and the 1000 mg dose of d-α-tocopherol equals in size but not in activity two 500 mg acetaminophen (Tylenol®, Advil®) tablets.

Configurations of d-α-Tocopherol Stereoisomers	Biological Activity (IU/mg) Compared to d-α-Tocopherol (%)		Dosages of d-α-Tocopherol	
			in IU	in mg
2*R*,4*R*,8*R*	1.5	100	1.499 ~ 1.5	1.0
2*S*,4*R*,8*R*	0.46	31	1.0	0.667
2*R*,4*R*,8*S*	1.34	89	100	66.7
2S,4*R*,8*S*	0.55	37	400	267
2*R*,4*S*,8*S*	1.09	73	600	400
2*S*,4*S*,8*R*	0.31	21	800	537
2*R*,4*S*,8*R*	0.85	57	1000	667
2*S*,4*S*,8*S*	1.10	73	2000	1334
			3000	2000
			4000	2668
			~4500	3000
			~4800	3200
			~5247	3500

The biologically most important stereoisomer is RRR-α-tocopherol or, more precisely, the 2*R*,4*R*,8*R* stereoisomer, in practice also denoted as d-α-tocopherol. This natural 100% isomer is one single compound. All other stereoisomers are less active [**Table 7A-1**]. Synthetic vitamin E is the all-racemic mixture of dl-α-tocopherol composed of all eight stereoisomers. This racemate is unfortunately sometimes also used in clinical trials. Aside from the different activities of the various vitamin E stereoisomers and the racemate, it is also important to be aware of the metabolisms of various isomers in the human body [3–5].

In the human body, on oral consumption, the all-*rac*-d-α-tocopherol, i.e., the mixture of all stereoisomers, is first delivered to the intestine and then transferred to the liver. The liver regulates the selective absorption of only one stereoisomer, namely RRR-α-tocopherol using the specific RRR-α-tocopherol transfer protein (α-TTP), which is encoded by the gene ttp, located at the 8q13.1-13.3 region of chromosome 8. The protein α-TTP was isolated and crystallized and the DNA sequence was determined [3–5]. After absorption, the α-TTP-d-α-tocopherol complex is transferred to the plasma membranes where alpha-tocopherol is released and absorbed by lipoproteins [3–5]. All other isomers are present in the plasma only in small amounts [5]. The plasma contains d-α-tocopherol in the range 11–37 μmol/liter, the other isomers about 1–5 μmol/liter [5]. The half-life of d-α-tocopherol in plasma is about 48 hours, those of the other isomers are much shorter. These isomers are metabolized similarly to xenobiotics via ω-oxidation by cytochrome P450, β-oxidations, conjugations, and excretions without utilization by the human body [3–5].

d-α-Tocopherol is also found in the human skin in the dermis and epidermis at 15 and 30 nmol/g of tissue, respectively, 20–25 nmol/mL in plasma, 45 nmol/g in the heart, and 356 nmol/g in fat tissue [6]. The UV radiation of the human skin causes a considerable destruction of the vitamin [7]. Hence, the inclusion of vitamin E into sunscreen formulations may have only a very limited benefit. (See **Section 5**.)

In many medicinal studies and in personal care products, tocopheryl acetate and succinate are used because of their higher stability than the regular unprotected tocopherols. In these compounds, the vital phenolic group, which is essential for the antioxidative properties, is protected by conversion to the esters, and, hence cannot function, unless the protective group is deblocked. The ineffectiveness of tocophenyl esters has been described in many publications [8–13].

Furthermore, the all-important α-tocopherol transfer protein, α-TTP, has different affinities for various forms of tocopherols. Thus, in the case of RRR-α-tocopherol, the affinity is 100%, while with α-tocopheryl acetate it is only 2%. Accordingly, the ester is actually not absorbed and not utilized by the human body. Another very important factor that is often overlooked in medicinal studies is the necessity to maintain vitamin E as an active antioxidant. It is well established that α-tocopheryloxy radical, which is formed in reactions with reactive oxygen species and other oxidants, is a resonance-stabilized radical and inactive as antioxidant. (See **Section 5**.) However, this radical can be converted into the original tocopherol by continuous reduction with ascorbic acid. The reduction of the oxidized vitamin E species can be readily achieved, because the redox potential of vitamin C is below that of vitamin E. This synergistic "chaperone" effect by vitamin C is of great value. Thus, it was shown on various occasions that reactions using vitamin E and C separately produced no desired effect, while reactions using both vitamins produced excellent results. It is important to use vitamin C in excess of vitamin E [10–14].

A group of children, who had been receiving anticonvulsant drug therapy over a long period of time, received 400 IU/day of vitamin E supplementation as an added therapy, resulting in a noticeable reduction in seizures and improvements in seizure control [15].

Patients with early symptoms of Parkinson's disease received daily 3200 IU of vitamin E and 3000 mg of vitamin C for about 66 months when therapy with levodopa was required to treat the symptoms. Nevertheless, patients on the antioxidants therapy progressed for two and a half years longer than the untreated patients before levodopa was required [16].

A similar group with Parkinson's disease received 400–3200 IU/day of vitamin E for an average of seven years. The disease was significantly less severe in vitamin E supplemented patients [17].

In a large number of trials with Alzheimer patients using vitamin E supplements, it was concluded that supplementations with vitamin E cause a slowdown of the progression of the disease in patients with moderately severe impairments, in particular in cases where vitamin E doses of IU 2000/day were administered [18].

In a double-blind trial, 341 patients with Alzheimer's disease were treated for two years either with a mixture of 2000 IU of vitamin E and seligiline 10 mg/day, or selegiline alone, using for diagnosis the delaying of the primary outcome of disease progression, such as either the inability to perform basic activities, need for institutionalization, or death. The primary endpoint was 53% lower in the group of patients who received the vitamin E supplementation alone, 34% who were treated with selegiline alone, and 31% with patients who took a mixture of vitamin E and selegiline, as compared to the group on placebo [19, 20].

The effect of UV radiations on the delayed type of hypersensitivity (DTH) was investigated with 32 healthy 60-year-old adults using as supplements either 800 mg/day of vitamin E for 30 days or a placebo. In the group with vitamin supplementation, a significant improvement in the DTH response was noticeable in most but not all participants [21]. In a double-blind study with 74 participants aged 65 years and older, a supplementation of the diet with 100 mg/day of vitamin E had no significant effect [22].

In a case-control study, 356 patients with macular degeneration and 520 controls, all aged 55–80 years, who received carotenoids were found to have a 43% lower risk for the age-related degeneration as compared to controls, whereby zeaxanthin and lutein were most strongly associated with a decreased risk [23].

In a study with 152 participants who had cataracts and 152 cataract-free patients, a 50% decrease in cataract risk resulted in persons who regularly used vitamin E supplementation [24].

In a similar study with 764 participants, the risk of nuclear opacification decreased by 57% in persons who regularly took vitamin E supplements [25].

In a study with 976 participants who were 40 years old and older, it was found that persons with plasma vitamin levels in the lowest quartile had a double risk of the age-related macular degeneration, while persons with higher plasma levels of vitamin E and C and β-carotene were protected against the age-related macular degeneration. Nevertheless, there was no correlation between the age-related macular degeneration and the use of vitamin supplements [26].

The daily oral administration to 40 volunteers for 50 days of a mixture of 2 grams of vitamin E and 3 grams of vitamin C caused a significant suppression of the UV light induced sunburns (erythema, MED), whereas vitamin E in the absence of vitamin C was ineffective. Thus, it is obvious that both vitamins are synergistically effective [10].

An analogous trial using 1000 IU of vitamin E and 2 grams of vitamin C per day caused an increased median protection against erythema, while the use of either vitamin E or C resulted in no significant protection. Hence, it is evident that both vitamins cause synergistically the suppression of the erythema effect [14].

Healthy volunteers received orally 400 IU/day supplementation of α-tocopheryl acetate during a period of six months without protection against the UVB induced sunburn reaction (erythema) [13, 27].

In another study, 20 volunteers received 500 IU of RRR-α-tocopherol either alone or in combination with 25 mg of carotenoids per day for a period of 12 weeks. The erythema was produced by using a blue-light solar simulator. The erythema suppression was somewhat more pronounced with a combination of β-carotene and vitamin E, although the difference was statistically insignificant [28].

A toxicity study was conducted by the National Institute of Arthritis, Metabolism, and Digestive Diseases with 28 adults over a period of 3 years. The administration of vitamin E ranged between 100 and 800 IU, causing no side effects in either the kidneys, liver, muscles, blood cells, or the thyroid gland, or coagulations [29].

Clinical trials were conducted with vitamin E administered to patients for up to 11 years with doses ranging from 200 IU to more than 3000 IU per day. These regimes were well tolerated by patients with only 0.8% minor side effects, such as gastrointestinal disturbances, dermatitis, and fatigue [30].

Administration to patients of vitamin E ranging between 600 and 1200 IU daily caused no detectable side effects. A minimal dose of 400 IU was required to achieve a decrease in susceptibility to LDL oxidation [31]. Intravenous injections of 1000 mg of α-lipoic acid into patients with Type II diabetes caused an enhancement of the insulin-stimulated glucose disposal by about 50% [32]. Analogous results were obtained with a 500 mg supplementation of α-lipoic acid for 10 days. In this case the effect was 30% [33].

Clinical improvements were achieved with Type I and Type II diabetes patients by administering 600 mg of α-lipoic acid per day for two weeks, followed by 300 mg/day for 10 weeks, and then, either a 1571 IU administration of vitamin E for 10 weeks, or 100 mcg/day of selenium for 12 weeks [34–36]. A vitamin E supplement of 900 mg/day for 3 weeks was well tolerated by 25 Type II diabetic patients without side effects in liver and renal functions [37]. In another trial, 18 patients orally received 3200 mg of vitamin E per day for 9 weeks, resulting in only minor side effects, such as diarrhea and intestinal cramps [38].

In several trials, it was found that administration to patients of at least 100 IU of vitamin E per day over a period of 2 years resulted in less coronary artery disease progression and a 37% lower relative risk of coronary disease as compared to patients on placebo [39, 40].

A group of 11178 patients aged 67–105 years who took simultaneously vitamin E and C were found to have a 53% decreased risk of coronary heart disease mortality, while the use of vitamin E alone decreased the risk of coronary heart disease mortality by 47% [41]. The results of a randomized, double-blind, placebo-controlled secondary prevention trial of the benefits and risks of antioxidant vitamins (vitamins E and C, and β-carotene) among 8000 women with preexisting CVD have also been reported [42].

A double-blind, randomized, and placebo-controlled trial with 103 patients was conducted by orally administering 525 IU of α-tocopherol 48 hours before, 24 hours before, and in the morning prior to the coronary procedures. The conclusions of this study were that oral vitamin E administrations are prophylactive against the contrast-induced nephropathy in patients with chronic kidney diseases undergoing coronary procedures [43].

A randomized, double-blind, placebo-controlled trial with 231 patients, who have had either coronary angiography or intervention, were given 3 grams of ascorbic acid at least 2 hours before the procedure, 2 grams at night, and 2 grams in the morning after the procedure. The conclusion was that the preventive oral administration of ascorbic acid may protect against the contrast-medicated nephropathy in high risk patients with venal disfunctions and in patients undergoing coronary procedures [44].

The results of antioxidant supplements for the prevention of mortality were obtained from many randomized trials involving 232550 participants, including healthy participants and participants with various diseases such as gastrointestinal, cardiovascular, neurogical, ocular, dermatological, venal, endocrinological, rheumatoid, and unspecified, using the antioxidants vitamin A, C, E, β-carotene, and selenium versus placebo. The goal was to establish the effectiveness of these antioxidants for the prevention of mortality in healthy patients and in patients with various diseases. The conclusions were that these antioxidant supplements had no preventive effects, and that vitamins A and E and β-carotene may have a negative effect [45].

A randomized, double-blind, placebo-controlled study involving 14641 male physicians was conducted to establish whether the antioxidants vitamins E and C could cause a decrease in risk of major cardiovascular events in men. The oral supplements were 400 IU of vitamin E administered every other day and 500 mg of vitamin C daily. After 8 years of follow-up, it was found that 1245 major cardiovascular events occurred. The conclusions were that, compared to placebo, both vitamins E and C had no effect on the incidents of major cardiovascular events [46].

A similar randomized, controlled trial was conducted with healthy women using 600 IU of natural-source vitamin E on alternate days for 10.1 years for the prevention of cardiovascular disease and cancer. The conclusions were that such supplements with vitamin E provide no benefit for major cardiovascular events and cancer and have no influence on the total mortality [47].

A randomized factorial trial was conducted with 8171 female health professionals during a period of 9.4 years using a mixture of ascorbic acid, 500 mg/day, vitamin E, 600 IU every other day, and β-carotene, 50 mg every other day. The goal was to establish the effects of these antioxidants on the combined outcome of the myocardial infarction, stroke, coronary revascularization, and cardiovascular disease death among the female participants. The conclusion was that there were no significant overall effects of these antioxidants on the cardiovascular events among women at high risk of cardiovascular disease death [48].

Furthermore, the supplementation with vitamin C, vitamin E, or β-carotene offers no overall benefits in the primary prevention of total either cancer incidence, or cancer mortality in participating women [49].

A small number of 43 patients with mild dementia, i.e., Alzheimer's disease, that was progressing very slowly, were treated over a period of 48 month with supplements of 600 mg/day of α-lipoic acid. The treatment resulted in a stabilization of cognitive functions [50, 51].

In non-melanoma cell carcinoma prevention trials, the participants were segregated into three groups based on their serum concentrations of carotenoids, α-tocopherol, and selenium, and were monitored for incidents, histologically confirmed basal cell carcinoma (BCC), and squamous cell carcinoma (SCC) for a period of 8 years. The conclusions were that selenium concentrations are associated with an approximately 60% decrease in subsequent cancer incidents for BCC and SCC, while serum concentrations of carotenoids and α-tocopherol are not associated with later skin cancer incidents [52, 53].

A double-blind, randomized, placebo-controlled trial was conducted involving 35533 male participants over a period of 7–12 years to investigate the effect of selenium and vitamin E on the risk of prostate and other cancers. Selenium, 200 micrograms per day, was administered as L-selenomethionine and vitamin E, 400 IU, as the all-racemic α-tocopheryl acetate. The main outcome was pursued for prostate cancers, and secondary outcome for lung, colorectal, and overall primary cancers, and Type 2 diabetes mellitus. The outcome was that neither selenium nor vitamin E alone, nor in combination, at the doses employed, had any preventive effects on the population of healthy men [54]. However, since in this trial [54] vitamin E was used as racemic α-tocopheryl acetate, a diminished activity was to be expected [8–13, 55].

A randomized, double-blind, placebo-controlled preventive trial was conducted testing the possible effects of β-carotene, retinol, and α-tocopherol supplementation on cancer incidences in adult male smokers. Cancer survival was examined by the Kaplan–Meier method. There were diagnosed 1891 men with prostate cancer and 395 persons died from this disease. The high serum levels of α-tocopherol were associated with improved prostate cancer survivals, while β-carotene and retinol had no influences [56]. In a ten-year cohort study with 35242 men, it was found that the risk for advanced prostate cancer significantly decreased with greater daily supplementations of Vitamin E [57].

Negative results were obtained in a large, long-term trial for the prevention of prostate and total cancer in men using oral supplementation of 500 mg/day of vitamin C and 400 IU of vitamin E every other day. The conclusions of this trial were that neither vitamin C nor vitamin E supplementations reduced the risk of prostate and total cancers [58].

Meta-analyses involving 19 randomized trials were conducted with 135967 participants during a period of about 38 years. Nine of the trials investigated vitamin E supplementations combined with other materials, such as vitamin C, β-carotene, selenium, Aspirin™, garlic oil, fish oil, hormones, selegiline, zinc, copper, and others. The dosages of vitamin E ranged between 16.5 IU to 2000 IU per day with a median dosage of 400 IU/day. The vitamin sources and specific configurations were not well defined probably because of a diversity of biological activities that were reported from various studies and then related to the all-racemic α-tocopheryl acetate. Clinical results with vitamin E and the risk for all mortality data were apparently provided by institutions from nine countries: USA, Canada, England, Italy, Israel, China, Australia, Finland, and France. The pooled, all-cause mortality risk data in the so-called high dosage level, ≥ 400 IU/day, were often small and performed in patients with chronic diseases. The conclusions were as quoted, "High dosage (≥ 400 IU/day) vitamin E supplements may increase all-cause mortality and should be avoided." [59]

It is important to be aware that vitamin E is a lipophilic substance. This property has been usually ignored in administering vitamin E to participants in numerous medical trials. In a simple experiment, it was shown that an administration of 300 mg (447 IU) of vitamin E every day with food to a group of participants over a period of only 15 days resulted in an increase of plasma vitamin E in participants to 84% as compared to 29% increase in the group of participants who received vitamin E without food. Furthermore, the lipid peroxide scavenging activity increased in the group with lipophilic supplementations by 14%, while no change occurred in the group that received vitamin E without food [60].

By analyzing the at randomly selected examples of various medicinal studies [15–58], one arrives at the conclusion that vitamin E and C are well tolerated by humans even at high dosages of 3200 mg/day over long periods, such as ten years and longer [1, 29–31, 37, 38]. It is evident that, to achieve good results, vitamin E should be used in conjunction with vitamin C [10–14]. The concerns about the toxicity of vitamin E and C are unfounded on the basis of the following considerations. In analyzing various clinical studies and trials it is evident that no attention has been paid to the modality of oral intake of vitamin E. This detail can be of paramount importance for the outcome of clinical investigations. Since vitamin E is a lipophilic substance and is processed in the human body via the lipophilic pathways by the α-tocopherol transfer protein (α-TTP) [3–5], it is important that vitamin E should be consumed with lipophilic food stuff [60] for maximum utilization by the human body and not just with plain water, e.g., with olive oil in conjunction with vitamin C as part of a salad instead of vinegar. Thus, it is possible to make assessments of the lethal levels of these vitamins on the basis of LD_{50} values that were obtained with other mammals [**Table 7A-2**]. On the basis of these results, the lethal dosages for a 70 kg (154 lb) human can be estimated to be about 600 mL (1 pint) of vitamin E and about 1 liter (~1 quart, ~1 kg) for vitamin C. These estimates mean that vitamin E is rated as slightly toxic to moderately toxic, as, for example, the common table salt, and vitamin C is slightly to practically nontoxic [**Table 7A-2**]. α-Lipoic acid is in the toxicity category of vitamin E and β-carotene [**Table 7A-2**] [61]. It is of interest that, in various medicinal studies, no international units were used for α-lipoic acid and β-carotene. In most studies, 50 mg of β-carotene were used for oral supplementations. The international units for β-carotene are known, i.e., one IU = 0.6 μg = 0.0006 mg (USA) and 0.3 μg (Canadian). In the case where one would prefer to consume natural carrots instead of β-carotene, one would have to consume with each oral supplement about 758 grams of carrots, since 100 g of carrots contain 6.6 mg of β-carotene. In some studies, the antioxidant selenium has been used with promising results. In general, it seems that in case-control studies, more meaningful results were obtained than in cohort studies and meta-analysis studies. The inspection of many clinical studies reveals a large number of inconsistencies and contradictory results and interpretations on the same topics [62, 63]. This is actually not surprising in view of the manifold of experimental designs and result evaluations. In this connection, for example, the meta-analysis [59] contains many incongruities. Thus, one of the problems is that, since the biological activities of vitamin E compounds differed among isomeric forms in various studies, the biological activities of vitamin E compounds are reported relative to all-racemic α-tocopheryl acetate. The biological ineffectiveness of tocopheryl acetate and tocopheryl succinate has been reported on many occasions over the years [8–13]. The study has been extensively criticized, and cited in an excellent review [5]. On the basis of results obtained from randomly selected clinical studies, which have been conducted over long periods of time, it is now possible to make assessments about the usefulness and efficacies of endogenous antioxidants in the prevention and possible cure of various diseases. The most extensively investigated have been the various isomers of vitamin E including all-racemic mixtures and esters, such as acetates and succinates either alone or in combination with other antioxidants, such as β-carotene, other carotenoids, and most importantly in conjunction with vitamin C. Although all kinds of vitamin E have been used in various investigations, only use of the natural d-α-tocopherol (2*R*,4*R*,8*R*) could be expected to give optimum results. The dosages of vitamin E varied considerably. The tendencies have been to use 400–800 IU (267–537 milligrams) and seldom exceeding 1000 IU (667 mg). However, the best results were obtained with high dosages ranging between 2000 and 3000 mg (about 4800 IU) in conjunction with an excess of ascorbic acid [10–14, 29, 30].

Table 7A-2. Physical and biological properties of vitamin C, vitamin E, β-carotene, α-lipoic acid, Aspirin™, and other anti-inflammatory drugs. The data are useful in appraisals of various trials.

Acidities of Aspirin™ and other organic acids widely distributed in nature. These are weak acids with only slight tendencies to release protons.		
Acetic acid	1.75×10^{-5}	$pK_a = 4.76$
Ascorbic acid (vitamin C)	5.23×10^{-5}	$pK_a = 4.17$
Lactic acid	1.39×10^{-4}	$pK_a = 3.86$
Aspirin™ (acetylsalicylic acid)	3.27×10^{-4}	$pK_a = 3.48$
Citric acid	7.4×10^{-4}	$pK_a = 3.13$
Salicylic acid	1.05×10^{-3}	$pK_a = 2.98$

Analgesic potencies of anti-inflammatory drugs		Weak
Acetaminophen (Tylenol®)	$LD_{50} = 200$ mg/kg, rat	↓
Aspirin™ (acetylsalicylic acid)	$LD_{50} = 180$ mg/kg, rat	↓
Diflunisal	$LD_{50} = 7.2$ mg/kg, rat	↓
Indomethacin	$LD_{50} = 2.56$ mg/kg, rat	Strong

Toxicities LD_{50} mg/kg orally/rat	**Categories**
d,l-αTocopherol	4000 4
d-αTocopherol	>7000–10,000 5
d,l-αTocopheryl acetate, all-racemic mixture	10,000 5
d-α-Tocopheryl succinate	7000 5
β-Carotene 0.6 IU/mg	>5000 5
α-Lipoic acid	1130–2000 4
Ascorbic acid (vitamin C)	11,900 5
Aspirin™ (acetylsalicylic acid)	1400 4
Ibuprofen (Advil®)	1255 4
Acetaminophen (Tylenol®)	338 (mouse) 3
Diflunisal	439 (mouse) 4
Salt (NaCl)	3000 4
Sodium bicarbonate	4220 4

	MW
R,*R*,*R*-α-Tocopherol	471
Ascorbic acid	176
β-Carotene	537
Aspirin™	180

Toxicity Ratings in Humans [42,43]	**Categories**
1. Extremely toxic	<1–5 mg/kg
2. Highly toxic	5–50 mg/kg
3. Very toxic – Moderately toxic	50–500 mg/kg
4. Moderately toxic – Slightly toxic	500–5000 mg/kg
5. Sligthly toxic – Practically nontoxic	5000–15000 mg/kg
6. Practically nontoxic-Harmless	>15000 mg/kg

Oral Lethal Doses for a 70 kg [154 lbs) Person
[42,43]

Category 3	30 mL
Category 4	600 mL (~1 pint)
Category 5	1000 mL (~1 quart)

Another promising antioxidant is α-lipoic acid. In a biological environment, α-lipoic acid is in equilibrium with dihydrolipoic acid, which is actually the antioxidant. α-Lipoic acid was used as 600 mg oral supplement and as an intravenous injection using a 1000 mg dose.

The oral supplementation with β-carotene, other carotenoids, selenium, and other antioxidants, either alone or in combination with vitamin E produced no convincing results.

Conclusions

The administration of α-lipoic acid, either orally or intravenously, and vitamin E, specifically the natural stereoisomer RRR-d-α-tocopherol (2*R*,4*R*,8*R*), administered orally in high dosages together with ascorbic acid, could function either in preventions of certain diseases, or more likely, as mitigating and/or ameliorating agents and retarding agents in disease progressions, but not as rapidly acting drugs.

Summary

Failures to obtain unambiguous results in various clinical studies can be attributed to the use of either low dosages, e.g., 100–600 IU of vitamin E, use of esters, such as acetates and succinates as racemates, or in the absence of vitamin C. For optimum results, the tocopherol stereoisomer 2*R*,4*R*,8*R* should be used exclusively at high dosages, above 3000 IU, in the presence of a large excess of vitamin C. Vitamin E oral supplementations should not be consumed in the traditional way with water but with lipophilic food stuffs, such as olive oil, in conjunction with a large excess of vitamin C.

References

1. Pryor W. A. (2000) Vitamin E and heart disease: basic science to clinical intervention trials. *Free Radical Biol. Med.* **28**: 141–164.
2. Horwitt M. K. (1986) Promotion of vitamin E. *J. Nutr.* **116**: 1371–1377.
3. Min C. K. (2007) Structure and function of alpha-tocopherol transfer protein: implications for vitamin E metabolism and AVED. *Vitam Horm.* **76**: 23–43.
4. Qian J., Atkinson J. and Manor D. (2006) Biological consequences of heritable mutations in the alpha-tocopherol transfer protein. *Biochemistry* **45**: 8236–8242.

5. Traber M. G. (2007) Vitamin E regulatory mechanisms. *Annu. Rev. Nutr.* **27**: 347–362.
6. Friedrich W. (1988) *Vitamins*. Walter de Gruyter, Berlin.
7. Thiele J., Traber M. G. and Packer L. (1998) Depletion of human stratum corneum vitamin E: an early and sensitive *in vivo* marker of UV induced photooxidation. *J. Invest. Dermatol.* **110**: 756–761.
8. McVean M. and Lieber D. C. (1999) Prevention of DNA photodamage by vitamin E compounds and sunscreens: roles of ultraviolet absorbance and cellular uptake. *Mol. Carcinog.* **24**: 169–176.
9 Berton T. R., Conti C. J., Mitchell D. L., Aldaz C. M., Lubet R. A. and Fischer S. M. (1998) The effect of vitamin E acetate on ultraviolet-induced mouse skin carcinogenesis. *Mol. Carcinog.* **23**: 175–184.
10. Fuchs J. and Kern H. (1998) Modulation of UV-light-induced skin inflammation by d-alpha-tocopherol and L-ascorbic acid: a clinical study using solar simulated radiation. *Free Radical Biol. Med.* **25**: 1006–1012.
11. Fuchs J. (1998) Potentials and limitations of the natural antioxidants RRR-alpha-tocopherol, L-ascorbic acid and β-carotene in cutaneous photoprotection. *Free Radical Biol. Med.* **25**: 848–873.
12. Pinnell S. (2003) Cutaneous photodamage, oxidative stress and topical antioxidant protection. *J. Am. Acad. Dermatol.* **48**: 1–19.
13. Stahl W. and Sies H. (2001) Protection against solar radiation-protective properties of antioxidants. In: *Sun Protection in Man*, pp 561–572, Giacomoni, P. U. (ed.), Elsevier Science, Amsterdam.
14. Eberlein-König B., Placzek M. and Przybilla B. (1998) Protective effect against sunburn of combined systemic ascorbic acid (vitamin C) and d-α-tocopherol (vitamin E). *J. Am. Acad. Dermatol.* **38**: 45–48.
15. Ogunmekan A. O. (1988) Is there a role of vitamin E therapy in epilepsy? *Int. Clin. Nutr. Rev.* **8**: 50–52.
16. Fahn S. (1991) An open trial of high-dosage antioxidants in early Parkinson's disease. *Am. J. Clin. Nutr.* **53**: 380S–382S.
17. Factor S. A. and Weiner W. J. (1989) Retrospective evaluation of vitamin E therapy in Parkinson's disease. *Ann. N. Y. Acad. Sci.* **570**: 441–442.
18. Doody R. S., Stevens J. C., Beck C., Dubinsky R. M., Kaye J. A., Gwyther L., Mohs R. C., Thal L. J., Whitehouse P. J., DeKosky S. T. and Cummings J. L. (2001) Practice parameter: management of dementia (an evidence based review). Report of the quality standards subcommittee of the American Academy of Neurology. *Neurology* **56**: 1154–1166.

19. Sano M., Ernesto C., Thomas R. G., Klauber M. R., Schafer K., Grundman M., Woodbury P., Growdon J., Cotman C. W., Pfeiffer E., Schneider L. S. and Thal L. J. (1997) Controlled clinical trial of selegiline, alfa-tocopherol or both as treatment for Alzheimer's disease. *N. Engl. J. Med.* **336**: 1216–1222.
20. Grundman M. (2000) Vitamin E and Alzheimer disease: the basis for additional clinical trials. *J. Clin. Nutr.* **71**: 630S–636S.
21. Meydani S. N., Barklund M. P., Liu S., Meydani M., Miller R. A., Cannon J. G., Morrow F. D., Rocklin R. and Blumberg J. B. (1990) Vitamin E supplementation enhances cell-mediated immunity in healthy elderly subjects. *Am. J. Clin Nutr.* **52**: 557–563.
22. De Waart F. G., Portengen L., Doekes G., Verwaal C. J. and Kok F. J. (1997) Effect of 3 months vitamin E supplementation on indices of the cellular and humoral immune response in elderly subjects. *Br. J. Nutr.* **78**: 761–774.
23. Seddon J. M., Ajani U. A., Sperduto R. D., Hiller R., Blair N., Burton T. C., Farber M. D., Gragoudas E. S., Haller J., Miller D. T., Yannuzzi L. A. and Willett W. (1994) Dietary carotenoids, vitamin A, C and E and age-related macular degeneration. *J. Am. Diet. Assoc.* **272**: 1413–1420.
24. Robertson J. M., Donner A. P. and Trevithick J. R. (1989) Vitamin E intake and risk of cataracts in humans. *Ann. N. Y. Acad. Sci.* **570**: 372–382.
25. Leske M. C., Chylack L. T., He, Q., Wu S. Y., Schoenfeld E., Friend J. and Wolfe J. (1998) Antioxidant vitamins and nuclear opacities: the longitudinal study of cataract. *Ophthalmology* **105**: 831–836.
26. West S., Vitale S., Hallfrisch J., Munoz B. and Bressler N. M. (1994) Are antioxidants or supplements protective for age-related macular degeneration? *Arch. Ophthalmol.* **112**: 222–227.
27. Werninghaus K., Meydani M., Bhawan J., Margolis R., Blumberg J. B. and Gilchrest B. A. (1994) Evaluation of the photoprotective effect of oral vitamin E supplementation. *Arch. Dermatol.* **130**: 1257–1261.
28. Stahl W., Heinrich U., Jungmann H., Sies H. and Tronnier H. (2000) Carotenoids and carotenoids plus vitamin E protect against ultraviolet light-induced erythema in humans. *Am. J. Clin. Nutr.* **71**: 795–798.
29. Farrell P. M. and Bieri J. G. (1975) Megavitamin E supplementation in man. *Am. J. Clin. Nutr.* **28**: 1381–1386.

30. Salkeld R. M. (1979) Safety and tolerance of high dosage vitamin E administration in man: a review of the literature. *Fed. Regist.* **44**: 16172.
31. Jialal I., Fuller C. J. and Huet B. A. (1995) The effect of alpha-tocopherol supplementation on LDL oxidation. *Arterioscler., Thromb., Vasc. Biol.* **15**: 190–198.
32. Jacob S., Henriksen E. J., Schiemann A. L., Simon I., Clancy D. E., Tritschler H. J., Jung W. I., Augustin H. J. and Dietze G. J. (1995) Enhancement of glucose disposal in patients with type 2 diabetes by alpha-lipoic acid. *Arzneim. Forsch.* **45**: 872–874.
33. Jacob S., Henriksen E. J., Tritschler H. J., Augustin H. J. and Dietze G. J. (1996) Improvement of insulin-stimulated glucose disposal in type 2 diabetes after repeated parenteral administration of thioctic acid. *Exp. Clin. Endocrinol. Diabetes* **104**: 284–288.
34. Kahler W., Kuklinski B., Ruhlmann C. and Plotz C. (1993) Diabetes mellitus – a free radical-associated disease. Results of adjuvant antioxidant supplementation. *Z. Gesamte Inn. Med. Ihre Grenzgeb.* **48**: 223–232.
35. Haak E., Usadel K. H., Kusterer K., Amini P., Frommeyer R., Tritschler H. J. and Haak T. (2000) The effects of alpha-lipoic acid on microcirculation in patients with peripheral diabetic neuropathy. *Exp. Clin. Endocrinol. Diabetes* **108**: 168–174.
36. Nagamatsu M., Nickander K. K., Schmelzer J. D., Raya A., Wittrock D. A., Tritschler H. J. and Low P. A. (1995) Lipoic acid improves nerve blood flow, reduces oxidative stress and improves distal nerve conduction in experimental diabetic neuropathy. *Diabetes Care* **18**: 1160–1167.
37. Paolisso G., D'Amore A. D., Galzerano D., Balbi V., Giugliano D., Varricchio M. and D'Onofrio F. (1993) Daily vitamin E supplements improve metabolic control but no insulin secretion in elderly type II diabetic patients. *Diabetes Care* **16**: 1433–1437.
38. Anderson T. W. and Reid D. B. W. (1974) A double-blind trial of vitamin E in angina pectoris. *Am. J. Clin. Nutr.* **27**: 1174–1178.
39. Hodis H. N., Mack W. J., LaBree L., Cashin-Hemphill L., Sevanian A., Johnson R. and Azen S. P. (1995) Serial coronary angiographic evidence that antioxidant vitamin intake reduces progression of coronary artery atherosclerosis. *J. Am. Med. Assoc.* **273**: 1849–1854.
40. Rimm E. B., Stampfer M. J., Ascherio A., Giovannucci E., Colditz G. A. and Willett W. C. (1993) Vitamin E consumption and risk of coronary heart disease in men. *N. Engl. J. Med.* **328**: 1450–1456.

41. Losonczy K. G., Harris T. B. and Havrlik R. J. (1996) Vitamin E and vitamin C supplement use and risk of all-cause and coronary heart disease mortality in older persons: the established populations for epidemiologic studies of the elderly. *Am. J. Clin. Nutr.* **64**: 190–196.
42. Manson J. E., Gaziano J. M., Spelsberg A., Ridker P. M., Cook N. R., Buring J. E., Willett W. C. and Hennekens C. H. (1995) A secondary prevention trial of antioxidant vitamins and cardiovascular disease in women: Rationale, design, and methods. *Ann. Epidemiol.* **5**: 261–269.
43. Tasanarong A., Piyayotai D. and Thitiarchakul S. (2009) Protection of radiocontrast induced nephropathy by vitamin E (alpha-tocopherol): a randomized controlled pilot study. *J. Med. Assoc. Thailand* **92**: 1273–1281.
44. Spargias K., Alexopoulos E., Kyrzopoulos S., Iokovis P., Greenwood D. C., Manginas A., Voudris V., Pavlides G., Buller C. E., Kremastinos D. and Cokkinos D. V. (2004) Ascorbic acid prevents contrast-medicated nephropathy in patients with renal dysfunction undergoing coronary angiography or intervention. *Circulation* **110**: 2837–2842.
45. Bjelakovic G., Nikolova D., Gluud L. L., Simonetti R. G. and Gluud C. (2008) Antioxidant supplements for prevention of mortality in healthy participants and patients with various diseases. *Cochrane Database Syst. Rev.* (2): CD007176.
46. Sesso H. D., Buring J. E., Christen W. G., Kurth T., Belanger C., MacFadyen J., Bubes V., Manson J. E., Glynn R. J. and Gaziano J. M. (2008) Vitamins E and C in the prevention of cardiovascular disease in men: the physicians' health study II randomized controlled trial. *J. Am. Med. Assoc.* **300**: 2123–2133.
47. Lee I. M., Cook N. R., Gaziano J. M., Gordon D., Ridker P. M., Manson J. E., Hennekens C. H. and Buring J. E. (2005) Vitamin E in the primary prevention of cardiovascular disease and cancer: the Women's Health Study: a randomized controlled trial. *J. Am. Med. Assoc.* **294**: 56–65.
48. Cook N. R., Albert C. M., Gaziano J. M., Zaharris E., MacFadyen J., Danielson E., Buring J. E. and Manson J. E. (2007) A randomized factorial trial of vitamins C and E and beta-carotene in the secondary prevention of cardiovascular events in women: results from the women's antioxidant cardiovascular study. *Arch. Intern. Med.* **167**: 1610–1618.
49. Lin J., Cook N. R., Albert C., Zaharris E., Gaziano J. M., Van Denburgh M., Buring J. E. and Manson J. E. (2009) Vitamins C and E

and beta-carotene supplementation and cancer risk: a randomized controlled trial. *JNCI, J. Natl. Cancer Inst.* **101**: 14–23.

50. Holmquist L., Stuchbury G., Berbaum K., Muscat S., Young S., Hager K., Engel J. and Munch G. (2007) Lipoic acid as a novel treatment for Alzheimer's disease and related dementias. *Pharmacol. Ther.* **113**: 154–164.
51. Hager K., Kenklies M., McAfoose J., Engel J. and Munch G. (2007) α-Lipoic acid as a new treatment option for Alzheimer's disease – a 48 months follow-up analysis. *J. Neural Transm., Suppl. A* **72**: 189–193.
52. Dorgan J. F., Boakye N. A., Fears T. R., Schleicher R. L., Helsel W., Anderson C., Robinson J., Guin J. D., Lessin S., Ratnasinghe L. D. and Tangrea J. A. (2004) Serum carotenoids and alpha-tocopherol and risk of nonmelanoma skin cancer. *Cancer Epidemiol, Biomarkers Prev.* **13**: 1276–1282.
53. Van der Pols J. C., Heinem M. M., Hughes M. C., Ibiebele T. I., Marks G. C. and Green A. C. (2009) Serum antioxidants and skin cancer risk: an 8-year community-based follow-up study. *Cancer Epidemiol., Biomarkers Prev.* **18**: 1167–1173.
54. Lippman S. M., Klein E. A., Goodman P. J., Lucia M. S., Thompson I. M., Ford L. G., Parnes H. L., Minasian L. M., Gaziano J. M., Hartline J. A., Parsons J. K., Bearden J. D. 3rd, et al. (2009) Effect of selenium and vitamin E on risk of prostate cancer and other cancers: the selenium and vitamin E cancer prevention trial (SELECT). *J. Am. Med. Assoc.* **301**: 39–51.
55. Gensler H. L., Aickin M., Peng Y. M. and Xu M. (1996) Importance of the form of topical vitamin E for prevention of photocarcinogenesis. *Nutr. Cancer* **26**: 183–191.
56. Watters J. L., Gail M. H., Weinstein S. J., Virtamo J. and Albanes D. (2009) Associations between α-tocopherol, β-carotene, and retinol and prostate cancer survival. *Cancer Res.* **69**: 3833–3841.
57. Peters U., Littman A. J., Kristal A. R., Patterson R. E., Potter J. D. and White E. (2008) Vitamin E and selenium supplementation and risk of prostate cancer in the vitamins and lifestyle (VITAL) study cohort. *Cancer, Causes Control* **19**: 75–87.
58. Gaziano J. M., Glynn R. J., Christen W. G., Kurth T., Belanger C., MacFadyen J., Bubes V., Manson J. E., Sesso H. D. and Buring J. E. (2009) Vitamin E and C in the prevention of prostate and total cancer in men: the Physicians; Health Study II randomized controlled trial. *J. Am. Med. Assoc.* **301**: 52–62.

59. Miller E. R. III, Pastor-Barriuso R., Dalal D., Riemersma R. A., Appel L. J. and Guallar E. (2005) Meta-analysis: high-dosage vitamin E supplementation may increase all-cause mortality. *Ann. Intern. Med.* **142**: 37–46.
60. Iuliano L., Micheletta F., Maranghi M., Frati G., Diczfalusy U. and Violi F. (2001) Bioavailability of vitamin E as function of food intake in healthy subjects. *Arterioscler., Thromb., Vasc. Biol.* **21**: e34–e37.
61. Cremer D. R., Rabeler R., Roberts A. and Lynch B. (2006) Safety evaluation of alpha-lipoic acid (ALA). *Regul. Toxicol. Pharmacol.* **46**: 29–41.
62. Tatsioni A., Bonitsis N. G. and Ioannidis J. P. (2007) Persistence of contradicted claims in the literature. *J. Am. Med. Assoc.* **298**: 2517–2526.
63. Siontis G. C., Tatsioni A., Katritsis D. G. and Ioannidis J. P. (2009) persistent reservations against contradicted percutaneous coronary intervention indications: citation content analysis. *Am. Heart J.* **154**: 695–701.

B. Evaluation of Aspirin™ and Other Nonsteroidal Anti-inflammatory Drugs as Anticancer Drugs

i. Comparisons of Aspirin™ with Other NSAIDs

The selected nonsteroidal anti-inflammatory drugs (NSAIDs) comprise a great variety of classes of organic compounds, such as Aspirin™, benoral, Tylenol® (acetaminophen, *p*-acetaminophenol), diflunisal, salicylazosulfapyridine, diclofenac, fenamic acid, carprofen, fenbufen, ibufenac, flurbiprofen, ibuprofen, ketoprofen, naproxen, tolmetin, indomethacin, sulindac, flufenamic acid, and tolfenamic acid [1, 2]. All, except Tylenol®, have in common a carboxyl group; however, only a small number have the carboxyl group located at the aromatic benzene ring, namely, in Aspirin™, benoral, diflunisal, and salicylazosulfapyridine. In all other drugs, the carboxyl group is linked to aliphatic groups, and, among the salicylic acid derivatives, only Aspirin™ and benoral have an acetylated aryloxy group. While Aspirin™ has an unprotected carboxylic acid group, the acid group in benoral is esterified with the phenolic group of acetaminophen. Acetaminophen has no carboxylic and acetyl groups, but it is an antioxidative phenol. Thus, in benoral are combined the chemotherapeutic benefits of Aspirin™ and acetaminophen, and there exists a considerable literature on this topic [1, 2].

Salicylic acid, the major metabolite of Aspirin™ is widely distributed in nature [1–3]. Salicylic acid often functions as the main defense mechanism in various plants against oxidative stress by regulating the formation and inhibition of certain reactive oxygen species [4–8]. Thus, salicylic acid was found to induce the formation of superoxide anion radical ($O_2\cdot^-$) and hydrogen peroxide, while at the same time, to cause inhibition of the formation of hydroxyl radicals which are usually derived from hydrogen peroxide [8]. Salicylic acid can also function as an antioxidant, but unlike vitamin E, it accepts the hydroxyl radical (HO·) resulting in the production of 2,3- and 2,5-dihydroxybenzoic acids and catechol [4–8]. Salicylic acid is also widely distributed in the blood of animals and mammals, and occurs naturally in humans, e.g., in urine as the metabolite salicyluric acid, a salicylic acid–glycine conjugate [2–3]. In general, salicylic acid is strongly bonded to the circulating albumin. The acetyl group of acetylsalicylic acid, i.e., Aspirin™, is of paramount importance for the activity of Aspirin™, and it can become covalently attached to a variety of proteins, glucoproteins, lipids, and other biomolecules and, in particular, to the active sites of cyclooxygenase and lipoxygenase enzymes, and to leucotrienes, prostaglandins, and thromboxanes [2–18]. Aspirin™ acetylation of cyclooxygenase irreversibly destroys the enzyme activity. The resulting salicylic acid is inactive. The biological half-life of salicylic acid in the therapeutic plasma is about 3 hours; however, it can range according to the dose employed. The other NSAIDs cause inhibition of the enzyme; however, they are metabolized at the same time and excreted, leaving the enzyme intact [17].

The elimination rate of the NSAID from the enzyme depends on the half-life of the NSAID, i.e., at about six to seven times the half-life of the drug. Thus, for example, in the case of ibuprofen, with a half-life of 3 hours, the residence time at the enzyme could be about 18 hours [17].

Acetylation by Aspirin™ can also be involved in the tricarboxylic acid Krebs cycle by reaction of Aspirin™ with coenzyme A to give acetyl-CoA to start the Krebs cycle [2]. The acetyl group is usually derived from pyruvic acid for the Krebs cycle. Hence, it is, therefore, very important not to equate the modes of chemotherapeutic actions of NSAIDs with that of Aspirin™ [2, 10, 13–15, 17]. The chemotherapeutic actions of Aspirin™ and of other NSAIDs in the human body involve the inhibition of excessive oxidative transformation of the arachidonic acid pathways leading to harmful conditions [9–13]. The excess of reactive oxygen species (ROS) in the human body occurs when the regular biological antioxidative mechanisms of enzymes and vitamins fail to adequately control the formation of ROS.

ii. Pathways of the Arachidonic Acid Metabolism under Oxidative Stress

The pathways to products of the metabolism of arachidonic acid are important oxidative processes in the development of inflammatory sites in the human body. Arachidonic acid [**Fig. 7B.ii-1**] is an essential fatty acid and a precursor of the biosynthetic formation of leucotrienes, prostaglandins, and thromboxanes [2, 17].

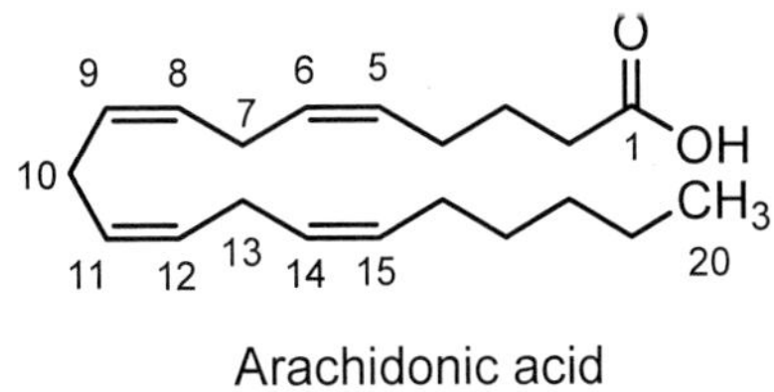

Fig. 7B.ii-1. Structure of arachidonic acid.

The oxidations of arachidonic acid are induced by the cyclooxygenase (COX-1, COX-2) and lipoxygenase (LOX) enzymes, and proceed by free radical type mechanisms via the pentadienyl free radical that is produced by abstraction of doubly allylic hydrogens located at positions 7, 10, and 13, followed by rearrangement to give resonance-stabilized radicals at positions 5, 8, 12, and 15. The reactions of these radicals proceed with molecular oxygen ($\cdot{}^3O_2\cdot$), which is a diradical species in the ground state, to give arachidonic acid hydroperoxides. These hydroperoxides readily decompose either thermally to give the corresponding alkoxy radicals and hydroxyl radicals (HO·) or more likely by Fenton-type reactions to give alkoxy radicals and hydroxide anions (HO^-). The alkoxy radicals of arachidonic acid can undergo various reactions, such as abstraction of hydrogen atoms from various biological entities to give hydroxy compounds, i.e., arachidonic acid alcohols, which can be further oxidized to the keto derivatives. The hydroxyl radicals are an extremely reactive species and can undergo additions to double bonds and abstractions of hydrogen atoms from various entities. (See **Section 4**.) This arachidonic acid cascade, as it is often called, results in the formation of a series of endogenous metabolites, such as hydroperoxyeicosatetraenoic acid (HPETE), hydroxyeicosatetraenoic acid (HETE), leucotrienes LTA_4 and LTB_4, and the peptidoleucotrienes LTC_4, LTD_4, and LTE_4, which are formed via the lipoxygenase pathways [2, 10, 14, 17].

The leucotrienes are potent bronchoconstrictors, chemostatic agents, and mediators in inflammatory processes, and are involved in hypersensitivity reactions. This group of endogenous metabolites formed via the influence of lipoxygenase (LOX) pathways is related to prostaglandins and thromboxanes, which are formed via the cyclooxygenase pathways [2, 10, 11, 13, 17].

In **Sch. 7B.ii-1** and **Sch. 7B.ii-2** are shown the mechanistic interpretations of pathways for the formation of leucotrienes and prostaglandins by free radical oxidations of arachidonic acid with molecular oxygen $\cdot{}^3O_2\cdot$. These oxidations are mediated by four lipoxygenase, 5-, 8-, 12- and 15-LOX, and two cyclooxygenase, COX-1 and COX-2, enzymes without considerations of possible regio- and stereocontrol leading to *S* and *R* configurations of the end products that can occur in a biological environment. Of course, the racemates can be resolved into *S* and *R* enantiomers. Analogous oxidations occur in nature with various unsaturated fatty acids. On the basis of the synthetic pathways, various naturally occurring leucotrienes and prostaglandins can be synthesized. The most studied prostaglandin, F_{2a} (**1**), is closely related to prostaglandin PGE_2 (**2**), and both are derived from the same precursors in nature and in the synthetic routes [**Sch. 7B.ii-1** and **Sch. 7B.ii-2**].

Thus, the cyclooxygenase-induced cyclizations involving the radicals at positions 8 and 12 of the arachidonic acid result in the formation of the cyclopentane ring structures with a keto group at position 9 and hydroxy groups at positions 11 and 15, and derivatives with the hydroxy group at positions 9, 11, and 15. These prostaglandins, PGE_2, $PGF_{2\alpha}$, PGD_2, and PGI_2 (prostacyclin), are biologically important lipidic acids with properties such as dilation of arteries, stimulation of muscles, bronchial dilation, menstruation, inflammatory reactions, inhibition of gastric secretion, platelet aggregation, induction of labor, increase of occular pressure, and kidney functions. Finally, the group of thromboxanes, compounds derived from the endoperoxides of prostaglandins cause platelet aggregations, contraction of arteries, and other biological effects. These compounds are found in platelets, leucocytes, lung tissue, kidney, and the umbilical artery. They are important mediators of the actions of polyunsaturated acids that are transformed by cyclooxygenase enzymes. Thromboxane A_2 (TXA_2) contains an unusual oxetane-oxane ring structure, and tromboxane B_2 (TXB_2) contains a six-membered-ring system with a hemiacetal component that can undergo hydrolytic and other reactions. Tromboxane TXA_2 causes vasoconstrictions and induces platelet aggregations [17].

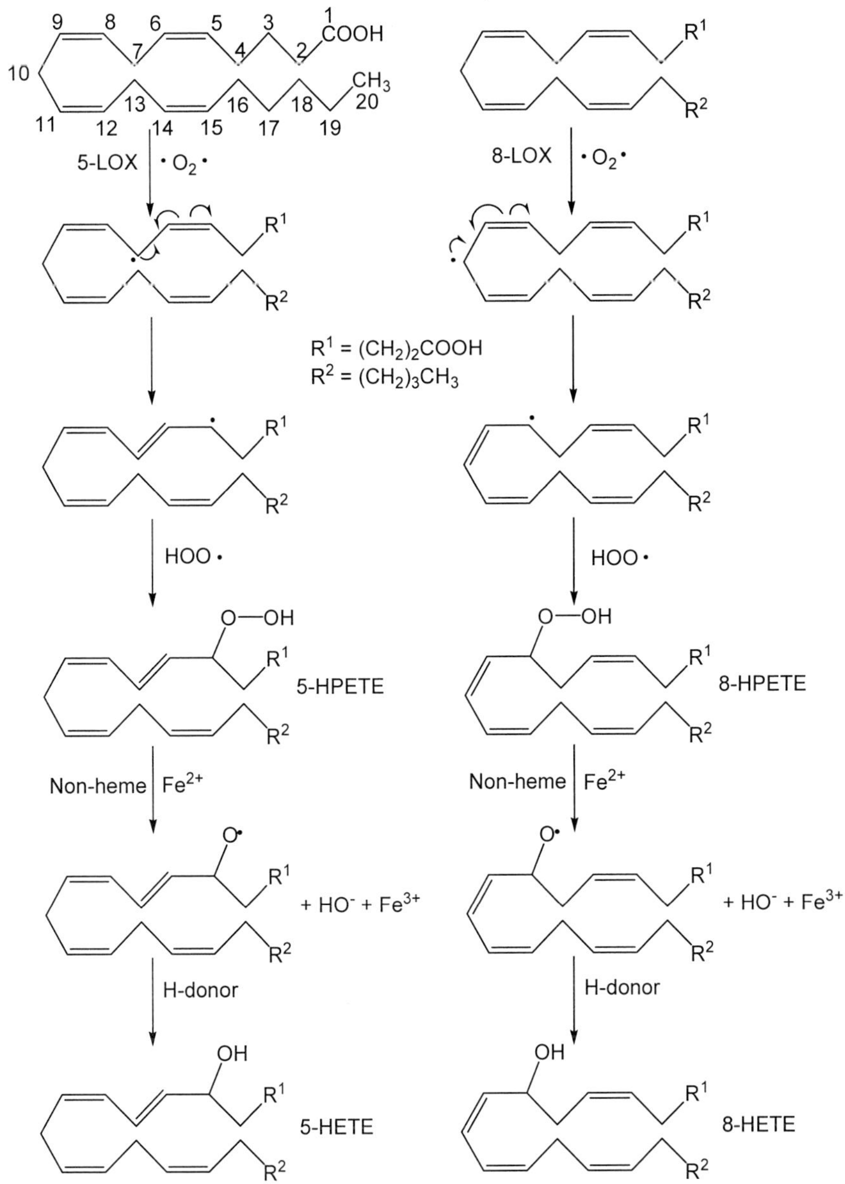

5-LOX
8-LOX
$R^1 = (CH_2)_2COOH$
$R^2 = (CH_2)_3CH_3$
HOO •
5-HPETE
8-HPETE
Non-heme Fe^{2+}
$+ HO^- + Fe^{3+}$
H-donor
5-HETE
8-HETE

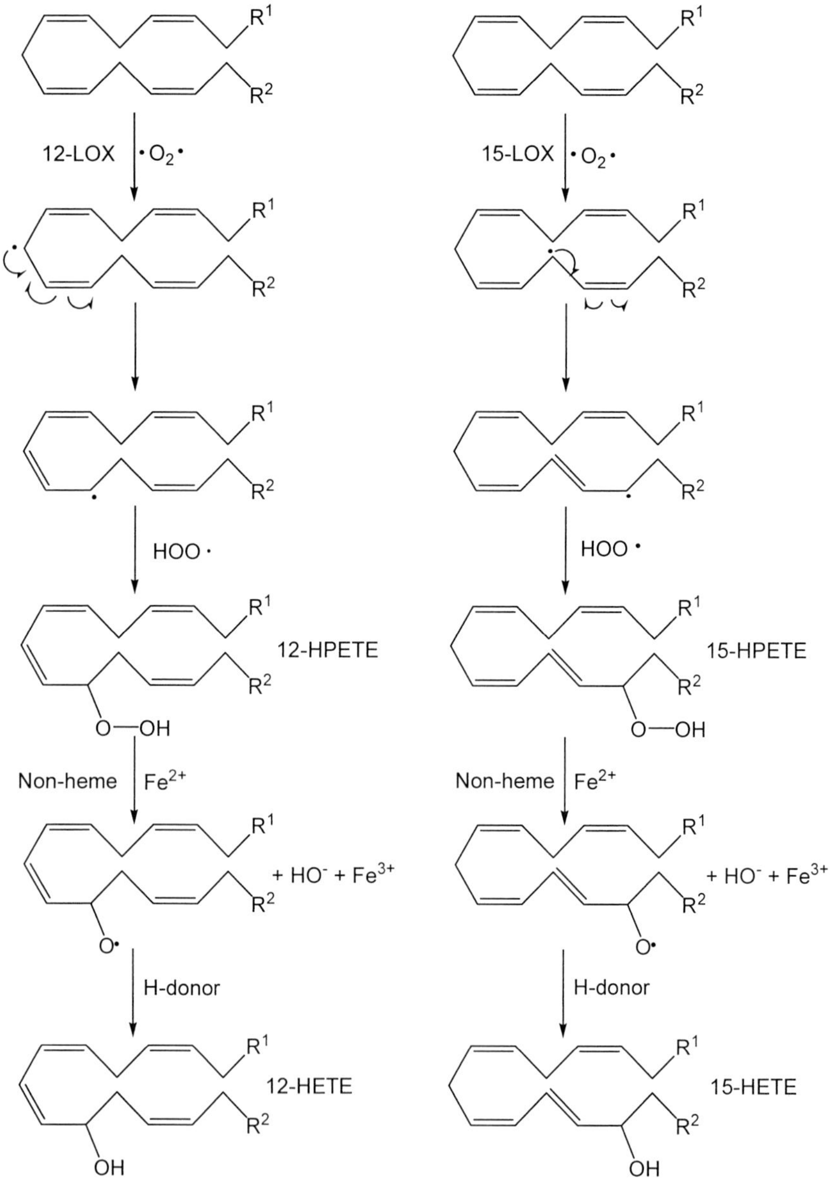

Sch. 7B.ii-1. Pathways to leucotrienes 5-, 8-, 12-, and 15-hydroperoxyeicosatetraenoic acids (HPETEs) and 5-, 8-, 12-, and 15-hydroxyeicosatetraenoic acids (HETEs).

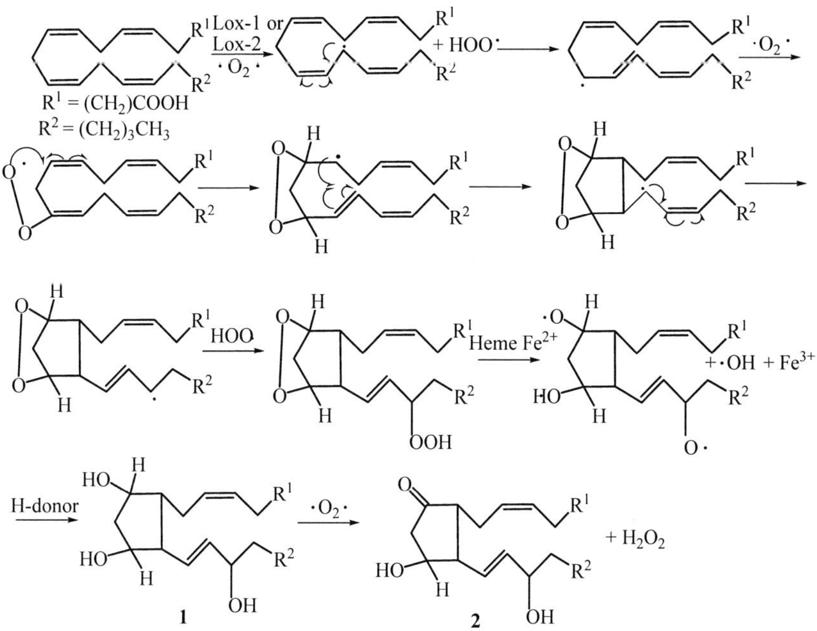

Sch. 7B.ii-2. Pathways to prostaglandins 9,11,15-trihydroxy-5,9-dien-1-oic acid, F_{2a} (**1**), and 11,15-dihydroxy-9-oxo-5,13-dien-1-oic acid, PGE_2 (**2**).

The general mechanisms of action of Aspirin™ and other NSAIDs involve the inhibition of cyclooxygenase enzyme activities and prevention of biosyntheses of prostaglandins and thromboxanes, although the detailed mechanisms are different for Aspirin™ and other NSDAIDs. There are two cyclooxygenase enzymes denoted as COX-1 and COX-2. The inhibition of COX-1 and COX-2 by Aspirin™ action occurs at different concentrations of the drug. The selective acetylation of COX-1 can be achieved with low doses of Aspirin™ ranging between 30–50 mg/day. This acetylation of the platelet COX-1 causes a complete inactivation of COX-1 and inhibition of TXA_2 biosynthesis. The inactivation processes apparently occur equally well in women and men [19, 20].

Aspirin™ and other NSAIDs, in particular methyl and trolamine salicylates, have been extensively used topically as analgesics and counterirritants against dermal inflammations that are mediated, in part, by the metabolites of arachidonic acid. The rates of absorption and penetration of the human skin by inflammatory drugs depend on the structures and lipophilicities of the drugs and other factors [17].

On the basis of clinical studies, it is certain that Aspirin™ supplementations can be used to prevent myocardial infarction and ischemic stroke with 75–100 mg doses [21]. It is believed that the efficacy of Aspirin™ is achieved by a complete inactivation of COX-1 and suppression of TXA_2 [13, 22, 23]. Aspirin™ is also effective as an antithrombotic agent in reducing the risk of vascular nonfatal myocardial stroke and the risk of vascular death by using doses ranging from 75 to 325 mg and 500 to 1500 mg, whereby no statistically significant difference in effect was achieved with various dosages [19, 22–25].

The other NSAIDs are less effective than Aspirin™ in the inhibition of the platelet COX-1 and lead to only insignificant suppression of TXA_2. However, the drug naproxen is an exception, since, with a dose of 500 mg bid (L. bis in die, meaning twice a day), about 90% inhibition of COX-1 and suppression of TXA_2 can be achieved [26, 27].

The inhibition of COX-2 with NSAIDs varies between 50 and 90%, while, at the same time, the suppression of TXA_2 is negligible. There are various selectivity and dose levels for individual NSAIDs that are similar to those of the synthetic coxibs [28, 29]. These inhibitors, such as celecoxib, etoricoxib, valdecoxib, rofecoxib, parecoxib, and lumiracoxib contain no acetylating group, no phenolic hydroxy groups, and no carboxylic groups, except for lumiracoxib, which is an analog of diclofenac. Rofecoxib (Vioxx®) has a lactone group that can undergo a γ-hydrolytic ring-opening to a hydroxy acid derivative. Celecoxib and valdecoxib have in their structures a sulfonamide group that is found in many carbonic anhydrase inhibitors, such as sulfonamide drugs.

Coxibs were associated with about a 42% increase in the incidence of serious cardiovascular events, i.e., 0.9% to 1.2% per year relative to placebo, and similar to those associated with traditional NSAIDs of about 0.9% per year [28]. The cardiovascular effects of NSAIDs, except naproxen, have similar prothrombic, cardio-toxic properties of synthetic coxibs. In particular, it was found that rofecoxib (Vioxx®) and valdecoxib can cause an increased risk of myocardial infractions (heart attacks) and stroke. Consequently, these two coxibs were withdrawn from the market in spite of the worldwide popular use of Vioxx® in more than 80 countries [28–30].

iii. Medicinal Evaluations of Aspirin™ and other NSAIDs as Anticancer Drugs

A very large number of clinical trials, such as case-control studies, cohort-studies, and meta-analyses have been conducted over the years with Aspirin™ and other non-steroidal anti-inflammatory drugs (NSAIDs) in order to firmly establish the efficacy and safety of these drugs either in the prevention or cure of myocardial infractions, ischemic stroke, vascular death, and other major diseases including cancers. A small number of abstracts selected at random are included in this discussion.

In a meta-analysis of four randomized clinical trials, the effects of Aspirin™ were evaluated with 2967 participants for the secondary prevention of colorectal carcinomas. The participants aged 58 years were 60% male. Doses of Aspirin™ ranged between 81 and 325 mg/day, and the follow-up period was about 33 months. At the end of this period, 2698 participants were screened by colonoscopy with the following results. Adenomas were detected in 424 (37%) of 1156 participants on the placebo regime and 507 (33%) of 1542 participants who took any dosage of Aspirin™. The conclusion was that the use of Aspirin™ is effective in the prevention of colorectal adenomas in persons with a history of these lesions [31].

The American Heart Association proposed the use of Aspirin™, acetaminophen, tramadol, and narcotin analgesics for patients with concurrent osteoarthritis and heart disease. In the case of Aspirin™ use, increasing the dose from 75–100 mg to 650–1300 mg/day was proposed [32].

A cohort study was conducted with 82911 women over a period of twenty years providing supplementations of either 0.5 to 1.5 standard Aspirin™ tablets, 2 to 5 tablets per week, 6 to 14 tablets per week, or more than 14 tablets per week. The side effect was gastrointestinal bleeding, even in women who were on placebo, i.e., 0.77 incidents/1000 persons, 1.07 who used 2 to 5 tablets of Aspirin™ per week, 1.40 who used 6–14 tablets of Aspirin™ per week, and 1.57 cases for persons who took more than 14 tablets of Aspirin™ per week. The conclusion was that the use of Aspirin™ reduces the risk of colorectal cancer. The degree of gastrointestinal bleeding is a dose-related risk [33].

A randomized controlled investigation was conducted with 39876 women aged 45 and older who had no previous occurrence of cancers or cardiovascular and other major diseases. They were treated by oral administration either with a low dose of 100 mg of Aspirin™ or a placebo every other day over a period of 10.1 years. At the end of the trial period, the conclusion was that the treatment with Aspirin™ under the chosen conditions had no effect on the lowering of the risk of total breast, colorectal, and other site-specific cancers, except that a protective effect for lung cancer could not be ruled out [34].

A cohort study was conducted with 1279 men and women participants who were diagnosed with stage I, II, and III of colorectal carcinoma. After

11.8 years of follow-up studies, there were 193 (35%) of total death and 81 (15%) of colorectal cancer-specific deaths among 549 participants who regularly used Aspirin™ as compared to 287 (39%) of total deaths and 141 (19%) of colorectal cancer-specific deaths among 730 participants who were not users of Aspirin™. The effect of Aspirin™ differed considerably, depending on the level of cyclooxygenase-2 (COX-2) expression in cancers. Thus, Aspirin™ use was only effective against cancers that were overexpressed with COX-2. Aspirin™ was not associated either with a weak or an absent expression of COX-2 [35].

In a cohort study involving 22507 women participants during a period of 10 years with supplementations of Aspirin™ and non-Aspirin™ non-steroidal anti-inflammatory drugs (NSAIDs), the outcome was different from that of the previous study, namely that the use of Aspirin™, but not that of non-Aspirin™ NSAIDs, was associated with a lower risk of cancer incidents and mortality, and was more pronounced for nonsmokers and former smokers than active smokers [36].

In a randomized study, 1121 participants received a placebo or Aspirin™ either 81 or 325 mg per day for three years when colonoscopy tests were conducted. After additional 3–5 years, the participants had colonoscopy tests again. Analogous procedures were adopted with other NSAIDs. The risk assessment of adenoma among frequent users of NSAIDs was about 27%, while for the placebo group and the group with infrequent users the risk was 40%. The conclusion was that the frequent use of either Aspirin™ or NSAIDs could enhance the preventive effect against colorectal adenoma [37].

In a randomized double blind trial, 945 patients participated who had adenomas removed six months prior to the trial. Aspirin™, 300 mg/day, and folate, 0.5 mg/day, were administered to 434 patients over a period of 3 years, and 419 patients received a placebo. The results were that 99 patients (22.8%) of the 434 patients who received Aspirin™ had a recurrence of the adenomas as compared to 121 patients (28.9%) of the 419 patients who received the placebo. A total of 104 patients developed an advanced colorectal adenoma, and 41 (9.4%) of these patients received Aspirin™, while 63 (15.0%) were in the placebo group. The folate supplementation had no effect on the adenoma recurrence. Thus, regular use of Aspirin™ caused a reduced risk of colorectal adenoma recurrence, and could function as a preventive drug [38].

A group of 272 patients participated in four randomized, placebo-controlled trials. The patients were randomly divided into two groups, who received 160 mg and 300 mg doses of lysine acetylsalicylate, a salt of Aspirin™, respectively, or a placebo after removal of at least three adenomas or one adenoma 6 mm in diameter. The supplementations with either dose of Aspirin™ were found to cause a 37% reduction in the risk of any recurrence of adenoma and a 70% reduction in the risk of a recurrence of adenoma larger than 5 mm in diameter. Thus, the use of Aspirin™ can prevent colorectal neoplasia through inhibition of the cyclooxygenase enzyme [39].

Based on a large number of various studies, assessment was made that regular use of Aspirin™ is associated with a reduced risk of colorectal cancers, and, based on limited evidence, the use of Aspirin™ has a favorable effect on the cancers of the esophagus, stomach, breast, ovary, and lung. The effects of Aspirin™ on cancers of the pancreas, prostate, bladder, non-Hodgkin lymphomas, and myeloma are uncertain [40, 41].

In spite of the beneficial effects of regular Aspirin™ use on cancers of the gastrointestinal tract, in particular colorectal cancers and adenomas, it can also cause in some patients gastrointestinal bleeding and even hemorrhagic stroke [10, 12, 13]. Gastrointestinal complications (gastropathy) in anti-inflammatory therapy have been recognized since the introduction of salicylates and Aspirin™ in 1874–1899. The rate of hospitalizations in the USA is about 1% and of mortality about 0.1% [17]. Actually, Aspirin™ is a very weak acid with a relatively weak analgesic potency [**Table 7A-2**], and is well tolerated by the majority of users, since this bleeding effect can be mitigated or even prevented by the commercial buffered formulations [17]. Some uncertainties exist about the level of dosages for long-term therapies with Aspirin™. The tendencies are to recommend the use for supplements the regular, e.g., 325 mg, tablets that can be obtained without prescription. These quantities are probably inadequate to achieve the desired results within a reasonable period of time, in particular, when the aim is the prevention and cure of certain cancers [33].

Since the toxicity of Aspirin™ is rated as slightly to moderately toxic with a lethal dose of about 600 g (600 mL, over one pint) for a 70 kg person [**Table 7A-2**] [42, 43], it is not unreasonable to assume that, for long-term treatments, high dosages of Aspirin™ in the range of at least 560 to 1300 mg/day or even higher could be used without any danger [13, 32, 33], although, at present, it is uncertain whether these elevated dosages would result in a pronounced advantageous effect.

The supplementations with Aspirin™ have other potential benefits than chemoprevention of colorectal cancers and other cancers [14, 31, 33–41]. Thus, Aspirin™ was shown to prevent about 10–20 fatal and non-fatal vascular events for every 1000 patients treated for one year [14, 19, 22, 26, 29]. Aspirin™ was used for cardioprotection in trials with coxib and NSAIDs for osteoarthritis and rheumatoid arthritis [26]. It was recommended that the use of coxib supplementations without the use of a low dose of Aspirin™ should be avoided [26]. Aspirin™ has been shown on many occasions to have cardioprotective properties over a wide range of dosages ranging between 30 to 1500 mg/day [19, 25, 29]. Aspirin™ use was shown to reduce the risk of vascular events, such as myocardial infarction, stroke, and vascular death [13, 14, 29]. The prevention of myocardial infarction and ischemic stroke was achieved with a wide range of dosages between 30 and 1500 mg, and, for antithrombotic events, the dosages ranged between 75 and 100 mg. No statistically significant differences in vascular events were found using lower, 75–325 mg, and higher, 500–1000 mg, doses [13, 25, 29].

Aspirin™ is effective as supplementation for the following disorders: acute myocardial infarction and acute ischemic stroke with a 160 mg/day dose; in the case of chronic stable and unstable angina, 75 mg/day; for arterial fibrillation, 325 mg/day; and for antithrombotic effects, 75–100 mg/day [13, 14, 29]. Aspirin™ has been used for cardioprotection in studies with coxibs and NSAIDs against osteoarthritis, rheumatoid arthritis, and other cardiovascular events [13, 14, 25, 26, 29].

Coxibs, such as the weakest celecoxib (Celebrex™), are anti-inflammatory drugs mainly used for pain relief [24, 29]. It has been recommended that the use of supplementations with coxibs should be avoided without a prior administration of low doses of Aspirin™ [29]. At present, celecoxib (Celebrex™) is the only coxib that is available in the USA. Celecoxib is considered to be a specific inhibitor of COX-2. However, it was found that celecoxib can also tightly bind to a subunit of COX-1 [44]. This process interferes with the essential binding of Aspirin™ to COX-1, since Aspirin™ must bind to both units of the COX-1 dimer in order to fully inhibit the cyclooxygenase-1 enzyme [44]. Hence, it was proposed that, in order to safeguard patients against thrombotic and other cardiovascular events, the administration of Aspirin™ should occur prior to celecoxib administration. Apparently, the complete inhibition of COX-1 by Aspirin™ is achieved within about 30 minutes, i.e., within about the half-life time of 15–20 minutes of Aspirin™. It is believed that, during this short time, the acetylation of COX-1 by Aspirin™ is completed. The half-life times of celecoxib and non-selective NSAIDs are much longer, i.e., about 8–12 hours for celecoxib and 8–9 hours for non-selective NSAIDs, respectively, except for naproxen (12–15 hours). In contrast to Aspirin™, all of these drugs are not protective against various cardiovascular events [14, 29].

The coadministration of Aspirin™ and naproxen causes an inhibitory effect on the Aspirin™ in the COX-1 activity and function [26, 27]. However, there is no inhibition effect on Aspirin™ if naproxen is administered either 2 hours after Aspirin™ or in the reverse order [27].

It is not unreasonable to assume that there is plenty of time for the administration of celecoxib and other NSAIDs without interfering in the acetylation of COX-1 by Aspirin™. Because of the long half-times of celecoxib and other drugs, the administration of these drugs should occur bid (L. bis in die - twice a day).

The therapy with Aspirin™ for the prevention and cure of various diseases and certain cancers has one insuperable advantage overr NSAIDs and coxibs. Namely, Aspirin™, on acylation of the target, reverts to salicylic acid that is part of the human physiology. No other drug has such benign metabolism.

In conclusion, it is now well established [45–60] that the induction and progression of various diseases and, in particular, cancers are associated with chronic inflammations. The inflammations are caused by a chain of events involving free radical type reactions of reactive oxygen species with arachidonic acid and other aliphatic long chain acids, which are found in high-fat food consumptions, mediated by lipoxygenase and cyclooxygenase enzymes. Lipoxygenase enzymes 5-LOX, 8-LOX, 12-LOX, 15-LOX-1, and 15-LOX-2, as well as two cyclooxygenase isoenzyme dimers, the constitutive COX-1 and inducible COX-2 isoenzymes, have been identified. Two cyclooxygenase genes that encode the two COX isoenzymes have been cloned. The reactivity of these enzymes has been established. In recent years, in extensive studies, the structures, properties, and biological action of these entities have been explored. An analytical method was developed for the selective visualization of cyclooxygenase-2 in inflammations and cancers by fluorescent imaging agents. There is, no doubt, that the targets for systematic chemotherapeutic treatments for the prevention and cure of cancers are the lipooxygenase and cyclooxygenase enzymes, and Aspirin™ appears to be a promising non-toxic drug in these cases.

References

1. Rainsford K. D. and Path M. R. S. (eds.) (1984) *Aspirin and Salicylates*. Butterworth & Co. (Publishers), London.
2. Rainsford K. D. and Path M. R. S. (eds.) (1985) *Anti-Inflammatory and Anti-Rheumatic Drugs*, Vol. I–III, CRC Press, Boca Raton.
3. Paterson J. R., Baxter G., Dreyer J. S., Halket J. M., Flynn R. and Lawrence J. R. (2008) Salicylic acid sans aspirin in animals and

man: persistence in fasting and biosynthesis from benzoic acid. *J. Agric. Food Chem.* **56**: 11648–11652.

4. Kawano T. and Furuichi T. (2007) Salicylic acid as a defense-related plant hormone. In: *Salicylic Acid: a Plant Hormone*, pp 277–321, Hayat S. and Ahmad A. (eds.), Springer, The Netherlands.
5. Deschamps D., Fisch C., Fromenty B., Berson A., Degott C. and Pessayre D. (1991) Inhibition by salicylic acid of the activation and thus oxidation of long chain fatty acids. Possible role in the development of Reye's syndrome. *J. Pharmacol. Exp. Ther.* **259**: 894–904.
6. Tomita M., Okuyama T., Watanabe S. and Watanabe H. (1994) Quantitation of the hydroxyl radical adducts of salicylic acid by micellar electrokinetic capillary chromatography: oxidizing species formed by a Fenton reaction. *Arch. Toxicol.* **68**: 428–433.
7. Diez L., Livertoux M. H., Stark A. A., Wellman-Rousseau M. and Leroy P. (2001) High-performance liquid chromatographic assay of hydroxyl free radicals using salicylic acid hydroxylation during in vitro experiments involving thiols. *J. Chromatogr. B: Biomed. Sci. Appl.* **763**: 185–193.
8. Kawano T. and Muto S. (2000) Mechanism of peroxidase actions for salicylic acid-induced generation of active oxygen species and an increase in cytosolic calcium in tobacco cell suspension culture. *J. Exp. Bot.* **51**: 685–693.
9. Feng L., Xia Y., Garcia G. E., Hwang D. and Wilson C. B. (1995) Involvement of reactive oxygen intermediates in cyclooxygenase-2 expression induced by interleukin-1, tumor necrosis factor-alpha, and lipopolysaccharide. *J. Clin. Invest.* **95**: 1669–1675.
10. Thun M. J., Henley S. J. and Patrono C. (2002) Nonsteroidal anti-inflammatory drugs as anticancer agents: mechanistic, pharmacologic, and clinical issues. *JNCI, J. Natl. Cancer Inst.* **94**: 252–266.
11. Kiritoshi S., Nishikawa T., Sonoda K., Kukidome D., Senokuchi T., Matsuo T., Matsumura T., Tokunaga H., Brownlee M. and Araki E. (2006) Reactive oxygen species from mitochondria induce cyclooxygenase-2 gene expression in human mesangial cells: potential role in diabetic nephropathy. *Diabetes* **52**: 2570–2577.
12. Martinez M. E. and Greenberg E. R. (2007) More aspirin for less cancer? *JNCI, J. Natl. Cancer Inst.* **99**: 582–583.
13. Patrono C. and Rocca B. (2008) Aspirin: promise and resistance in the new millennium. *Arterioscler., Thromb., Vasc.* Biol. **28**: 25–32.

14. Patrono C. and Baigent C. (2009) Low-dose aspirin, coxibs, and other NSAIDs: a clinical mosaic emerges. *Mol. Interventions* **9**: 31–39.
15. Pedersen A. K. and FitzGerald G. A. (1984) Dose-related kinetics of aspirin. Presystemic acetylation of platelet cyclooxygenase. *N. Engl. J. Med.* **311**: 1206–1211.
16. Vane J. R. and Botting R. M. (1998) Anti-inflammatory drugs and their mechanism of action. *Inflammation Res.* **47** (Suppl. 2): 78–87.
17. Famaey J. P. and Paulus H. E. (eds.) (1992) *Therapeutic Applications of NSAIDs. Subpopulations and new formulations*. Marcel Dekker, New York.
18. Suhr Y.-J., Chun K.-S., Cha H.-H., Han S.-S., Keum Y.-S., Park K.-K. and Lee S.-S. (2001) Molecular mechanisms underlying chemopreventive activities of anti-inflamatory phytochemicals: down-regulation of COX-2 and iNOS through suppression of NF-kB activation. *Mutat. Res., Fundam. Mol. Mech. Mutagen.* **480–481**: 243–268.
19. Patrono C., Baigent C., Hirsh J. and Roth G. (2008) Antiplatelet drugs. American College of Chest Physicians evidence-based clinical practice guidelines, 8th ed. *Chest* **133**: 1995–2335.
20. Patrignani P., Filabozzi P. and Patrono C. (1982) Selective cumulative inhibition of platelet thromboxane production by low-dose aspirin in healthy subjects. *J. Clin. Invest.* **69**: 1366–1372.
21. Campbell C. L., Smyth S., Montalescot G. and Steinhubl S. R. (2007) Aspirin dose for the prevention of cardiovascular disease: a systematic review. *J. Am. Med. Assoc.* **297**: 2018–2024.
22. Baigent C., Sudlow C., Collins R. and Peto R. (2002) Antithrombotic Trialists' Collaboration. Collaborative meta-analysis of randomised trials of antiplatelet therapy for prevention of death, myocardial infarction, and stroke in high risk patients. *Br. Med. J.* **324**: 71–86.
23. Undas A., Brummel-Ziedins K. E. and Mann K. G. (2007) Antithrombotic properties of aspirin and resistance to aspirin: beyond strictly antiplatelet actions. *Blood* **109**: 2285–2292.
24. Maree A. O., Curtin R. J., Dooley M., Conroy R. M., Crean P., Cox D. and Fitzgerald D. J. (2005) Platelet response to low-dose enteric-coated aspirin in patients with stable cardiovascular disease. *J. Am. Coll. Cardiol.* **46**: 1258–1263.
25. Patrono C., García Rodrígues L. A., Landolfi R. and Baigent C. (2005) Low-dose aspirin for the prevention of atherothrombosis. *N. Engl. J. Med.* **353**: 2373–2383.

26. Capone M. L., Tacconelli S., Sciulli M. G., Grana M., Ricciotti E., Minuz P., Di Gregorio P., Merciaro G., Patrono C. and Patrignani P. (2004) Clinical pharmacology of platelet, monocyte, and vascular cyclooxygenase inhibition by naproxen and low-dose aspirin in healthy subjects. *Circulation* **109**: 1468–1471.
27. Capone M. L., Sciulli M. G., Tacconelli S., Grana M., Ricciotti E., Renda G., Di Gregorio P., Merciaro G. and Patrignani P. (2005) Pharmacodynamic interaction of naproxen with low-dose aspirin in healthy subjects. *J. Am. Coll. Cardiol.* **45**: 1295–1301.
28. Kearney P. M., Baigent C., Godwin J., Halls H., Emberson J. R. and Patrono C. (2006) Do selective cyclo-oxygenase-2 inhibitors and traditional non-steroidal anti-inflammatory drugs increase the risk of atherothrombosis? Meta-analysis of randomised trials. *Br. Med. J.* **332**: 1302–1308.
29. Fiorucci S., Santucci L. and Distrutti E. (2007) NSAIDs, coxibs, CINOD and H_2S-releasing NSAIDs: what lies beyond the horizon. *Dig. Liver Dis.* **39**: 1043–1051.
30. Praticò D. and Dogné J.-M. (2005) Selective cyclooxygenase-2 inhibitors development in cardiovascular medicine. *Circulation* **112**: 1073–1079.
31. Cole B. F., Logan R. F., Halabi S., Benamouzig R., Sandler R. S., Grainge M. J., Chaussade S. and Baron J. A. (2009) Aspirin for the chemoprevention of colorectal adenomas: meta-analysis of the randomized trials. *JNCI, J. Natl. Cancer Inst.* **101**: 256–266.
32. Antman E. M., Bennett J. S., Daugherty A., Furberg C., Roberts H. and Taubert K. A. (2007) Use of nonsteroidal antiinflamatory drugs. An update for clinicians: a scientific statement from the American Heart Association. *Circulation* **115**: 1634–1642.
33. Chan A. T., Giovannucci E. L., Meyerhardt J. A., Schernhammer E. S., Curhan G. C. and Fuchs C. S. (2005) Long-term use of aspirin and non-steroidal antiinflamatory drugs and risk of colorectal cancer. *J. Am. Med. Assoc.* **294**: 914–923.
34. Cook N. R., Lee I. M., Gaziano J. M., Gordon D., Ridker P. M., Manson J. E., Hennekens C. H. and Buring J. E. (2005) Low-dose aspirin in the primary prevention of cancer: the women's health study: a randomized controlled trial. *J. Am. Med. Assoc.* **294**: 47–55.
35. Chan A. T., Ogino S. and Fuchs C. S. (2009) Aspirin use and survival after diagnosis of colorectal cancer. *J. Am. Med. Assoc.* **302**: 649–658.
36. Bardia A., Ebbert J. O., Vierkant R. A., Limburg P. J., Anderson K., Wang A. H., Olson J. E., Vachon C. M. and Cerhan J. R. (2007) As-

sociation of aspirin and nonaspirin nonsteroidal anti-inflammatory drugs with cancer incidence and mortality. *JNCI, J. Natl. Cancer Inst.* **99**: 881–889.

37. Grau M. V., Sandler R. S., McKeown-Eyssen G., Bresalier R. S., Haile R. W., Barry E. L., Ahnen D. J., Gui J., Summers R. W. and Baron J. A. (2009) Nonsteroidal anti-inflammatory drug use after 3 years of aspirin use and colorectal adenoma risk: observational follow-up of a randomized study. *JNCI, J. Natl. Cancer Inst.* **101**: 267–276.
38. Logan R. F., Grainge M. J., Shepherd V. C., Armitage N. C. and Muir K. R. (2008) Aspirin and folic acid for the prevention of recurrent colorectal adenomas. *Gastroenterology* **134**: 29–38.
39. Chan A. T. (2010) COX-2 expression in adenoma: an imperfect marker for chemoprevention. *Gut* **59**: 568–569.
40. Bosetti C., Gallus S. and La Vecchia C. (2006) Aspirin and cancer risk: an updated quantitative review to 2005. *Cancer, Causes Control* **17**: 871–888.
41. Bosetti C., Gallus S. and La Vecchia C. (2009) Aspirin and cancer risk: an updated quantitative review to 2005. *Recent Results Cancer Res.* **181**: 231–251.
42. Gosselin R. E., Smith R. P., Hodge H. C. and Braddock J. E. (eds.) (1984) *Clinical toxicology of commercial products*. Williams & Wilkens, Baltimore.
43. Klaassen C. D. (ed.) (2001) *Casarett and Doull's Toxicology: the basic science of poisons*. McGraw-Hill Medical Publishing Division, New York.
44. Rimon G., Sidhu R. S., Lauver D. A., Lee J. Y., Sharma N. P., Yuan C., Frieler R. A., Trievel R. C., Lucchesi B. R. and Smith W. L. (2010) Coxibs interfere with the action of aspirin by binding tightly to one monomer of cyclooxygenase-1. *Proc. Natl. Acad. Sci. U. S. A.* **107**: 28–33.
45. Yoshimura R., Matsuyama M., Takemoto Y., Tsuchida K., Kawahito Y., Sano H. and Nakatani T. (2004) Relationship between lipoxygenase and human testicular cancer. *Int. J. Mol. Med.* **13**: 389–393.
46. Fürstenberger G., Krieg P., Müller-Decker K. and Habenicht A. J. (2006) What are cyclooxygenases and lipooxygenases doing in the driver's seat of carcinogenesis? *Int. J. Cancer* **119**: 2247–2254.
47. Soumaro L. T., Iida S., Uetake H., Ishiguro M., Takagi Y., Higuchi T., Yasuno M., Enomoto M. and Sugihara K. (2006) Expression of 5-lipoxygenase in human colorectal cancer. *World J. Gastroenterol.* **12**: 6355–6360.

48. Smith W. L., DeWitt D. L. and Garavito R. M. (2000) Cyclooxygenases: structural, cellular, and molecular biology. *Annu. Rev. Biochem.* **69**: 145–182.
49. Chandrasekharan N. V. and Simmons D. L. (2004) The cyclooxygenases. *Genome Biol.* **5**: 241.
50. Brown J. R. and DuBois R. N. (2005) COX-2: a molecular target for colorectal cancer prevention. *J. Clin. Oncol.* **23**: 2840–2855.
51. Carvello M. and Montalto G. (2006) Cyclooxygenases in hepatocellular carcinoma. *World J. Gastroenterol.* **12**: 5113–5121.
52. Menter D. G., Schilsky R. L. and DuBois R. N. (2010) Cyclooxygenase-2 and cancer treatment: understanding the risk should be worth the reward. *Clin. Cancer Res.* **16**:1384–1390.
53. Baba Y., Nosho K., Shima K., Goessling W., Chan A. T., Ng K., Chan J. A., Giovannucci E. L., Fuchs C. S. and Ogino S. (2010) PTGER2 overexpression in colorectal cancer is associated with microsatellite instability, independent of CpG island methylator phenotype. *Cancer Epidemiol., Biomarkers Prev.* **19**: 822–831.
54. Yuan C., Sidhu R. S., Kuklev D. V., Kado Y., Wada M., Song I. and Smith W. L. (2009) Cyclooxygenase allosterism, fatty acid-mediated cross-talk between monomers of cyclooxygenase homodimers. *J. Biol. Chem.* **284**: 10046–10055.
55. Vecchio A. J., Simmons D. M. and Malkowski M. G. (2010) Structural basis of fatty acid substrate binding to cyclooxygenase-2. *J. Biol. Chem.* **285**: 22152–22163.
56. Uddin M. J., Crews B. C., Blobaum A. L., Kingsley P. J., Gorden D. L., McIntyre J. O., Matrisian L. M., Subbaramaiah K., Dannenberg A. J., Piston D. W. and Marnett L. J. (2010) Selective visualization of cyclooxygenase-2 in inflammation and cancer by targeted fluorescent imaging agents. *Cancer Res.* **70**: 3618–3627.
57. Schetter A. J., Heegaard N. H. H. and Harris C. C. (2010) Inflammation and cancer: interweaving microRNA, free radical, cytokine and p53 pathways. *Carcinogenesis* **31**: 37–49.
58. Mateos J. L. (2010) Selective inhibitors of cyclooxygenase-2 (COX-2), celecoxib and parecoxib: a systematic review. *Drugs Today* **46** (Suppl A): 1–25.
59. Schneider C., Pratt D. A., Porter N. A. and Brash A. R. (2007) Control of oxygenation in lipoxygenase and cyclooxygenase catalysis. *Chem. Biol.* **14**: 473–488.
60. Buczynski M. W., Dumlao D. S. and Dennis E. A. (2009) Thematic review series: proteomics. An integrated omics analysis of eicosanoid biology. *J. Lipid Res.* **50**: 1015–1038.

CHAPTER EIGHT

CONCLUSIONS

1. There is a consensus that, although solar radiation has the all-encompassing effects which are essential for the sustenance of life on this planet, it also has malign streaks, i.e., it is a prooxidant, a mutagen, and a carcinogen to living matter.
2. The solar radiation that reaches the earth surface consists of UVB (280–320 nm), UVA1 (340–400 nm), and UVA2 (320–340 nm) radiations. About 70% of the energy UVB radiation is scattered and absorbed by the stratum corneum, and 30% reaches the epidermis and superficial dermis. About 30% of the energy of the UVA radiations is absorbed by the epidermis and 20% by the dermis.
3. Specifically, the energies of UV radiations are absorbed in the human skin by chromophores of urocanic acid, melanins, heterobases of DNA, NADH, flavins, unsaturated lipids, amino acids with aromatic nuclei, and other entities.
4. The energies of the chromophores are elevated by UV radiations involving n,π^* and π,π^* transitions to the excited states. The excited states can undergo various reactions, such as isomerizations, condensations, rearrangements, degradations, and reactions with molecular oxygen, which is a diradical in the ground state and an excellent quencher of triplet states.
5. The reactions with oxygen produce a cascade of reactive oxygen species (ROS), such as peroxyradical anion ($O_2{\cdot}^-$), hydroxyl radical ($HO{\cdot}$), hydrogen peroxide (H_2O_2), hydroperoxyl radical ($HOO{\cdot}$), singlet oxygen ($^1O_2$), and other species. These oxidizing species are exceedingly detrimental to biological systems, causing a variety of oxidative and degradative processes.
6. Urocanic acid and melanins are natural, endogenous sunscreens that have evolved over long periods of time, whereby the main protection of human skin is rendered by the eumelanins and less by pheomelanins. However, this protection is rather low. Thus, depending on the type of human skin, the sun protection factor for urocanic acid is about 2 and that for melanins is, on average, about 4. Further-

more, prolonged irradiation in the presence of oxygen results in the degradation of urocanic acid and melanins with formation of reactive oxygen species.

7. UVB and UVA2 radiations of the human skin cause damages to the DNA, producing nucleotide fragments. Interactions of these fragments with the tyrosinase enzyme produce constitutive and induced pigmentations of melanin.
8. UVA1 and UVA2 radiations induce another type of pigmentation. Thus, these radiations in small doses produce in about 15 minutes the so-called immediate pigmentation darkening (IPD) with grayish skin coloration that disappears in about two hours. Higher doses of UVA radiations produce the brownish persistent pigmentation darkening (PPD). The pigmentations occur by photooxidative processes of melanin and provide no protection against UV radiation induced damage of the skin.
9. After more than eighty years of commercial sunscreen use, it appears, that these radiation filters, when applied to the human skin as recommended at 2 mg/cm^2, can reduce the number of new keratoses, cause some remissions of existing keratoses, provide limited protection against skin aging, and provide protection against erythema, the so-called sunburns.
10. Uncertainties exist about the very desirable complete protection by sunscreen agents against the UV light induced skin cancers, such as squamous cell carcinoma (SCC), basal skin carcinoma (BSC), and malignant melanomas. Although reduced incidences of SCC have been reported, no such results were obtained with BCC and malignant melanoma.
11. SCC and BCC occur almost exclusively at cutaneous sites that receive most of the sun exposures. The metastasis of SCC is infrequently observed. The non-melanoma cancers can occur at any part of the human body, but primarily at the head, neck, hands, and forearms, i.e., on sites that are most readily exposed to solar radiations.
12. The majority of melanomas, >90%, are cutaneous lesions. However, melanomas can also occur on the retina, i.e., ocular melanoma, on mucous membranes, the nasopharyngeal sinuses, the vulva, and the anal canal. These non-cutaneous melanomas are usually detected at more advanced stages and are seldom curable.
13. Skin cancers are the most common type of all cancers. Thus, in the USA for example, more than one million of new skin cancer cases are diagnosed per year, whereby melanomas amounted in 2010 to about 69260 cases diagnosed with 8700 deaths, women and men included,

that is 4% of all skin cancer cases diagnosed. Women have a lower incidence of melanomas than men. The melanomas account for about 90% of skin cancer related mortalities.

14. The five year survival rates with melanoma are between 95 and 67 percent, depending on the advanced stages of the disease. The survival rate for non-melanoma cancers is about 99%.
15. After a regional spread of the disease, the survival rate for melanoma drops to about 35% and for non-melanoma cancers to about 50%.
16. After the spread of growth to distant organs, the survival rate for melanoma is about 2% and for non-melanoma about 10%. Since skin cancers are readily clinically detectable, the death rates for SCC and BCC are about 2%.
17. The protective capacity of sunscreens against the UV light induction of BCC and melanoma has not been firmly substantiated. One of the reasons could be that solar inductions of BCC and melanoma occur during childhood and adolescence, while the clinical manifestations appear, after years of dormancy, in a person's advanced years.
18. It has also been observed that persons who have outdoor occupations, and hence receive chronic exposures to UV radiations of the sun, acquire a tan and have, in general, a reduced risk of BCC and melanoma inceptions than persons who spend most of their time indoors with intermittant exposures to solar radiation.
19. Skin cancers are clinically treated with surgery, radiation therapy, and chemotherapy. For the chemotherapy of malignant melanoma, there are a number of drugs available belonging to various classes of organic compounds, including the rather toxic alkylating drugs, such as 1-(2-chloroethyl)-3-cyclohexylnitrosourea (CCNU).
20. It was found that the spin-labeled analogs of the clinically used antimelanoma drug CCNU, such as 1-(2-chloroethyl)-3-(1-oxyl-2,2,6,6-tetramethylpiperidinyl)-1-nitrosourea (SLCNU-1), have lower toxicities and higher activities than those of the clinically used parent drug. This effectiveness has been attributed to the lower carbamoylating and higher alkylating properties of the spin-labeled analogs than those of the unlabeled clinically used drug.
21. Furthermore, it was found that combinations of clinically used antimelanoma drugs, such as cisplatin and cyclophosphamide, and nitric oxide donor compounds result in therapeutically enhancing synergistic effects.
22. One of the beneficial properties of solar radiation is the generation of vitamin D in the human body, while sunscreens have a detrimental effect.

23. It was found that applications of sunscreen agents and avoidance of sun exposure can result in a drastic lowering of vitamin D levels in the human body, and that the required levels of vitamin D cannot be restored by dietary means but only by oral supplementations with vitamin D.
24. Low levels of vitamin D can have grave consequences such as risks of various diseases, including cancers.
25. It is also important to be aware that persons with dark skins are at a greater risk of developing D deficiencies than persons with lighter skins.
26. Nationwide, the healthcare costs associated with vitamin D deficiencies are much higher than those incurred by skin cancers.
27. The failures of protection by sunscreens against skin cancers and other biological maladies can be attributed, in part, to the intrinsic properties of sunscreens under UV radiations, and, in part to the unavoidable noncompliance by users to adhere to the unattainable requirements to spread an even layer of 2 mg/cm^2 over the whole UV light exposed skin.
28. In practice, it has been estimated that the thickness of layers on the skin are, at best, about 0.5 mg/cm^2, resulting in a sun protection factor (SPF) of about 2–3 using sunscreens with SPFs of 15–30. Therefore, the rendered protection is no better than the hereditary protection by melanins, at no cost.
29. Under these conditions, it was estimated that an SPF of 15 actually results in an SPF value of about 2 with a percent UV transmission, i.e., the amount of radiation that reaches the skin, of about 50%. The same considerations in the case of SPF 30 result in an SPF value of 2.3 with a percent UV transmission of 43%; for an SPF 50, the actual SPF value would be 2.6 with a percent transmission of 38%, and an SPF 100 would be reduced to an SPF 3.2 and a percent transmission of 21%.
30. The SPF values that are supplied with sunscreen products are poorly understood by the users, and are commercially exploited in marketing by advertising the merits of higher and higher SPF values than 30, implying highly improved properties of the sunscreen product that is actually not justified. In some countries, the advertising of SPF values higher than 30 is disallowed.
31. UVA and UVB radiations can cause immunosuppression even at suberythermal doses. The photoinduced immunosuppression is of concern since it is believed that, as a consequence of immunosuppression, mutation of the p53 gene can occur resulting in loss of apoptosis

control by the gene. Furthermore, the Langerhans cells contact hypersensitivity (CHS) and other biologically important entities are affected.

32. It appears that the sun protection factor (SPF) has no relevance to these events, since it might be possible to estimate on the basis of SPF values the periods of exposure to the sun without a visible erythema, while no information can be obtained about the possible onset of immunosuppression and other biological events that may occur prior to the erythema.
33. UVA and UVB radiations of the human skin induce structural and cellular changes in skin tissues through formation of radicals and reactive oxygen species (ROS), whereas UVA radiations at 320–400 nm induce the formation of radicals and ROS in the lower parts of the dermis.
34. The UV radiation induced harmful oxidative reactions are not unique to sunscreen products, since compounds of various classes with similar conjugated chromophores can undergo such reactions. Of particular importance is being aware that a large number of orally administered drugs and their metabolites readily migrate to the human skin and are exposed to UV radiations.
35. The extent of radical and ROS formation and the protection of the human skin by sunscreen agents can be quantitatively measured in vivo at the human skin by electron paramagnetic resonance spectrometry and expressed as the radical sun protection factor (RSP).
36. The RSP can be used similarly to SPF for the determination of increases in time for sun exposure of the skin with sunscreen to generate the same number of radicals and ROS as compared to unprotected skin.
37. Another sun protection factor, the p53 labeling index, has been proposed, and is obtained in vivo by an assessment of the sunscreen effectiveness in preventing the UV radiation induced DNA damage.
38. There are mounting concerns about the biological properties of sunscreens, excipients, and various skin care products that have been detected on many occasions in humans, other mammals, and the environment.
39. All sunscreen compounds and skin care products are formulated with about 30–50 different excipients that consist, not only of well-defined organic and inorganic compounds, but also of ill-defined plant extracts and polymers.
40. Sunscreens are often included in skin care products. Thus, for example, the sunscreen 2-hydroxy-4-methoxybenzophenone (oxybenzone,

benzophenone-3) can often be found in facial creams, moisturizers, conditioners, lipsticks, anti-aging creams, and other commercial products.

41. During the past decades, extensive results have been published about the allergic and photoallergic properties of sunscreen agents, including oxybenzone, excipients, and their degradation products. In general, the tendency has been either to minimize or to ignore these facts.
42. Sunscreens and skin care products contain also DMDM hydantoin, imidazolidinyl urea, and diazolidinyl urea, that degrade over time with liberation of carcinogenic formaldehyde which has been linked to possible risks of breast cancer, reproductive functions, and the development of melanoma.
43. UV irradiation of the frequently used sunscreens 4-*tert*-butyl-4-methoxydibenzoylmethane, 4-methylbenzylidene camphor, 2-ethylhexyl 4-methoxycinnamate, and benzophenone-3 facilitates the permeation of these compounds through the human skin into deeper nucleated layers of the dermis, where living cells are encountered, and are then detected in the human plasma and urine. The permeations are facilitated by the lipophilicities and low molecular weights (below 500) of these compounds.
44. Furthermore, it was found that the sunscreens 2-ethylhexyl 4-methoxycinnamate, 2-ethylhexyl salicylate, 3,3,5-trimethylcyclohexyl salicylate (homosalate), 2-ethylhexyl 4-dimethylaminobenzoate (2-ethylhexyl dimethyl PABA), benzophenone-3, and benzophenone-4 can function as skin permeation enhancers of insecticides, herbicides, and other xenobiotics.
45. It was also shown that when all three sunscreens, octocrylene, 2-ethylhexyl 4-methoxycinnamate and benzophenone-3, penetrate the nucleated layers of the human skin on UV irradiation, the levels of the generated ROS increase above the levels that normally are formed by irradiation of epidermal chromophores in the absence of sunscreens.
46. There have been extensive investigations of the estrogenic activities and endocrine disruptive properties of sunscreens, excipients, and cosmetic skin products, fragrances, and their metabolites.
47. A large number of these substances have been tested for estrogenic activities and immune system modulatory effects in vitro and in vivo by topical applications using rats, fish, aquatic invertebrates, and human volunteers.
48. These substances have been detected in adipose tissues, brain, plasma, and testes in rats. It was concluded that similar absorptions can occur in humans.

49. Thus, in the USA, benzophenone-3 was found in the urine of about 97% of human volunteers. Three to five hours after topical application of oxybenzone to human volunteers, with and without UV irradiation, it was excreted and was detected in the urine of 98% of six- to eight-year-old girls. The levels of oxybenzone were higher in girls and women than in boys and men.
50. The estrogenic sunscreens, 4-methylbenzylidene camphor and 3-benzylidene camphor, which are part of various skin care cosmetics, were tested for transdermal passages from mothers to offsprings through breast milk. It was found that 79% of women used these cosmetics and 76% of milk samples contained these fillers.
51. Low levels of the sunscreens 2-ethylhexyl 4-methoxycinnamate, 4-*tert*-butyl-4'-methoxydibenzoylmethane, and octocrylene have been detected in Swiss lakes and rivers.
52. Sunscreen compounds have been found in swimming pools, untreated and treated wastewaters, and sewage sludges that originate from private households and industrial activities.
53. Various parabens (alkyl 4-hydroxybenzoates) are routinely included in sunscreen products and skin care cosmetics. These compounds have acute and chronic toxic effects on fish and algae.
54. The very lipophilic benzotriazole filters were found distributed throughout the marine food chains in the Arika sea waters of Japan. These compounds accumulate in oysters and marine mammals. High concentrations of triazoles were also discovered in mussles in Korean, Hong-Kong, and Japanese waters.
55. Polycyclic musk fragrances, which are used in perfumes, cosmetics, and laundry detergents, were found in many organisms collected in Japanese coastal waters and in seals and dolphins in US waters.
56. Sunscreen filters and ingredients were shown to cause substantial bleaching of corals. It is estimated that about 10% of the worldwide coral reefs are affected. Furthermore, the affected corals release viruses to the surrounding waters, thus promoting viral infections.
57. Another area of concern is the unchecked proliferation of nanosize materials for a variety of profitable applications, including sunscreens, excipients, and skin care products. Specifically, it was found that carbon nanosize materials can, similarly to asbestos, cause lung inflammation and mesothelioma cancer. However, to date, no negative effects have been reported for nanosize UV filters, including the inorganic sunscreens titanium dioxide and zinc oxide, which do not permeate through the human skin and are not toxic.

58. In spite of these unfavorable reports, no governmental enforceable standards, guidelines, and regulations exist for these products that are readily available "over the counter" to anyone without prescription.
59. Glycoproteins derived from the Maillard reaction and Amadori and Heyns rearrangements are widely distributed in the human body. Maillard condensations also occur in food processing at elevated temperatures. The initial glycation products are further converted by oxidative and non-oxidative pathways to the so-called advanced glycation end products (AGEs).
60. The UV light induced reactions of AGEs with molecular oxygen produce a cascade of reactive oxygen species (ROS) and other products. The processes are associated with aging and various diseases, such as diabetes, macular degeneration, Alzheimer's, Parkinson's, cardiovascular, and other diseases.
61. A large number of persons with light-colored skin are using the so-called sunless self-tanning agents to obtain darker skin pigmentations. One of the self-tanning agents is dihydroxyacetone (DHA). It is important when using this self-tanning agent to avoid prolonged exposures to solar radiations shortly after the application of DHA to the skin.
62. The reasons for this precaution are based on the following results. The Maillard reaction of DHA, which is a mini-ketosugar, with amino acids in the skin layers followed by Heyns rearrangement, produces glycoproteins. The UV irradiation of this product in the presence of oxygen (air) produces a cascade of reactive oxygen species (ROS) in the human skin that can cause dermatological damage.
63. The amount of reactive oxygen species in the human skin can be measured by electron spin resonance spectroscopy. The value that is obtained was designated the radical sun protection factor (RSF). This method was used to establish that the UV radiation of DHA-treated skin generates quantities of ROS that are far above those found in the skin not treated by DHA.
64. Sunscreen agents are not a special class of compounds endowed with unique facilities to absorb the energy of solar radiations. Thus, sunscreen agents and many other compounds of various classes, such as topically and orally used medications, many antioxidants found in plants and the endogenous environment, melanins, urocanic acid, advance glycation end products, porphyrins, flavins, and many other compounds, just to mention a few, contain common, well-defined, and conjugated chromophores that can undergo photophysical and photochemical reactions.

65. UV light induces chromophores to undergo n,π* and π,π* transitions to the excited singlet state, followed by intersystem crossing (ISC) to the excited triplet state. At this stage, various reactions can occur, such as isomerizations, fragmentations, self-condensations to cyclobutane derivatives, and condensation with DNA heterobases to give cyclobutane derivatives.
66. The triplet state species can be readily quenched by molecular oxygen, which is a diradical in the ground state and the best quencher of excited triplets, resulting in a cascade of reactive oxygen species.
67. Hence, since any organic substance containing such chromophores could function as a sunscreen agent, it is a fallacy to promulgate the contention that commercially produced sunscreen agents are a special class of compounds endowed with unique facilities for the prevention of skin cancers and other maladies. Because of these conclusions, it is doubtful whether a further frantic search and proliferation of sunscreen products is justified. Clearly, the effectiveness of sunscreens has been overrated.
68. The development of new organic sunscreen agents should only be considered with restraint, since a discovery of products with unexpected revolutionary new properties is in doubt. Instead, more attention should be devoted to inorganic materials, such as titanium dioxide, zinc oxide, and other oxides.
69. The human safety, stability, and percutaneous absorptions of inorganic sunscreens titanium dioxide and zinc oxide have been thoroughly investigated using nanosize particles of these oxides. There seems to be a consensus that these UV filters are very stable and, unlike some organic sunscreens, are not degrading and not penetrating into the human skin beyond the upper stratum corneum. These sunscreen filters absorb the energies of UVA and UVB radiation. Cerium dioxide (CeO_2) was proposed as an additional inorganic UV filter with similar absorptions. These filters must be encapsulated to prevent reactions with molecular oxygen.
70. Photostabilities of frequently used commercial sunscreen filters have been investigated using UVA and UVB radiations in the presence of vitamin E and compared with nitroxide (nitroxyl, aminoxyl) radical inhibitors. It was found that considerable reduction in oxidative damage to the sunscreens resulted only in the presence of aminoxyl radical inhibitors, while with vitamin E there was either no effect or a lesser effect as compared to the aminoxyl inhibitors.
71. Since vitamin E is a rather unstable compound under these conditions, blocked vitamin E compounds, such as ether and ester derivatives,

have been frequently used. However, these compounds have been found to be either only marginally effective or inactive.

72. Results obtained in many investigations over the years could not provide unambiguous information on the efficiencies of topically and orally administered exogenous antioxidants for the prevention of photoinduced damage to biological systems, including cancers.
73. In recent years, spin-labeled sunscreens, possessing aminoxyl radicals in their structures, have been synthetized. Thus, 4-methoxycinnamic acid was esterified with 4-hydroxy-2,2,6,6-tetraethylpiperidin-4-yl-1-oxyl (TEMPOL) to give spin-labeled 1-oxyl-2,2,6,6-tetramethylpiperidin-4-yl 4-methoxy-cinnamate. These novel sunscreens containing an antioxidant are aimed at reducing the photodamage to traditional sunscreens caused by UV radiations.
74. In the past fifty years, a number of investigations with very large numbers of participants have been conducted, such as case-control studies, cohort studies, meta-analyses, and randomized controlled trials in order to establish the usefulness of various endogenous antioxidants as possible drugs for various diseases, including cancers. The following antioxidants have been mainly investigated: vitamin E, vitamin C, vitamin A, α-lipoic acid, β-carotene, other carotenes, and, occasionally, selenium.
75. Analyzing at random selected results from various medicinal studies of vitamin E, it appears that, in order to obtain meaningful results, a high dosage of vitamin E should be used, such as 3200 mg (~4500 IU) per day, in conjunction with a large excess of vitamin C. The reason for the need of an excess of vitamin C is its function as a "chaperon" to vitamin E by continuously restoring the reducing capacity of vitamin E.
76. Although all kinds of vitamin E have been used in trials, reliable results can be expected and have been obtained only with the natural dα-tocopherol, (2*R*,4*R*,8*R*).
77. Another promising antioxidant appears to be α-lipoic acid, which was used in trials either as a 600 mg oral supplement or as an intravenous injection using a 1000 mg dose.
78. In conclusion, the antioxidants vitamin E and lipoic acid could function either in the prevention of certain diseases, or more likely as mitigating, ameliorating, and retarding agents in disease progression, but not as rapidly acting drugs.
79. It is now well established that the induction and progression of various diseases, and in particular cancers, are associated with chronic inflammations. The inflammations are caused by a chain of events in-

volving free radical type reactions of molecular oxygen and ROS with arachidonic acid and with other aliphatic long-chain unsaturated acids, which are formed in high-fat food consumptions, mediated by lipoxygenase and cyclooxygenase enzymes.

80. It is not unreasonable to assume that anti-inflammatory drugs like Aspirin™ (acetyl salicylic acid), other anti-inflammatory drugs (NSAIDs), and coxibs such as Celebrex®, could be used for the prevention and possible cure of inflammatory diseases by inhibiting the formation of reactive oxygen species catalyzed by lipooxygenase and cyclooxygenase enzymes.
81. Based on very large numbers of various studies, an assessment can be made that regular use of Aspirin™ is associated with a reduced risk, and even cure, of colorectal cancers, and based on still-limited evidence, when administered regularly over long periods of time, may have a favorable retarding effect on other cancers.
82. Furthermore, Aspirin™ has been shown on many occasions to have various cardioprotective properties over a wide range of dosages, and it has been recommended that it should be coadministered with the anti-inflammatory drugs that lack this property and often cause heart problems.
83. In conclusion, it appears certain that the key targets for the prevention and possible cure of cancers are the lipoxygenase and cyclooxygenase enzymes, and Aspirin™ is a promising nontoxic drug candidate for further evaluation with other diseases including cancers.

CHAPTER NINE

RECOMMENDATIONS

It is recommended that:

1. In line with IARC recommendations, the approval process of sunscreen products should follow the same safety requirements as those used by the FDA for the approval of orally administered medicines, i.e., detailed accounts must be provided by the producers about the biological properties of all ingredients in their products.
2. The FDA and other regulatory agencies should initiate investigations into the systemic absorptions of sunscreen and cosmetic product ingredients and their estrogenic and endocrine disruptive properties, since it was shown that benzophenone-3 and 3-(4'-methylbenzylidene) camphor apparently possess these properties.
3. It should be the general practice to include a disclaimer on product labels of commercial sunscreen products that the product should not be considered for the prevention of skin cancers, and that the product is only deemed effective for ameliorating erythema, i.e., inflammation and sunburn effects when applied according to recommended guidelines.
4. All sunscreen agents and ingredients in sunscreen formulations and skin care cosmetics, which were found to permeate the human skin and were detected in humans, should be immediately withdrawn from commercial products pending further investigations.
5. The FDA and other regulatory agencies should undertake detailed evaluations of the frequently used ingredients (parabens, DMDM hydratoin, imidazolidinyl urea, and diazalidinyl urea) in sunscreens and skin care cosmetics. The parabens were detected in cancerous breast tissues and the ureas are degraded with formation of cancerous formaldehyde. US members of Congress have instructed the FDA to pursue this matter.
6. The use of Sun Protection Factor (SPF) numbers on commercial products should be abandoned since they convey to the user of sunscreens a false sense of security. Instead, a device should be devel-

oped, which could be supplied with the products that would enable the users to assess, by color changes, the degree of severity of solar radiation at the prevailing exposure conditions, similarly to the UV color index which was developed by the World Health Organization, United Nations Environmental Program. Other factors, such as the Radical Sun Protection Factor (RSF) and additional proposed factors should be considered for inclusion.

7. The formulations of sunscreens should include the enzymes photolyases and endonucleases, which, unlike sunscreens, can remove the photoproducts of the DNA and even prevent damage to the immunosuppression process. These ingredients should be listed on the commercial product packaging.
8. It should be established whether the precursors and precancerous lesions contain specific markers, mutated entities, such as cancer-induced pluripotent stem cells, which can be identified and followed during the whole evolutionary process until eventually they are clinically diagnosed as malignant cancerous growth.
9. Regulatory agencies, such as the FDA, should pursue the reports on pollution from household and industrial effluents and sludges containing sunscreens and cosmetic product contaminants which were detected in humans and their urine excreta; on pollution of aquatic environments, such as rivers, lakes, and marine mammals; and on the destruction of coral reefs worldwide by sunscreen products.
10. Organic sunscreens should be forsaken altogether, and only the inorganic compounds titanium dioxide (TiO_2) and zinc oxide (ZnO) should be used, with further consideration for cerium dioxide (CeO_2). These compounds are stable and do not migrate through the human skin even in the form of nanosize particles, are used in sunscreens and cosmetic products, and are particularly suited for persons with skin sensitive to organic sunscreens. According to the Environmental Working Group (EWG), they have the best safety record.
11. Organic nanosize sunscreens, excipients, and cosmetic skin care products should be investigated for possible harmful properties since it was found that certain nanosize carbon materials can cause lung inflammations and even mesothelioma similarly to asbestos.
12. Persons who use the "sunless" tanning agent dihydroxyacetone (DHA) should avoid exposures to UV radiations immediately following the application of DHA because of excessive UV light induced formation of ROS.
13. Persons who have vitamin D deficiencies because of irregular sun exposures, diligent use of sunscreens, or have inherited dark skin col-

orations should take oral vitamin D supplementations and not rely on dietary regimes which are ineffective.

14. The proven effectiveness of spin-labeled antimelanoma drugs, and the synergistic effects of nitric oxide donor compounds with clinically used antimelanoma drugs should be further explored in Phase I, II, and III trials.
15. The use of vitamin E and its ethers and esters in sunscreen formulations and skin care cosmetics should be discontinued and replaced with the more effective aminoxyl radical antioxidants.
16. For oral administration of vitamin E, only d-α-tocophenol should be used together with lipophilic food, such as olive oil and an excess of vitamin C.
17. Aspirin™ be administered together with anti-inflammatory drugs, such as Celebrex™, in order to prevent cardiovascular complications.

CHAPTER TEN

ADDENDUM: SYNOPSIS: AN EXTENDED NARRATIVE OF THE REVIEW

SOLAR-ENERGY-ABSORBING SUBSTANCES AND OXIDATIVE STRESS AND INFLAMMATORY DISEASES

A. Skin Cancers

Although solar radiation has all-encompassing benign effects that are essential for the sustenance of life on this planet, it has also malign streaks, i.e., it can function as a pro-oxidant, a mutagen, and a carcinogen. The most important consequences of these properties of solar radiation are the induction of cutaneous cancerous growth in humans, other mammals, and other species.

In recent years, more than one million new skin cancer cases have been diagnosed per year in the USA, as compared to about 1.3 million cases of all other cancers combined. Hence, the incidence of skin cancers is about one half of all other cancers that have been diagnosed per year. Fortunately, the death rates for skin cancers, including melanomas, are low as compared to most other cancers. The most prevalent skin cancers are the basal cell carcinoma (BCC), the squamous cell carcinoma (SCC), and melanomas. The non-melanoma skin cancers are mainly found on the head, neck, hands, and forearms; however, they can also appear on any other part of the skin.

Actually, four histologic types of cutaneous melanomas are known, i.e., lentigo maligna melanoma, superficial spreading melanoma, nodular melanoma, and acral lentiginous melanoma. The first three melanomas are the more common cancers of the skin. The lentigo maligna melanoma is definitely caused by cumulative life-long exposures to solar radiation. In the other melanomas, the inductions of the diseases are not certain. The melanomas are composed of more than 90% cutaneous lesions. However, they can also occur as non-cutaneous growth in the retina, mucous membranes, and other parts of the body. In the United States, about 60,000 to 70,000 cases of melanoma are diagnosed annually, resulting in about 8,000–9,000 deaths.

Although, over the years, the incidence of melanoma was on average about 4% of that of non-melanoma cancers, the melanoma cancers caused about three times as many death as the non-melanoma cancers.

Melanoma was barely known at the beginning of the twentieth century. Thus, in 1935, the chance of suffering from melanoma was about 1 in 1500, while 35 years later the ratio was about 1 in 70. Anecdotally, the increase in incidences of melanoma coincides with the increase of sales and consumption of sunscreen products. These figures are frequently quoted in various articles stressing the apparently unabated growth of incidences of melanoma, and a possible role of sunscreen agents in the proliferation of skin cancers, seemingly without consulting some pertinent statistical data.

At this juncture, it might be worthwhile to consider the bare facts of this issue. Thus, the incidence of melanoma over the past thirty years in the USA among the "whites", i.e., people with light-colored skin, rose during the period 1975 to 2006 from about 8 to 24 per 100,000, while the rates for persons of African origin remained unchanged at approximately 1 to 2 per 100,000, and for people with other types of colored skin such as Hispanics, Asia/Pacific Islanders, American Indians, and Alaska natives, the incidence remained unchanged during the period 1993 to 2003, from 2 to 5 per 100,000. It is also of interest that the incidence of melanoma among the white male and female populations of age groups 50–54 to 85 declined during the years 2001 to 2003 in comparison to the period 1992 to 1994. Further, it is also significant that, in spite of the steep increase of incidences of melanoma in white populations, the mortality rate in the USA remained practically unchanged during the period 1975 to 2008, between 2 and 2.5 per 100,000 for the white population, and even lower for people with colored skin, between 1 and 2 per 100,000.

Sometimes alarmist statements can be found in the press, such as "one person with melanoma dies every 68 minutes." However, it amounts actually to a death of 7624–8700 per one million incidences per year in the USA, which is one of the lowest of all cancers. Thus, such statements convey a possible epidemic that is not real. It is further instructive to assess and make comparisons of the percentages of patients who will succumb to the respective cancers based on the diagnosed cases in the USA in 2008. In the following evaluation, the first entries in the brackets are the incidences per year, the second entries are the associated deaths, and the third entries are the percentages of those who died of a particular cancer:

pancreatic (37,170, 33,370, 90%), esophageal (16,470, 14,280, 87%), lung (220,020, 162,610, 74%), multiple myeloma (19,920, 10,690, 54%), acute leukemias (44,270, 21,710, 49%), ovarian (21,650, 15,520, 72%), gastric (21,000, 10,880, 52%), non-Hodgkin lymphoma (66,120, 19,160, 29%), colorectal/anal (148,810, 49,960, 34%), kidney (54,390, 13,010, 24%), cervical (11,070, 3,670, 33%), urethelial (68,810, 14,100, 21%), breast (182,460, 40,480, 22%), endometrial (39,080, 7,400, 19%), prostate (186,320, 28,600, 15%), all skin cancers (one million diagnosed, 8,700 deaths, ~ 1%; based on 69,180 incidences of melanoma cases and associated deaths of 8,700 in 2009, the mortality rate would be about 12.8%).

Thus, in spite of their highest incidences of all cancers, skin cancers are among the lowest in mortality. Furthermore, in contrast to most other cancers, skin cancers and their precursors can be early visually detected and readily clinically diagnosed. Most melanomas and nearly all non-melanoma skin cancers, which are diagnosed at an early stage, can be readily cured by surgery, radiation, and chemotherapy. The five-year (a period of time that is considered a cure) survival rates are 87% for melanoma when it is localized and 99% for non-melanoma cancers. In the case of a regional spread, the survival figures are 35% for melanoma and 50% for non-melanomas, while, for a delayed treatment resulting in a distant spread to other organs, i.e., metastasis, the survival figures for melanoma are only 2% and for the non-melanomas <10%. However, metastasis occurs only in about 2% of SCC patients and in about 0.1% of BCC patients.

The clinical treatments of melanoma at advanced states of the disease by a combination of drugs, such as dacarbazine (DTIC), cisplatin, and carmustine (BCNU), usually result in median survivals below 12%. In contrast, non-melanoma cancers can be successfully treated in many cases with 5-fluorouracil (5-FU). In recent years, substantial exploratory research has been conducted in search for new drugs against various cancers including melanoma. Of particular interest, but somewhat neglected, are the so-called spin-labeled drugs, i.e., clinically well-established drugs, such as DTIC, chloroethylnitrosoureas, and rubomycin, containing the nitroxyl (aminoxyl) moiety. Characteristically, these spin-labeled drugs have a lower toxicity and a higher activity in vivo than the unlabeled clinical parent drugs. These results have been attributed to their lower carbamoylation and higher alkylation properties than those of the clinical drugs.

A further important result was achieved by a combination of clinically used drugs against melanomas, such as cyclophosphamide (Endoxan), with a nitric oxide donor compound producing a positive synergistic effect. This result is actually not surprising considering the well-known and important roles of nitric oxide in biological systems.

It is not unreasonable to assume that all skin cancers would be preceded by some lesions, i.e., pathologically altered tissues of the skin, which might be viewed as precursors or precancers. While in cases of SCC and melanoma such recognizable precursors are observed, in the case of BCC and melanoma no such precursors can be found. BCC and SCC are very common slow-growing cancers that rarely metastasize. The precursors of SCC are dysplasias in the form of actinic (solar) keratosis, which appear at the sun-exposed areas of the skin and are well identifiable in clinical oncology. Patients with solar keratosis can have a 30–50% deficit in DNA repair of photoproducts. These solar keratoses often regress. SCC appearances may occur twenty or forty years after the initial appearances of dysplasias, and they seldom, if ever, regress. The mechanism of regression is not fully understood. However, it is believed that the cause of regression could be the recovery of the immune system, coupled with a possible induction of apoptosis, since the solar keratosis and SCC are frequently found in patients on immunosuppressive drugs. The p53 gene, which regulates the cell cycle and cell death, i.e., apoptosis, and the PTCH gene, which is part of the signaling pathways, are mutated in BCC and SCC. The p53 is also mutated in dysplasias and in at least one half of all human cancers. Dysplasias can be clinically treated with 5-fluorouracil, which, apparently, is somehow involved as an apoptosis-inducing agent.

Many conclusions on the propagation of skin cancers are based on experiments with small, short-lived mammals, usually with specially bred mice, because one can obtain results in a much shorter time than with human volunteers. Thus, one can observe the evolution of a cancer in a small mammal over a period of two years, while it would require a period of up to 60 to 80 years with human volunteers. Clearly, it is risky to form definite conclusions on the basis of experiments with small mammals.

The precursors of melanoma may appear at an early age of one to five years, either as melanocytic naevi (Greek naevi, i.e., moles, birthmarks), which increase in numbers and disappear by the ages of 15 to 25, or as dysplastic naevi, i.e., atypical moles which can have malignant characteristics. The typical benign moles, i.e., melanocytic naevi are regularly shaped with tan or brown color. Persons with this type of moles are at some risk of eventually developing melanoma. Atypical moles, i.e., dysplastic naevi are large and irregularly shaped with tan and brown color. Persons with this type of moles are at about 80% risk of developing melanoma. These pigmented lesions may appear in childhood at ages 5 to 6 years. The number of naevi is directly proportional to the exposure to sunlight during the early ages of life. Moles usually regress by the ages of 15 to 25, and, at advanced ages, the moles are usually absent. Thus, it was found that, each year, out of 7000 cases with common naevi and 80 with dysplastic naevi, only one melanoma case is diagnosed. About 5 percent of melanomas also regress. Since it is believed that melanomas are caused in part by a convoluted mechanism involving immunosuppression, the regression is probably associated with the restoration of the immune system and apoptosis. The progression of naevi to the melanomas is a slow process and may commence at the age of 30 or later.

Many mammalian melanomas contain mutations and inactivations in the p53 gene and in the tumor-suppressor gene CDKN2A, involving methylation processes of the cytosine sites, resulting in the formation of 5-methylcytosines, which are converted into thymines by a deamination process.

Although the cancer precursors, such as solar keratoses, moles, papillomas, naevi, and other lesions of the skin, and, finally, manifestation of the cancerous growth, can be clinically well diagnosed and treated, the ultimate question is whether all these visual signs and possible markers, such as the mutated genes, are propagated during the whole process over many decades until the appearance of the cancerous lesions, or is one, at present, following the wrong trails. How can one be sure that skin cancer formation is prevented by elimination of the precursors, such as keratinocytes and naevi? It is possible that besides these and other markers, which may or may not develop into the cancerous state after decades of incubation following induction by solar radiation, there exist precancerous cell types, such as cancerous stem cells, which cannot be detected and clinically treated at the present time. Unlike normal healthy cells, which are continuously dividing, producing progeny copies, and eventually dying out, the cancerous stem cells can undergo differentiation, divide only occasionally, can remain in a resting phase for prolonged periods of time, and are not affected by regular treatments with anticancer drugs. It is possible that these stem cells, which comprise only a small fraction of all cells, are determining the outcome of skin cancers, and the bulk of other cells are inconsequential. The challenge, then, is to be able clinically to recognize these cancerous stem cells and to devise methods for clinical treatments already at the early states of cutaneous cancer development, i.e., at the precursor or precancerous stages.

B. Effects of Sunscreen Use

The human skin is one of the larger organs of the human body, and, by evolutionary design, it is supposed to provide a barrier against the external environment which contains a variety of chemical species including pollutants, xenobiotics, and free radicals. There have been estimates that, in the industrialized countries, the inhabitants might be exposed to an atmosphere containing up to several thousands of various chemical species. Since the skin is also exposed at all times to high concentrations of molecular oxygen and to solar ultraviolet radiation, it is susceptible to oxidative stress involving reactive oxygen species (ROS), a condition where an imbalance occurs between antioxidant and prooxidant equilibria in favor of the latter, resulting in damaging conditions to the endogenous biological environment. It is now well established that ROS are the cause of inflammations leading to chronic inflammations, which are associated with various diseases including cancers.

The epidermis of the human skin is the first layer of defense, composed of lipid-soluble antioxidants, such as vitamin E, vitamin C, carotenoids, glutathione, the enzymes superoxide dismutase, catalase, glutathione reductase, glutathione dismutase, and water. The presence of these endogenous agents can reduce or even prevent lipid peroxidation processes of the skin, depending on the prevailing levels of these agents. However, the chronic, cumulative solar ultraviolet radiations with their strong prooxidant properties can overwhelm the protective capabilities of the antioxidant systems of the skin resulting in erythema, i.e., reddening, sunburn effects, aging of the skin, and inflammations which can lead to various diseases including cancers. Topical applications to the skin of antioxidants, such as vitamin E, vitamin C, and carotenoids can reduce the lipid peroxidation processes in the skin when applied before irradiation. In commercial sunscreen formulations, one often finds vitamin E acetate and vitamin E succinate because of their higher stability than that of the free vitamin E. These derivatives have been found to be either inferior or ineffective as antioxidants since they are not readily metabolized on the skin.

The various effects of solar radiation on the human body will depend on the intensity of solar radiation at the skin, that, in turn, will be determined by prevailing conditions, such as time of day, season, altitude, parts of the body which are exposed to direct irradiation, duration of exposure, i.e., whether it is chronic or intermittent, and whether the skin is topically covered with cosmetics, sunscreen agents, medications, antioxidants, or orally administered medications that will, inadvertently, surface at the skin either unchanged or, most likely, as metabolites.

In addition, the ubiquitous porphyrins, which are present in all living matter, might be involved in photophysical and photochemical processes. Flavin-adenine nucleotides, which are present as prosthetic groups of many enzymes; various entities with quinone moieties, e.g., melanins and flavonoids that are part of many exogenous antioxidants; advanced glycation end products; and many other entities might also be involved in these processes. All these compounds have in common a unifying feature, i.e., they all have analogous well-defined chromophores, which have the facility to absorb the energy of the solar ultraviolet radiations. These chromophores are composed of conjugated carbon–carbon, carbon–oxygen, and carbon–nitrogen double bonds containing π and n electrons, whereby the chromophores can be arranged in molecules either linearly or as ring systems.

Solar radiation causes π,π^* and n,π^* transitions to give excited singlet and triplet species that can undergo photophysical and photochemical reactions, such as either energetically return to the ground state with emissions of fluorescence and phosphorescence radiations, or undergo reactions involving bond breaking and reactions with the ubiquitous oxygen, resulting in a cascade of biologically damaging reactive oxygen species, such as hydroxyl radicals ($HO\cdot$), peroxyanion radicals ($O_2\cdot^-$), singlet oxygen ($^1O_2$), hydrogen peroxide, and other oxidants.

The human epidermis and stratum corneum can attenuate the UVA and UVB radiations, whereby the UVB radiations are more effectively attenuated than the UVA radiations. The natural pigmentation of the skin is provided by melanins, which were predestined by evolution, together with urocanic acid, to function as natural sunscreen agents. However, they are inefficient sunscreen agents and can undergo further photodynamic reactions with molecular oxygen to give reactive oxygen species. Furthermore, their use cannot provide full protection against the induced changes by solar radiations leading to immune suppression, depletion of Langerhans cells, suppression of contact and delayed hypersensitivity, T cell mediated immune responses, formation of various photoproducts of DNA involving thymine, cytosine, and purine bases, formation of DNA–protein cross-links, depression of NK cell activity, lipid peroxidations, urocanic acid cis–trans isomerizations, photodeactivation of enzymes, and other damaging reactions to biological entities.

Recently, an eye-catching statement was published calling sunscreens “the snake oil of the 21st century.” Although this statement might be excessive, nevertheless, it can be justified in view of the bold claims that are made about the effectiveness of sunscreen products, including their facility in preventing skin cancers.

The sunscreen products that are offered in the USA to the public "over the counter", i.e., without a doctor's prescription, belong mainly to seven classes of organic compounds—cinnamates, salicylates, benzophenones, anthranilates, dibenzoylmethanes, phenylbenzimidazole, *p*-aminobenzoic acid (PABA) and its derivatives—and the inorganic compounds titanium dioxide and zinc oxide.

In the USA, seventeen (17) representatives of these classes have been approved by the FDA. In Europe and worldwide, about twice as many analogues have been approved. In addition, there are several compounds in use which are camphor derivatives, and derivatives of heterocyclic classes of compounds, such as benzoxazole, benzimidazole, triazoles, triazenes, and miscellaneous.

Even a casual examination of the literature reveals that basically all major classes of sunscreen agents have been known for many years, although some products are advertised as new discoveries. Thus, 2-phenyl-1*H*-benzimidazole, which is used as a sulfonic acid derivative in sunscreen agents in the USA, Australia, and Europe, has been known since 1926 and used as an anthelmintic for sheep. In 2006, the FDA approved for use in the USA the water-soluble shortwave UVA filter terephthalidine-3,3'-dicamphor-10,10'-disulfonic acid (ecamsole, Mexoryl® SX). This approval is not a great revelation, since the compound was patented about 23 years ago. Complaints have been raised in the press that the approval of sunscreen products by the FDA is too demanding, thus preventing the introduction of new products, especially for the prevention of skin cancers, a claim that is overly contentious. It is further claimed that the application of a drug standard to sunscreen products would be inadmissible since the costs would be prohibitive and could not be recouped through sales by the pharmaceutical industry, as is the case for internally applied medications.

This type of argument is made by neglecting the facts that the discovery, development, and in vivo testing on humans in Phase I, II, and III clinical trials, which are required by the FDA for approval of internal medications, involve incomparably higher efforts, costs, and risks than the development of topically used, readily procurable sunscreen products that will not require such extensive trials.

About 30–50 of the so-called excipients are used in formulations of sunscreen products. In Latin, excipere means to take up or take out. This term is used to define an inert substance that provides a "vehicle", e.g., for a drug. It seems to be a poor choice of a term for complex mixtures of substances that are found in formulations of sunscreens, such as alcohols, esters, acids, proteins, carbohydrates, antioxidants, and other classes of ingredients. Thus, the alcohols can be oxidatively converted into toxic aldehydes, esters can undergo transesterifications, acids can undergo decarboxylations, and aromatic compounds can undergo photophysical and photochemical reactions induced by solar radiation. Some ingredients can decompose with the liberation of formaldehyde which is mutagenic. The formulations can also contain colorants and fragrances often without structural specifications. During the past decades, troubling results were obtained with some sunscreen agents and excipients, such as allergic and photoallergic reactions, possible estrogen activities and endocrine disruptive properties, permeations through the human skin, and their functions as carrier of xenobiotics through the skin, and detection in the breast milk of women and in the urine of adults and children. Furthermore, sunscreen agents have been detected in domestic and industrial wastewaters, in swimming pools, in lakes, rivers, and oceans, and in some destroyed coral reefs. Thus, to consider these substances as inert seems to be an oversimplification. In an approval process using drug standards, the excipients would also have to undergo a more careful scrutiny than has been the practice at present. Some of the more common sunscreens are also included in skin care products, such as lipsticks and facial creams. A large number of investigations have been conducted in vitro and in vivo with humans and other mammals, usually mice, concerning the possible protection rendered by topical applications of sunscreens to the skin against solar radiation induced pathological effects, including skin cancers.

A bewildering number of diverse and conflicting conclusions can be found concerning the efficacy of the use of sunscreen products. This diversity of results has been attributed to experimental designs and, in particular, to the use of "sunlamps", which contain significant portions of energies of non-solar UV spectra. Thus, sunlamps emitting UV light at wavelengths below 245 nm can cause immunosuppression followed by defects of other biological entities.

The consensus seems to be that sunscreen agents, if applied to the human skin at the prescribed coverage by the FDA of 2 mg/cm^2 thickness under well-controlled experimental conditions, can reduce and even prevent the erythema, i.e., sunburn effect, reddening, and inflammation of the skin, and possibly reduce the risk of SCC incidence, but not those of BCC and melanoma. These results are of particular significance for persons with light-colored skin. The incidents of skin lesions among persons with dark-colored skin are considerably lower.

Interestingly and somewhat surprisingly, in many cases, the use of sunscreens resulted in significantly higher risks of developing melanoma. Again, these results have been attributed to experimental designs. However, another explanation could be that sunscreen agents might undergo photolytic reactions resulting in products of degradation, rearrangements, dimerizations, and photodynamic reactions, i.e., reactions with molecular oxygen to give reactive oxygen species that are harmful to biological entities. In particular, UVA radiation is damaging to DNA, producing reactive oxygen species and resulting in the formation of cyclobutane pyrimidine dimers and other products, peroxidations, and carcinogenesis. The peroxidations can be ameliorated but not prevented by the use of endogenous and exogenous antioxidants, such as vitamin E, vitamin C, and other antioxidants. However, vitamin E and vitamin C might have, beside this benign effect, also a malign property since they could conceivably also function as prooxidants. The use of sunscreens has been found to reduce the number of DNA cyclobutane dimers. However, organic sunscreens were found to permeate through the human skin and to function as carriers of xenobiotics. In contrast, the inorganic sunscreens titanium dioxide and zinc oxide, when encapsulated, do not permeate through the skin and are not toxic. UV irradiation of unencapsulated titanium dioxide and zinc oxide sunscreens can produce strand breaks in DNA caused by the formation of reactive oxygen species. The formation of ROS has also been found with various organic sunscreen compounds, such as 2-ethylhexyl PABA, benzophenone-3, and phenylbenzimidazole. These results are not surprising since all of these compounds have conjugated chromophores that are essential for promotion to excited singlet and triplet species and further reactions with molecular oxygen to give ROS.

Ultraviolet solar radiation enhances the growth of melanoma. The mechanism of this enhancement is not fully understood; however, it is known that solar radiation can function not only as an initiator but also as a promoter of cancer development. In statistically designed studies, it has been found that the risk of developing melanoma was higher in users of sunscreens than in non-users, while in other studies the use of sunscreen agents was found to be ineffective.

However, one should be aware that solar radiation is mainly affecting persons with "light" skin, while persons with "dark" skin are much less susceptible, and the mortality rate from melanoma is very low, about 1 per 100,000 in the USA.

The effects of intermittent exposure to solar radiations are more prevalent in melanoma cases, than those from chronic exposures. Induction usually occurs during childhood, and sunlight can also function as a promoter in the following years. Persons with chronic solar exposures are at lower risks of developing melanoma than persons with intermittent exposures. Thus, melanoma incidences are more common in indoor working persons than outdoor workers, occurring on parts of the body that are only occasionally exposed to sunlight. Almost all BCC and SCC of human non-melanoma cancers occur on chronic exposures to sunlight, mainly on the head, neck, and hands. There is a clear association between the cumulative sun exposures and incidences of the non-melanoma cancers. In the case of BCC, the use of sunscreens had either no protective effect or a modest increase in BCC. A study involving 73,366 nurses exposed to sunlight outdoors in the summer resulted in an elevated risk of BCC as compared to non-users of sunscreen preparations. Actinic (solar) keratoses are considered to be precursors of SCC. In some studies, a protective effect by the use of sunscreens was found, whereas in other studies no effect could be detected. Thus, in experiments with human volunteers, the participants using sunscreens in one study had on average a 36% lower number of keratosis, while in another study a 25% higher number of keratosis was observed as compared with persons using a placebo. In a further study lasting two years with eight hours of daily solar exposures, there was no protective effect in persons who used sunscreens. In another study, the incidences of SCC were observed in 28 cases using sunscreens against 46 cases not using sunscreens. The topical application of antioxidants, such as vitamin E and vitamin C, to the mouse skin could not prevent the non-melanomas skin cancers, but could only ameliorate the condition.

UVA and UVB radiations are both potent immunosuppressors. The immunosuppression is probably relevant to the induction of skin cancers. In numerous studies, the efficacy of the use of sunscreens for the prevention of immunosuppression has been investigated. In addition, many other factors are believed to be involved in the progress of carcinogenesis, such as p53 gene mutations, contact hypersensitivity response (CHR), delayed-type hypersensitivity (DTH), depression of NK killer cell activity, Langerhans cell depletion, induced epidermal interleukin-10, urocanic acid trans–cis isomerization, and many other factors. The use of various sunscreen preparations with specially bred mice produced highly divergent results ranging between no protection to partial and even full protection. These results are not necessarily relevant to events which might be occurring at the human skin. Nevertheless, on the basis of these and other confusing results, the proclivity toward the use of sunscreen agents for the control of all malign effects induced by solar radiation at the human skin is overly optimistic.

The use of sunscreen agents has at best a prophylactic effect, i.e., cannot restore the damaged DNA, which was produced by solar radiation. In contrast, it has been found that the use of photolyase enzymes can mediate the restoration of the damaged DNA and can even prevent the UVB radiation induced immunosuppression.

CHAPTER ELEVEN

EPILOGUE: AN OVERVIEW AND OUTLOOK

Upon scanning of various chapters of our book, it will be evident that all topics, in spite of their great diversities, always contain discussions of reactive oxygen species (ROS) that, actually, should not to be surprising since all ROS are derived from molecular oxygen which is essential for the functioning and sustenance of life.

In this section, an attempt is made to prove the inevitable intertwining of ROS, chronic inflammations, and various diseases, including pain (dolor), itch (pruritus), and cancers. This interconnection is not a perception of recent years, but it had already been recognized in antiquity. Thus, the Greek physician Hippocrates, about 2400 years before present (BP), recognized the cancerous diseases and prescribed treatments. Another Greek physician Galeen(us), practicing in Rome about 1800 BP, introduced the term cancer (crab) based on the crab-like disfigurations of tissues in breast cancers. The inflammations associated with cancers and pain were recognized by Cornelius Celsus, also a physician in Rome, who associated inflammation with calor (heat), rubor (redness), tumor (swelling), and dolor (pain) [1, 2].

Chronic inflammations affect about 77 million Americans at a staggering cost of about 50 billion dollars, whereby 60% of cases, affecting mainly women, are attributed to arthritic pain, including fibromyalgia, and a chronic pain involving abnormal pain responses [3, 4]. At present, it appears that medical efforts to either cure or, at least, alleviate the persistent chronic pain by treatments with traditional analgesics seldom result in the relief of pain [4, 5, 6].

Thus, usually, treatments commence with oral administrations of nonsteroidal anti-inflammatory drugs (NSAIDs), such as Aspirin™, ibuprofen, and acetaminophen. These analgesics are frequently prescribed for the management of soft tissue injuries and acute pain. In cases of negative responses, combinations of weak narcotic analgesics are used, such as propoxyphen, oxycodone, percoset, codeine, and a large excess of Aspirin™ or acetaminophen. In cases of negative responses that are very common in chronic pain, strong opiates and opioids like methadone, codeine, and morphine are prescribed. All narcotics are habit-forming and should be used with caution [5, 6].

Similarly, corticosteroidal therapy with anti-inflammatory drugs, such as cortisone, dexamethasone, and methylprednisone has been clinically used for decades against chronic pain. In recent years, extensive efforts have been made to elucidate the very intricate mechanistic pathways leading to the sensation of pain. It appears that pain is elicited by neural activities that also affect the brain (neuropathic pain) [6].

Medicinal treatments with narcotic drugs can alleviate some of the pain. However, even over prolonged periods, this therapy cannot cure many diseases, including cancers. In order to achieve medicinal success with specific therapies, it is essential to understand the mechanisms of pathways in chronic inflammations which constitute the origins of diseases. In the past decades, considerable progress has been made in research covering a vast variety of topics pertaining to inflammations.

In this connection, similar difficulties have been encountered with itching diseases (itch, pruritus), which affect millions of people and, in cases of chronic inflammations, are frustratingly difficult to treat and cure. The question arises whether pain and pruritus have identical or separate inflammatory pathways. On the basis of recent research, it appears that the pathways of itch and pain are intertwined and the itch–pain regulatory neurons have receptors for both the itch and the pain which can function, depending on the kind of stimulation, either as pain or as itch responses.

Similar to inflammations, pruritus can be either an acute or a chronic disease, and either a cutaneous or systemic disorder. Hence, the antipruritic chemotherapy must be varied either for topical or systemic targets. A great variety of agents for the management of pruritus have been used, including opioids and UV light. However, there is no single universally effective treatment available for pruritus [7, 8, 9, 10, 11].

In recent years, extensive research efforts have been made in understanding the role of reactive oxygen species (ROS) and nitrogen species (RONS) in the progression of inflammatory processes leading to chronic pain and other pathologies including cancers [12–18].

ROS are formed by exogenous and endogenous pathways. The exogenous formation of ROS occurs in and at the human skin when exposed to solar UVA and UVB radiations. The human skin can harbor various substances derived from xenobiotics, sunscreen agents, cosmetic skin products, dermatological agents, orally administered anti-inflammatory drugs, contraceptive agents, antidepressants, cardiovascular drugs, anticancer drugs, and many other species.

All these compounds contain well recognizable chromophores and auxochromes, which readily absorb the energy of UV radiations. The energy absorbed by these substances causes a transfer of one electron to molecular oxygen, $\cdot{}^3O_2\cdot$, which is a diradical in the ground state, with the formation of the superoxide radical anion ($O_2\cdot^-$) [12, 15]. This species undergoes rapid protonation to give the hydroperoxyl radical (HOO·), followed by a dismutation reaction to hydrogen peroxide and molecular oxygen, and a cascade of reactions, including the ferrous ion catalyzed Fenton reaction, resulting in various radical and other species. Furthermore, if the energy of the photoexcited species exceeds 22.7 $kcal.mol^{-1}$, a conversion of molecular oxygen to singlet oxygen Δ^1O_2 can occur.

The reactive oxygen and nitrogen species are formed endogenously by various cells. Thus, in mitochondria, are continuously produced the superoxide anion radical ($O_2\cdot^-$), hydrogen peroxide (H_2O_2), and hydroxyl radical (HO·); by cytochrome p450 H_2O_2 and $O_2\cdot^-$; by macrophages $O_2\cdot^-$, H_2O_2, and nitric oxide (NO·); and by peroxysomes hydrogen peroxide. The mitochondrial reduction of molecular oxygen converts 95% of it to water and only 5% to superoxide anion radical ($O_2\cdot^-$). Furthermore, reactive nitrogen and oxygen species, such as peroxynitrite ($ONOO\cdot^-\ H^+$), nitrogen dioxide ($NO_2\cdot$), and singlet oxygen Δ^1O_2, are produced in various cells [12, 14].

The anticancer drugs etoposide and cisplatin can cause the formation of RONS and, depending on the level of RONS, the induction of apoptotic death of various cancers [12, 14].

In order to prevent excessive formation of ROS and RONS, the human body, guided by the evolutionary process, has developed an effective defense system that is comprised of enzymatic species, such as superoxide dismutase, catalase, glutathione peroxidase (GSH), GSH reductase, and various nonenzymatic compounds, such as ascorbic acid (vitamin C), d-α-tocopherol (vitamin E), glutathione (GSH), carotenoids, organic selenium compounds, flavonoids, and other species [12, 13].

Inflammations are medically distinguished between acute and chronic inflammations. Acute inflammations usually persist only for short periods of time and are regarded as "therapeutic inflammations", i.e., curable. Acute inflammations can become chronic inflammations, although chronic inflammations can be formed without proceeding through the acute stage [2, 14, 17, 18].

The properties and functions of chronic inflammations are greatly influenced by interactions with cytokines. There are proinflammatory cytokines, such as 1L-1, -6, -12, and -18, and anti-inflammatory cytokines, such as interferons. Thus, the inflammations can be either propagated or inhibited by cytokines, and the cancer genes can be either activated or deactivated. Cytokines can also affect cell death. The formation of cytokines is induced by the NF-kB pathways [1, 14].

Chronic inflammations are the source of most cancers, in particular, solid tumors, many chronic diseases, and other pathological conditions—such as hepatitis, bronchitis, gastritis, cardiovascular diseases, rheumatoid arthritis, kidney diseases, coronary artery diseases, neurodegenerative diseases, ischemia, advanced glycation endproducts diseases (AGEs), Parkinson's disease, Alzheimer's disease, Creutzfeldt–Jacobs disease, lens diseases, macular degeneration, and amyotropic lateral sclerosis (Lou Gehrig's disease)—that are attributed to oxidative stress involving ROS and RONS [1, 15, 19–23].

Thus, for example, in the brain of Alzheimer patients were found increased contents of iron and copper, apparently in ionized forms, which are involved in a Fenton-type reaction producing hydroxyl radicals (HO·) from hydrogen peroxide [22].

A number of carcinomas have been found to evolve within chronic inflammations induced by various infectious microorganisms, such as the bacterium *Helicobacter pylori* and the hepatitis B and C, Epstein–Barr, human herpes, human immune deficiency (HIV), and other viral species [1, 14].

Severe pain, in particular peralgesia (fibromyalgia), is medically defined as an augmented sensitivity to pain, which is derived from chronic inflammations, and it affects a large number of persons, particularly women [6]. To date, the medical profession has had great difficulties finding reliable alleviating treatments for this grave illness. Recently, in search of pain-relieving chemotherapies, it was discovered that the superoxide radical anion ($O_2\cdot^-$) and the derived species peroxynitrite ($ONOO\cdot^- H^+$) apparently have a decisive role in the development of pain diseases [12, 14, 15, 24, 26–28]. The reaction of superoxide anion radical with nitric oxide (NO·), a ubiquitous and important species in human metabolisms, results in the formation of a very toxic peroxynitrite species.

The inflammatory and other adverse health conditions are also caused by radical-type reactions of molecular oxygen with arachidonic acid and other long-chain unsaturated fatty acids, which are found in high-fat food products, mediated by lipoxygenases 5-, 8-, 12-, and 15-LOX, cytochrome p450 enzyme, and cyclooxygenases COX1 and COX2. These oxidations, mediated by lipoxygenases and cytochrome p450, produce metabolic leukotrienes, which are potent bronchoconstrictors and chemostatic agents.

The cyclooxygenases-induced cyclizations produce various prostaglandins, which are biologically important lipidic acids with properties, such as dilation of arteries, menstruation, bronchial dilation, gastric secretions, platelet aggregations, and other functions leading to diseases including cancers [12, 14, 23–26]. Derived from prostaglandins are a group of thromboxanes that cause vasoconstriction, platelet aggregation, constriction of arteries, and other functions. The induction and progression of various diseases, including cancers, are associated with chronic inflammations caused by ROS mediated by oxygenases.

Based on extensive long-term investigations involving a large number of volunteers, it was concluded that regular use of some NSAIDs and, in particular, Aspirin™ over long periods of time can cause a reduction of risk and even prevention of colorectal cancer [23, 24]. Derivatives of Aspirin™ were shown in animal tumor models and human cells to be effective against a number of cancers [12].

It has been found on many occasions that cancer cells are very sensitive to excessive oxidative stress by ROS, which can have a devastating effect on various cancers and in particular on hypoxic solid tumors. Hence, it is not unreasonable to treat the cancer tissue with toxic, oxygen-derived species. Thus, photodynamic therapy (PDT) involves a selective incorporation of photosensitizers into cancerous tissues, followed by irradiation with light of a suitable wavelength. The produced ROS, in particular the singlet oxygen species, cause a very effective destruction of cancerous tissues. PDT has been very successfully applied against esophageal, lung, bladder, head, neck, intrathoric, intraperitoneal, and even against brain cancers [2].

Chronic inflammations precede the initiations and progression of various diseases including cancers. The pathways in chronic inflammations leading to the development of diseases are mainly dominated by the nuclear NF-kB factor and the signal transducer and activator of transcription 3 (STAT3). Most genes that are linked to inflammations, proliferations, and metastasis are regulated by the activity of NF-kB and STAT3 [1, 12, 14, 29].

Hypoxic and acidic conditions in solid tumors cause an activation of the NF-kB factor but not STAT3. Carcinogens, such as asbestos and UV radiations, activate the NF-kB and STAT3 pathways. It was found that the NF-kB factor is also activated by a number of clinically used chemotherapeutic drugs, such as cisplatin, daunomycin, tamoxifen, paclitaxel, vinblastine, vincristine, 5-fluorouracil, and doxorubicin. Most agents that induce chronic inflammations and proliferations activate the NF-KB factor, and the NF-kB factor causes a resistance to anticancer chemotherapy [1].

A suppression of proinflammatory pathways that are regulated by NF-kB and STAT3 with suitable inhibitors could possibly be used to achieve either a reduction of the risk, or alleviation and even prevention and cure, of various diseases. Hence research targeting the development of inhibitors against the NF-kB and STAT3 factors would constitute a very promising approach for discoveries of novel chemotherapies [1].

Evolution has provided the human body with the means of self-destruction, i.e., the suicide of undesirable cancerous cells by apoptosis (Type I cell death) and autophagy (Type II cell death). The digestive autophagocytosis process is essential for the removal of portions of sick cells if healthy cells are to survive [13, 30–32]. The ROS generating drugs were shown to induce this process [30, 31]. It is remarkable that in all civilized societies suicide is considered a deplorable act, while in the evolutionary process this act is highly desirable and beneficial for the sustenance of health and life [1, 2, 13, 14].

Apoptosis is controlled by at least three genes, namely, the cancer suppressor gene p53, which promotes the induction of apoptosis, and two genes of the Bcl family, the Bcl-2 protein and the bax gene which exert an antiapoptosis effect. Apoptosis can occur spontaneously when induced by various entities, such as the tumor necrosis factor (TNF) and some anti-cancer drugs [2, 14, 31–33].

Autophagy can function as an alternative pathway to apoptosis for the elimination of undesirable cancerous growth when apoptosis is inactivated. Activation of the NF-kB factor causes a suppression of autophagy and, hence, contributes to a resistance against the anticancer therapy, while the suppressor gene p53 induces apoptosis and autophagy. There are several proinflammatory genes, such as the oncogene protein Bcl-2, which are regulated by the NF-kB and STAT-3 factors preventing apoptosis and exerting an enhancing effect on carcinogenesis [1, 2, 13, 14, 29–32, 34]. The chronic inflammatory environment contributes to cancer initiation, proliferation, and resistance to chemotherapy, whereby the reactive oxygen species (ROS) have decisive functions in these convoluted processes.

Cancer cells are very sensitive to oxidative stress and respond in different ways, depending on the levels of oxidative stress. Thus, conditions of slightly elevated levels of ROS above the normal levels in the human body are favorable for the development of various diseases, including cancers. Under hypoxic conditions, cancer cells can survive and proliferate [14], whereas at highly elevated levels, the ROS cause the induction of apoptosis and autophagy, whereby, specifically, the induction of autophagy is caused by a reaction with superoxide anion radical ($O_2 \cdot^-$), which is the first species in the formation of ROS from molecular oxygen.

Persistent elevated ROS levels at the cancer environment can cause the cancer cells to undergo the metastasis process, i.e., a relocation to other organs that are not directly connected to the original site. Metastasis is the major cause of patients' mortality [14, 35–38]. The growth of invasion and invasive agents were reviewed [2]. Thus, anti-invasive agents can block the cancer angiogenesis and, thereby, indirectly block metastasis.

Chemotherapies with well-established anticancer drugs, such as cisplatin, adriamycin, tamoxifen, temozolamide, cyclophosphamide, and other drugs, produce high levels of ROS and the induction of autophagy resulting in cell death. However, in other therapies with these drugs, in spite of the induction of ROS and autophagy, cell survival was observed. This result is difficult to interpret. Since the ROS and autophagy pathways are highly intertwined, these divergent results can perhaps be explained by the existence of diverse unknown factors involved in various cancer environments. Furthermore, to add more complexity to the matter, it is known that normal healthy cells containing p53 can undergo undesirable apoptosis in the presence of cytotoxic drugs.

Presently, it appears that ROS can function either in the protection or induction of autophagy, depending on the environmental conditions of cancer cells. Thus, the chemotherapeutic treatments of cancer patients would have to be devised in each individual case based on a detailed clinical evaluation of the properties of cancerous cells and their environments and adjusting the levels of ROS and autophagy to the desired levels for a cure.

At present, in the clinical therapy of chronic diseases, there are no means to control the levels of ROS that would be required in individual cases to induce either apoptosis or autophagy, resulting in the death of cancerous cells and the cure of patients. The timely clinical detection of cancer diseases in patients and subsequent treatments with radiation, surgery, and chemotherapy have been seldom successful in sustaining prolonged survivals.

These difficulties have been attributed to the formation of a small subset of pluripotent stem cells with antiapoptotic properties, which are involved in initiation, growth, and metastasis. These potent cells with an aberrant, antioxidant, self-renewal and survival capacities resist "classical" chemotherapy, and can remain dormant for prolonged periods of time, followed by spontaneous proliferation. This capacity for prolonged periods of dormancy could explain the fact that persons who conceive the melanoma in their childhood are diagnosed with the disease at an advanced age [32, 39–45].

At long last, based on the present scientific inquiry and disclosures, the outlook is bright for discoveries and developments of novel chemotherapeutic agents for the control of chronic inflammations, pain, pruritus, and various diseases including cancers. As a culmination of these achievements, the Nobel Prize Foundation has awarded the 2011 Nobel Prize in Physiology or Medicine to Bruce A. Beutler, Jules A. Hoffmann, and Ralph M. Steinman for their research "that has opened new avenues for the development of prevention and therapy against infections, cancer, and inflammatory diseases" [43–50]. The 2012 Nobel Prize for Physiology or Medicine was awarded to Sir John B. Gurdon and Shinya Yamanaka for their discovery that "mature, specialised cells can be reprogrammed to become immature cells capable of developing into all tissues of the body". The new developments in cell transplantation therapies focusing on induced pluripotent stem cells (iPS) are discussed in a recent review article [51].

References

1. Aggarwal B. B., Vijayalekshmi R. V. and Sung B. (2009) Targeting inflammatory pathways for prevention and therapy of cancer: short-term friend, long-term foe. *Clin. Cancer Res.* **15**: 425–430.
2. Gnewuch C. T. and Sosnovsky G. (2002) Critical appraisals of approaches for predictive designs in anticancer drugs. *Cell. Mol. Life Sci.* **59**: 959–1023.
3. Park, A. (2011) Healing the Hurt. Finding new ways to treat pain. *Time*: 63–71.
4. Suddath, C. (2011) Living with pain. *Time*: 72–79.
5. Famaey J. P. and Paulus H. E. (1992) *Therapeutic Application of NSAIDs*, Marcel Dekker, New York.
6. McEwen B. S. and Kalia M. (2010) The role of corticosteroids and stress in chronic pain conditions. *Metabolism* **59** (Suppl 1): S9–15.
7. Wolf L. K. (2011) Itching to know more about itch. *Chem. Eng. News* (July 4): 27–79.
8. Metz M., Grundmann S. and Ständer S. (2011) Pruritus: an overview of current concepts. *Vet. Dermatol.* **22**: 121–131.
9. Elmariah S. B. and Lerner E. A. (2011) Topical therapies for pruritus. *Semin. Cutaneous Med. Surg.* **30**: 118–126.
10. Cassano N., Tessari G., Vena G. A. and Girolomoni G. (2010) Chronic pruritus in the absence of specific skin disease: an update on

pathophysiology, diagnosis, and therapy. *Am. J. Clin. Dermatol.* **11**: 399–411.
11. Steinhoff M., Cevikbas F., Ikoma A. and Berger T. G. (2011) Pruritus: management algorithms and experimental therapies. *Semin. Cutaneous Med. Surg.* **30**: 127–137.
12. Rigas B. and Sun Y. (2008) Induction of oxidative stress as a mechanism of action of chemopreventive agents against cancer. *Br. J. Cancer* **98**: 1157–1160.
13. Pan J.-S., Hong M.-Z. and Ren J.-L. (2009) Reactive oxygen species: A double-edged sword in oncogenesis. *World J. Gastroenterol.* **15**: 1702–1707.
14. Hold G. L. and El-Omar E. M. (2008) Genetic aspects of inflammation and cancer. *Biochem. J.* **410**: 225–235.
15. Zhang N., Andresen B. T. and Zhang C. (2010) Inflammation and reactive oxygen species in cardiovascular disease. *World J. Cardiol.* **2**: 408–410.
16. Klaunig J. E., Kamendulis L. M. and Hocevar B. A. (2010) Oxidative stress and oxidative damage in carcinogenesis. *Toxicol. Pathol.* **38**: 96–109.
17. Lonkar P. and Dedon P. C. (2011) Reactive species and DNA damage in chronic inflammation: reconciling chemical mechanisms and biological fates. *Int. J. Cancer* **128**: 1999–2009.
18. Fang J., Seki T. and Maeda H. (2009) Therapeutic strategies by modulating oxygen stress in cancer and inflammation. *Adv. Drug Delivery Rev.* **61**: 290–302.
19. Kundu J. K. and Surh Y. J. (2008) Inflammation: gearing the journey to cancer. *Mutat. Res.* **659**: 15–30.
20. Jomova K. and Valko M. (2011) Advances in metal-induced oxidative stress and human disease. *Toxicology* **283**: 65–87.
21. Ko S. Y., Lin Y. P., Lin Y. S. and Chang S. S. (2010) Advanced glycation end products enhance amyloid precursor protein expression by inducing reactive oxygen species. *Free Radical Biol. Med.* **49**: 474–480.
22. Jomova K., Vondrakova D., Lawson M. and Valko M. (2010) Metals, oxidative stress and neurodegenerative disorders. *Mol. Cell. Biochem.* **345**: 91–104.
23. Rouzer C. A. and Marnett L. J. (2011) Endocannabinoid oxygenation by cyclooxygenases, lipoxygenases, and cytochromes P450: Cross-talk between the eicosanoid and endocannabinoid signaling pathways. *Chem. Rev.* **111**: 5899–5921.

24. Perrone M. G., Scilimati A., Simone L. and Vitale P. (2010) Selective COX-1 inhibition: A therapeutic target to be reconsidered. *Curr. Med. Chem.* **17**: 3769–3805.
25. Panigrahy D., Kaipainen A., Greene E. R. and Huang S. (2010) Cytochrome P450-derived eicosanoids: the neglected pathway in cancer. *Cancer Metastasis Rev.* **29**: 723–735.
26. Lee Y., Rodriguez C. and Dionne R. A. (2005) The role of COX-2 in acute pain and the use of selective COX-2 inhibitors for acute pain relief. *Curr. Pharm. Des.* **11**: 1737–1755.
27. Wang Z. Q., Porreca F., Cuzzocrea S., Galen K., Lightfoot R., Masini E., Muscoli C., Mollace V., Ndengele M., Ischiropoulos H. and Salvemini D. (2004) A newly identified role for superoxide in inflammatory pain. *J. Pharmacol. Exp. Ther.* **309**: 869–878.
28. Salvemini D., Little J. W., Doyle T. and Neumann W. L. (2011) Roles of reactive oxygen and nitrogen species in pain. *Free Radical Mol. Med.* **51**: 951–966.
29. Prasad S., Ravindran J. and Aggarwal B. B. (2010) NF-kappaB and cancer: how intimate is this relationship. *Mol. Cell. Biochem.* **336**: 25–37.
30. Dewaele M., Maes H. and Agostinis P. (2010) ROS-mediated mechanisms of autophagy stimulation and their relevance in cancer therapy. *Autophagy* **6**: 838–854.
31. Gibson S. B. (2010) A matter of balance between life and death: targeting reactive oxygen species (ROS)-induced autophagy for cancer therapy. *Autophagy* **6**: 835–837.
32. Acharya A., Das I., Chandhok D. and Saha T. (2010) Redox regulation in cancer: a double-edged sword with therapeutic potential. *Oxid. Med. Cell. Longevity* **3**: 23–34.
33. Levine A. J. and Puzio-Kuter A. M. (2010) The control of the metabolic switch in cancers by oncogens and tumor suppressor genes. *Science* **330**: 1340–1344.
34. Rabinowitz J. D. and White E. (2010) Autophagy and metabolism. *Science* **330**: 1344–1348.
35. Wu Y. and Zhou B. P. (2009) Inflammation: a driving force speeds cancer metastasis. *Cell Cycle* **8**: 3267–3273.
36. Rajput S. and Wilber A. (2010) Roles of inflammation in cancer initiation, progression, and metastasis. *Front. Biosci., Scholar Ed.* **2**: 176–183.
37. Pani G., Galeotti T. and Chiarugi P. (2010) Metastasis: cancer cell's escape from oxidative stress. *Cancer Metastasis Rev.* **29**: 351–378.

38. Reuter S., Gupta S. C., Chaturvedi M. M. and Aggarwal B. B. (2010) Oxidative stress, inflammation, and cancer: how are they linked? *Free Radical Biol. Med.* **49**: 1603–1616.
39. Vieira H. L., Alves P. M. and Vercelli A. (2011) Modulation of neuronal stem cell differentiation by hypoxia and reactive oxygen species. *Prog. Neurobiol.* **93**: 444–455.
40. Kawasaki B. T., Hurt E. M., Mistree T. and Farrar W. L. (2008) Targeting cancer stem cells with phytochemicals. *Mol. Interventions* **8**: 174–184.
41. Rowe A. A. (2011) Cancer Stem Cells. *Chem. Eng. News* (October 24): 41–44.
42. Kong H., Putnam A. and Schook L. B. (eds.) (2011) *Stem Cells and Revascularization Therapies*, CRC Press, Boca Raton.
43. Eisenstein M. (2012) The root of all evil. Two studies of tumor ancestry reveal evidence for discrete populations of cancer stem cells. *Nat. Methods* **9**: 942–943.
44. Driessens G., Beck B., Caauwe A., Simons B. D., and Blanpain C. (2012) Defining the mode of tumor growth by clonal analysis. *Nature* **488**: 527–530.
45. Chen B., Li Y., Yu T.-S., McKay R. M., Burns D. K., Kernie S. G., and Parada L. F. (2012) A restricted cell population propagates glioblastoma growth after chemotherapy. *Nature* **488**: 522–526.
46. Tedgui A., Owens A. P. III and Mackman N. (2011) 2011 Nobel Prize in Physiology or Medicine. Toll-like receptors, dendritic cells, and their roles in atherosclerosis. *Arterioscler., Thromb., Vasc. Biol.* **31**: 2767–2768.
47. Lemaitre B. and Hoffmann J. (2007) The host defense of *Drosophila melanogaster*. *Annu. Rev. Immunol.* **25**: 697–743.
48. Beutler B. A. (2009) TLRs and innate immunity. *Blood* **113**: 1399–1407.
49. Steinman R. M. (2010) Some active areas of DC research and their medical potential. *Eur. J. Immunol.* **40**: 2085–2088.
50. Ganesan S., Aggarwal K., Paquette N. and Silverman N. (2011) NF-KB/Rel proteins and the humoral immune responses of *Drosophila melanogaster*. *Curr. Top. Microbiol. Immunol.* **349**: 25–60
51. Nakamura M. and Okano H. (2013) Cell transplantation therapies for spinal cord injury focusing on induced pluripotent stem cells. *Cell Res.* **23**: 70–80.

APPENDIX 1

TRADEMARKS

Trademark	Trademark Owner
Advil®	WYETH LLC
Anthelios®	La Roche-Posay Laboratoire Pharmaceutique
Aspirin™	Bayer AG
CAS Registry Number℠	American Chemical Society
Celebrex®	G.D. Searle & Co.
Erbitux®	ImClone LLC
Erbitux® Cetuximab®	ImClone LLC
Escalol®	ISP Investments inc.
Eusolex®	Merck KGaA
Lilial®	Givaudan SA
L'OREAL®	L'Oreal, SA
Mexoryl®	L'Oreal, SA
Parsol®	DSM IP Assets B.V.
Temodar®	Merck Sharp & Dohme Corp.
Tinosorb®	BASF SE
Tylenol®	Johnson & Johnson
Tinuvin®	BASF SE
Uvinul®	BASF Corp.
Vioxx®	Tremeau Pharmaceuticals, Inc.